An Essential Guide to Cardiac Cell Therapy

An Essential Guide to Cardiac Cell Therapy

Edited by

Emerson C Perin MD PhD

Guilherme V Silva MD

James T Willerson MD

Texas Heart Institute
Houston, TX, USA

informa
healthcare

First published in the United Kingdom in 2006 by Informa Healthcare, 4 Park Square, Milton Park, Abingdon, Oxon OX14 4RN. Informa Healthcare is a trading division of Informa UK Ltd, Registered Office: 37/41 Mortimer Street, London W1T 3JH. Registered in England and Wales Number 1072954.

Tel.: +44 (0) 207 017 6000
Fax.: +44 (0) 207 017 6699
E-mail: info.medicine@tandf.co.uk
Website: http://www.informahealthcare.com

A CIP record for this book is available from the British Library.

Library of Congress Cataloging-in-Publication Data

Data available on application

ISBN10: 1 84184 471 3
ISBN13: 978 1 84184 471 8

Distributed in North and South America by

Taylor & Francis
6000 Broken Sound Parkway, NW, (Suite 300)
Boca Raton, FL 33487, USA

Within Continental USA
Tel: 800 272 7737; Fax: 800 374 3401

Outside Continental USA
Tel: 561 994 0555; Fax: 561 361 6018
E-mail: orders@crcpress.com

Distributed in the rest of the world by
Thomson Publishing Services
Cheriton House
North Way
Andover, Hampshire SP10 5BE, UK
Tel.: +44 (0)1264 332424
E-mail: tps.tandfsalesorder@thomson.com

Composition by C&M Digitals (P) Ltd, Chennai, India
Printed and bound in Great Britain by CPI Bath

Contents

Contributors

Eric W Alton MD FRCP
Royal Brompton Hospital
London, UK

Franca Stedile Angeli MD
Texas Heart Institute
Houston, TX, USA

Theodore A Bass MD
Cardiovascular Imaging Core Laboratories
University of Florida
Jacksonville, FL, USA

L Maximilian Buja MD
Texas Heart Institute
Houston, TX, USA

Noel Caplice MD PhD
Mayo Clinic College of Medicine
Rochester, MN, USA

Jonathan Clague MD
Royal Brompton Hospital
London, UK

Marco A Costa MD PhD
Cardiovascular Imaging Core Laboratories
University of Florida
Jacksonville, FL, USA

Luis de la Fuente MD
Instituto de Ciencias del Corazón
Hospital Clinico-Universitario
Valladolid, Spain

Arjun Deb MD
Mayo Clinic College of Medicine
Rochester, MN, USA

Nabil Dib MD MSC
Arizona Heart Institute
Phoenix, AZ, USA

Stefanie Dimmeler PhD
Molecular Cardiology, University of Frankfurt
Frankfurt, Germany

Francisco Fernández-Avilés MD PhD FESC FACC
Instituto de Ciencias del Corazón
Hospital Clínico-Universitario
Valladolid, Spain

Javier García-Frade MD PhD
Hospital Universitario del Río Hortega
Valladolid, Spain

Javier García-Sancho MD PhD
Instituto de Biología y Genética Molecular
Universidad de Valladolid
Valladolid, Spain

Yong-Jian Geng MD PhD
Texas Heart Institute
Houston, TX, USA

Manuel Gómez-Bueno MD
Instituto de Ciencias del Corazón
Hospital Clinico-Universitario
Valladolid, Spain

Amanda C Heinl-Green
Royal Brompton Hospital
London, UK

Silviu Itescu MD
Columbia University
New York, NY, USA

Pilar Jimenez-Quevedo MD
Texas Heart Institute
Houston, TX, USA

Frank D Kolodgie PhD
CVPath, International
Registry of Pathology
Gaithersburg, MD, USA

Maciej Kurpisz MD PhD
Institute of Human Genetics, Polish Academy of Sciences
Poznań, Poland

Elena Ladich MD
CVPath, International Registry of Pathology
Gaithersburg, MD, USA

Silvio Litovsky MD
University of Alabama
Birmingham, AL, USA

Javier Lopez
Texas Heart Institute
Houston, TX, USA

Edie M Oliveira MD MSc
Texas Heart Institute
Houston, TX, USA

Shaun R Opie
Arizona Heart Institute
Phoenix, AZ, USA

Harald C Ott MD
Center for Cardiovascular Repair
University of Minnesota
Minneapolis, MN, USA

María Jesús Peñarrubia MD PhD
Hospital Universitario del Río Hortega
Valladolid, Spain

Emerson C Perin MD PhD
Texas Heart Institute
Houston, TX, USA

Arshed A Quyyumi MD FRCP
Emory University School of Medicine
Atlanta, GA, USA

Ana Sánchez MD PhD
Instituto de Biología y Genética Molecular
Universidad de Valladolid
Valladolid, Spain

Pedro L Sánchez MD PhD FESC
Instituto de Ciencias del Corazón
Hospital Clinico-Universitario
Valladolid, Spain

José Alberto San Román MD PhD
Instituto de Ciencias del Corazón
Hospital Clinico-Universitario
Valladolid, Spain

Ricardo Sanz MD
Texas Heart Institute
Houston, TX, USA

Patrick W Serruys MD PhD FESC FACC
Erasmus MC, Thoraxcenter
Rotterdam, The Netherlands

Guilherme V Silva MD
Texas Heart Institute
Houston, TX, USA

Tomasz Siminiak MD PhD FESC FACC
University School of Medical Sciences
Poznań, Poland

Veerappan Subramaniyam MD
Emory University School of Medicine
Atlanta, GA, USA

Doris A Taylor PhD
Center for Cardiovascular Repair
University of Minnesota
Minneapolis, MN, USA

Carmen Urbich PhD
Molecular Cardiology, University of Frankfurt
Frankfurt, Germany

Marco Valgimigli MD
Erasmus MC, Thoraxcenter
Rotterdam, The Netherlands

Willem J van der Giessen MD PhD
Erasmus MC, Thoraxcenter
Rotterdam, The Netherlands

Deborah Vela MD
Texas Heart Institute
Houston, TX, USA

Renu Virmani MD
CVPath, International Registry of Pathology
Gaithersburg, MD, USA

James T Willerson MD
The University of Texas Health Science Centre at Houston
Texas Heart Institute
Houston, TX, USA

Andrew Zurick MD
Emory University School of Medicine
Atlanta, GA, USA

Introduction and Preface: Perspectives in Stem Cell Therapy

James T Willerson

All humans are products of stem cell biology. Each human develops from two cells, following the union of a father's sperm and mother's egg, which subsequently develop into all of the organs in the human body under the influence of programs that direct their differentiation, organization, and structural development. Thus, our general appearance, our intellect, and all of our organs are products of stem cell differentiation. From a fundamental understanding of the programs that direct the differentiation of stem cells will ultimately come the ability to regenerate each of the organs of the body from a person's own stem cells or from a universal stem cell created in vitro. Based on this perspective of human development, it is clear that stem cell biology will be a vital part of regenerative cardiovascular medicine.

Humans have rescue systems of stem cells that are activated following injury to organs – including a system to repair the heart and arteries. While the genius of such a system deserves recognition and respect, it is also apparent that it is relatively inadequate as far as recovery from experimental myocardial infarction is concerned. The recruited circulating and activated resident stem cells arrive too late and are present in too few numbers in the early evolution of the injury process to be completely protective. In the last several years, numerous experimental studies have attemtpted to amplify the intrinsic system of stem cell presence in animal models with experimentally created myocardial infarcts.[1–7] Fetal cells, adult circulating stem cells (often with $CD34^+$ and/or $CD133^+$ markers), stem cells derived from adipose tissue, and stem cells obtained from bone marrow have been administered into a coronary artery or by direct injection into the heart or into the venous circulation to monitor homing to experimentally created myocardial infarctions. In almost every case, these stem cells appear to assist in the recovery of heart function and to improve blood flow in and around the area of myocardial infarction. However, controversy persists concerning the ability of such stem cells to differentiate into new myocytes.[3–9]

Several previous studies have attempted to delineate the fate of injected stem cells following experimental myocardial infarction. In the last few years, we have performed studies with $CD34^+$ circulating human stem cells injected into the tail veins or the left ventricular cavities of severe combined immune-deficient (SCID) mice with experimentally created myocardial infarcts.[3,4] In these studies, the mice were euthanized 2 days after injection to determine whether the injected human stem cells homed to the area of infarction, and, if so, whether they developed into cells of interest. Our studies showed that the injected human circulating stem cells homed to the area of infarction in the murine heart; there, they developed into endothelial cells and smooth muscle cells, and fused to reversibly injured murine myocytes.[3,4] A smaller number differentiated into new myocytes.[3,4] Other groups have not always been able to demonstrate either the fusion process or the differentiation of stem cells into myocytes in experimentally injured animal hearts.[9]

However, we believe that this process does occur and can be observed when models are used that preclude rejection of the injected stem cells and allow a distinction to be made between injected stem cells and native myocytes in organs that have been experimentally injured. We and others have begun clinical studies using adult stem cells derived from a patient's own bone marrow.[10–13] In 2000, our group petitioned the Brazilian government to allow us to begin clinical studies with autologous bone marrow-derived mononuclear cells (BMMNCs) in patients with severe heart failure.[10] These patients had coronary heart disease and prior myocardial infarctions. They had undergone coronary artery bypass surgery and/or percutaneous coronary intervention procedures; nevertheless, they had developed large, dilated hearts and severe heart failure. All patients were receiving appropriate medical therapy.

Based on our earlier animal studies, we decided to take bone marrow aspirates from the iliac crests of these patients, separate the mononuclear cells, and reinject them into the patient's hearts by using a NOGA "electromechanical" catheter placed retrograde across the aortic valve. The NOGA catheter was used to identify sites of reversible injury as locations for injection of the BMMNCs.[10,14] We used single photon emission computed tomography (SPECT) studies to identify areas of reversible blood flow reduction. These studies were initiated at the Heart Hospital in Rio de Janeiro, Brazil, with Hans Dohmann and his colleagues.

We injected 2×10^6 BMMNCs transendocardially at 15 different sites where the NOGA catheter and SPECT studies suggested reversible injury.[10] We have not found evidence of harm in these patients at 3 years of follow-up.[15] Imaging and clinical studies have demonstrated improvement in clinical symptoms and in regional blood flow and contractile function.[10] This was the first study in patients with severe heart failure that used the NOGA catheter to map appropriate areas for injection of patients' own BMMNCs.[10] Subsequently, we obtained Food and Drug Administration (FDA) approval to proceed with similar studies in the USA at the Texas Heart Institute/St Luke's Episcopal Hospital in Houston, Texas. To date, we have randomized 24 patients in a treatment protocol similar to that used in Brazil. Patients are usually discharged from the hospital the day after the procedure. Regular follow-up visits include imaging procedures that evaluate changes in regional blood flow and function and in heart rhythm and clinical status. When we began these studies in Brazil, two different German groups, unknown to us at that time, were pursuing similar studies in patients with acute myocardial infarction, also using BMMNCs. These groups, however, were treating patients within several days of their infarcts by opening the infarct-related artery by angioplasty and injecting the patients' mononuclear cells directly into the artery.[11,12] Patients in the German studies, which were led respectively by Strauer[11] and by Dimmeler and Zeiher,[12,16,17] did not have heart failure. More recently, Wollert et al[13] have performed a randomized, controlled study in 60 patients with acute myocardial infarction using the German model of opening the infarct-related artery by angioplasty and injecting the BMMNCs directly into the infarct-related coronary arteries. The German-led studies demonstrated improvement in regional blood flow and function in the treated patients.[11–13] Similar to our own studies, the German studies did not identify untoward clinical effects.

Careful reflection upon the ability of humans to develop from two cells and the acceptance of experimental results in multiple animal models has led to these early stem cell studies in patients. Emerging clinical data appear to show at least modest benefits in patients with new myocardial infarcts, chronic coronary heart disease, and/or severe heart failure treated with BMMNCs. With these considerations in mind, the potential usefulness of stem cells in regenerative cardiovascular medicine appears promising.

An Essential Guide to Cardiac Cell Therapy has been written for physicians wishing to acquaint themselves with stem cell therapy for cardiac disease. The *Guide* includes chapters written to provide an understanding of stem cells and stem cell therapy. These chapters cover basic stem cell biology, treatment of "no-option" patients, the use of large animal models, and the basics of embryonic stem cells and cloning. The book also addresses the applications of stem cell therapy, covering areas such as the use of mesenchymal lineage progenitor cells, methods of stem cell delivery, and concerns from a clinical perspective. The immediate needs now are to identify the best stem cell type(s), the optimal ways to deliver stem cells, and the patients most likely to benefit from this form of therapy. The more distant but achievable goals are the regeneration of the heart (and other organs) and repair of injured blood vessels with stem cells. These studies bring us closer to the promise and future of stem cell biology.

References

1. Asahara T, Masuda H, Takahashi T, et al. Bone marrow origin of endothelial progenitor cells responsible for postnatal vasculogenesis in physiological and pathological neovascularization. Circ Res 1999;85:221–8.
2. Shintani S, Murohara T, Ikeda H, et al. Mobilization of endothelial progenitor cells in patients with acute myocardial infarction. Circulation 2001;103:2776–9.
3. Yeh ETH, Zhang S, Wu HD, et al. Transdifferentiation of human peripheral blood $CD34^{+}$-enriched cell population into cardiomyocytes, endothelial cells, and smooth muscle cells in vivo. Circulation 2003;108:2070–3.
4. Zhang S, Dachun W, Estrov Z, et al. Both cell fusion and transdifferentiation account for the transformation of human peripheral blood CD34-positive cells into cardiomyocytes in vivo. Circulation 2004;110:3803–7.
5. Oh H, Bradfute SB, Gallardo TD, et al. Cardiac progenitor cells from adult myocardium: homing, differentiation, and fusion after infarction. Proc Natl Acad Sci USA 2003:100:12313–18.
6. Beltrami AP, Barlucchi L, Torella D, et al. Adult cardiac cells are multipotent and support myocardial regeneration. Cell 2003;114:763–76.
7. Silva GV, Litovsky S, Assad JAR, et al. Mesenchymal stem cells differentiate into an endothelial phenotype, enhance vascular density, and improve heart function in a canine chronic ischemia model. Circulation 2005;111:150–6.
8. Orlic D, Kajstura J, Chimenti S, et al. Bone marrow cells regenerate infarcted myocardium. Nature 2001;410:701–5.
9. Murry CE, Soonpaa MG, Reinecke H, et al. Haematopoietic stem cells do not transdifferentiate into cardiac myocytes in myocardial infarcts. Nature 2004;428:664–8.
10. Perin EC, Dohmann HFR, Borojevic R, et al. Transendocardial, autologous bone marrow cell transplantation for severe, chronic ischemic heart failure. Circulation 2003;107:2294–302.
11. Strauer BE, Brehm M, Zeus T, et al. Repair of infarcted myocardium by autologous intracoronary mononuclear bone marrow transplantation in humans. Circulation 2002;106:1913–18.
12. Assmus B, Schächinger V, Teupe C, et al. Transplantation of Progenitor Cells and Regeneration Enhancement in Acute Myocardial Infarction (TOPCARE-AMI). Circulation 2002;106:3009–17.
13. Wollert KC, Meyer GP, Lotz J, et al. Intracoronary autologous bone-marrow cell transfer after myocardial infarction: the BOOST randomized controlled clinical trial. Lancet 2004;364:141–8.
14. Perin EC, Silva GV, Sarmento-Leite R, et al. Assessing myocardial viability and infarct transmurality with left ventricular electromechanical mapping in patients with stable coronary artery disease: validation by delayed-enhancement magnetic resonance imaging. Circulation 2002;106: 957–61.
15. Silva VG, Perin EC, Dohmann HFR, et al. Catheter-based transendocardial delivery of autologous bone-marrow-derived monunuclear cells. Tex Heart Inst J 2004;31:214–19.
16. Britten MB, Abolmaali ND, Assmus B, et al. Infarct remodeling after intracoronary progenitor cell treatment in patients with acute myocardial infarction (TOPCARE-AMI): mechanistic insights from serial contrast-enhanced magnetic resonance imaging. Circulation 2003;108:2212–18.
17. Schachinger V, Assmus B, Britten MB. Transplantation of progenitor cells and regeneration enhancement in acute myocardial infarction: final one-year results of the TOPCARE-AMI trial. J Am Coll Cardiol 2004;44:1690–9.

Acknowledgments

The Editors would like to acknowledge the editors in Scientific Publications at the Texas Heart Institute for their help in the preparation of manuscripts and Ms Rupal Malde, development editor at Informa Healthcare, for her efforts to keep the book moving toward production. Finally, we would like to thank all of the contributors, whose work made this book a reality.

PART 1

Understanding the Basics of Stem Cells

chapter 1

What Are Stem Cells and What Do They Do?

Emerson C Perin and Guilherme V Silva

Introduction

As mentioned in the Introduction to this book, *we are the product of stem cells*. Babies are born every day! Incredibly, every cell in our body has our full genetic code. Just like growing dinosaurs in the film *Jurassic Park*, we can (theoretically) regenerate ourselves or our organs or tissues using the information contained within one cell. Although the concept of regenerative medicine is tangible and easily understandable, the science behind it is not. But even in a largely evidence-based field such as medicine, the collective imagination has soared.

The need for a clearer understanding of the stem cell field is required because, in recent years, a greater awareness of the biologic potential of stem cells has entered mainstream medicine. For example, many of the effects seen in current clinical trials of stem cell therapy may not truly be the result of cell "regeneration," but, nonetheless, it is just as important (if not even more so) to understand those effects as it is to understand what intuitively one might think the mechanisms at work should be. As we learn in medicine over and over again, not everything is intuitive. That is why we need to make every effort to understand what stem cells are, what they do, and how they work. The field has grown exponentially because the potential of stem cell therapy is easily recognized; however, we have only begun to comprehend the complexities and simplicities associated with stem cell biology.

In this book, we will lay the framework for understanding what is known – like a flashlight beam in a dark room – and for identifying some key elements of current knowledge that will better guide our understanding of the field.

Cardiology and Stem Cells

Great strides have been made in understanding the pathophysiology of coronary atherosclerosis and developing new treatments for this disease. Yet, despite considerable research efforts and generous allocation of resources, coronary artery disease (CAD) remains the predominant cause of premature death in the USA.[1] Reflected in the presence of a broader population of sicker and more compromised patients, a paradoxical increase in heart failure deaths has occurred over the past several years. What is sorely needed is a therapy that could address the contractile capability of the myocardium beyond repair of the "plumbing" of its blood supply – both in the acute phase of heart failure (when the damage occurs) and in the chronic phase (when a progressive march towards cardiac remodeling ensues). Enter regenerative cardiology.

Until the 1990s, atherosclerosis was understood to be a disease process leading to intravascular lipid deposition and luminal narrowing. The identification of risk factors for CAD allowed several advances in the primary prevention of coronary atherosclerosis. The recognition of atherothrombosis as the primary event in acute coronary syndromes led to the development of antithrombotic drugs that have significantly improved outcomes after an acute myocardial infarction (AMI). Percutaneous and surgical revascularization – the current mainstays of CAD therapy – have broadened our understanding of coronary atherosclerosis by providing insights into its intimate relationship with inflammation and endothelial function. This has ultimately led to the development of drug-eluting stents and the modern treatment of CAD, although efforts to identify and treat vulnerable plaque will likely yield a more *preventative* approach toward maintaining patency of the coronary tree.

Yet, despite active research on the pathophysiology of coronary atherosclerosis, little attention was paid until very recently to the concept of cardiac repair. This was due mainly to the deeply entrenched notion that the heart is a terminally differentiated organ. This dogma has been directly challenged by the discovery of circulating endothelial progenitor cells,[2] by evidence that bone marrow cells could transdifferentiate into endothelial cells, smooth muscle cells, or myocytes,[3–6] and by initial experiments showing that bone marrow cells are indeed involved in the process of cardiac repair. This could lead to a new clinical application and, ultimately, an entirely new field of cardiology.

When the skin is cut, it is able to repair itself. Now that newly discovered resident cardiac stem cells have been implicated in a process of cardiac repair, it is clear that the myocardium is also capable of repairing itself. In addition, it is clear that this capacity for self-repair is *limited* in hearts that have sustained an acute injury (e.g., an AMI) or that are chronically failing as a result of volume/pressure overload. Indeed, it is likely that the heart's endogenous ability to regenerate itself is unequal to the task of repairing the large amounts of necrosis and apoptosis often associated with these two conditions. Augmentation of this self-repair process through the transplantation of exogenous adult stem cells is the basis for cardiac stem cell therapy. As this approach comes closer and closer to clinical reality, clinicians will need to understand the fundamental concepts underlying the preclinical and clinical applications of stem cell therapy in the field of cardiology. This chapter provides a primer on those basic principles.

What Is a Stem Cell?

Stem cells are self-replicating cells capable of generating, sustaining, and replacing terminally differentiated cells.[7,8] Stem cells can be subdivided into two large groups: embryonic and adult. Embryonic stem cells (ESCs) are present in the earliest stage of embryonic development – the blastocyst. ESCs are *pluripotent*. That is, they are capable of generating any terminally differentiated cell in the human body that is derived from any one of the three embryonic germ layers – ectoderm, mesoderm, or endoderm.[9] After a series of divisions and differentiations, all the organs of the human body are created from the original ESCs that form the blastocyst.

Adult stem cells are intrinsic to specific tissues of the postnatal organism into which they are committed to differentiate.[10] They have been studied in the field of hematology for four decades, ever since the successful clinical introduction of bone marrow transplantation. Theoretically, adult stem cells are capable of perpetual self-renewal, yielding mature differentiated cells that are (a) integrated into a particular tissue and (b) capable of performing the specialized function, or functions, of that tissue. Each type of differentiated cell has its own phenotype (i.e., observable characteristics), which includes its shape or morphology, its interactions with surrounding cells and extracellular matrix, the expression of particular proteins (*receptors*) on its surface, and its particular behavior.[9] Adult tissue-specific stem cells are present in organs that are capable of self-renewal, including the liver, pancreas, skeletal muscle, and skin.

Where Do Therapeutic Cardiac Stem Cells Come From?

Adult-derived stem cells

The *bone marrow* is the primary source for obtaining adult stem cells. It is a complex organ with a specific geometric organization and an intricate system of cell-to-cell interaction and signaling. It is composed of hematopoietic progenitors, osteocytes, osteoblasts, and supporting mesenchymal (stromal) cells. To date, the most important subpopulation of bone marrow cells utilized for cardiac stem cell therapy has been the bone marrow mononuclear cell (BMMNC) subfraction. This subset contains mesenchymal stem cells (MSCs, also called stromal cells), hematopoietic progenitor cells (HPCs), endothelial progenitor cells (EPCs), and more committed cell lineages, such as natural killer, T, and B lymphocytes. Adult MSCs ($<0.01\%$) and EPCs (1–2%) both represent a very small fraction of the total BMMNC subpopulation.

MSCs are an important and a promising cell type for cardiac therapy, although clinical studies using this cell type have only recently been initiated. Chapter 3 discusses the basics of mesenchymal lineage progenitor cells.

On the other hand, EPCs have had significant clinical application in the realm of acute myocardial infarction. The more basic aspects of EPCs are discussed in Chapter 4, while Chapters 9, 13, and 15 expand on the clinical utilization of this important cell type.

Skeletal myoblasts

Even though skeletal myoblasts are not true stem cells, these skeletal muscle precursors can be harvested and expanded to allow therapeutic utilization. Chapters 9 and 14 present further details about the use of this cell type.

Embryonic stem cells

ESCs are derived from the cell mass of blastocysts in mice and humans. When cultured in the presence of leukemia inhibitory factor (LIF) or on the top layer of mitotically inactivated mouse embryonic fibroblasts, ESCs can proliferate indefinitely. Ethical issues involving the use of human ESCs have slowed research in several countries, including the USA.

Alternative sources of adult-derived stem cells

MSCs have also been isolated from adipose tissue, placental tissue, and umbilical cord blood. EPCs have also been isolated from fetal liver umbilical cord blood and from the peripheral circulation.[11]

What Characteristics Make Stem Cells Therapeutically Useful?

Traditionally, the bone marrow's hematopoietic system has been described as an organized hierarchic system with multipotent self-renewing cells at the top, committed progenitor cells in the middle, and lineage-restricted precursor cells that give rise to terminally differentiated cells at the bottom. There is now some evidence that adult stem cells (including hematopoietic stem cells, HSCs) may retain a degree of developmental plasticity that allows them to differentiate across boundaries of lineage, tissue, and germ layers. For example, MSCs are extremely plastic. They can develop into terminally differentiated mesenchymal phenotypes – including bone,[12,13] cartilage,[14] tendon,[15,16] muscle,[17,18] adipose tissue,[19,20] and hematopoiesis-supporting stroma – both in vitro and in vivo. MSCs can differentiate not only into tissues of the mesenchymal lineage but also into cells derived from other embryonic layers, including neurons and epithelia in the skin, lung, liver, intestine, kidney, and spleen.

Bone marrow-derived stem cells have long been known for their secretory capacity. In culture medium, BMMNCs are capable of releasing large quantities of angiogenic growth factors, such as vascular endothelial growth factor (VEGF), basic fibroblast growth factor (bFGF), and angiopoietins, which are associated with the generation of new blood vessels.

Bone marrow-derived stem cells are recruited from the bone marrow by exposure to certain pathophysiologic stimuli. Hypoxia or ischemia may enhance the local release of chemoattractant factors, and it is thought that bone marrow cells are mobilized as a result of cytokine and growth factor signaling.[10] Tissue ischemia and hypoxia in turn increase vascular permeability and promote the expression of adhesion proteins. These events may facilitate the homing process.[11] Although this homing mechanism is not completely understood, the microenvironment surrounding injured tissue (e.g., myocardium) is thought to play a role in the transdifferentiation of stem cells.

How Are Stem Cells Identified and Characterized?

Each adult stem cell subtype can be identified by its cell surface *receptors*. These are capable of selectively binding or adhering to particular *signaling* molecules. Differences in structure and binding affinity allow for a remarkable multiplicity of receptors. Normally, cells utilize these receptors and the molecules that bind to them as a means of communicating with other cells and performing the proper function of the tissue they belong to (e.g., contraction, secretion, or synaptic transmission). Each type of adult stem cell has a certain receptor or combination of receptors (i.e., *marker*) that distinguishes it from other types of stem cells (Table 1.1).

Stem cell markers are often given letter and number codes based on the molecules that bind to them (Table 1.1). For example, a cell that exhibits the stem cell antigen 1 receptor on its surface is identified as Sca-1^{+}. Cells that exhibit Sca-1 but not CD34 antigen or lineage-specific antigen (Lin) are identified as CD34^{-}Sca-1^{+}Lin^{-}. This particular combination of surface receptors marks such cells as MSCs.

Because different researchers have given the same bone marrow cells different names, the nomenclature can be confusing. Further complicating matters is the overlapping of surface marker designations within some cell subtypes. Most surface markers have proved inadequate for identifying stem cells, as these markers may also be found on non-stem cells. Moreover, a particular marker may be expressed only under certain culture conditions or at a certain stage of the cell's lifespan. Bone marrow stem cells are also highly plastic, so one subtype may give rise to others.

The strengths and weaknesses of utilizing cell surface markers to identify stem cells are best exemplified by the EPCs. "Immature," or "primitive," EPCs are known to have a surface marker profile similar to that of HSCs, and both cell types are thought to result from a common precursor, the hemangioblast (Figure 1.1). Within the bone marrow, both immature EPCs and HSCs express the surface markers CD34, CD133 (also known as AC133 or prominin) and VEGF receptor 2 (VEGFR-2, also known as KDR/FLK-1). Similarly, in the peripheral circulation, the more primitive cell population with the capacity for differentiating into EPCs also expresses these markers; however, once those primitive cells become more committed toward the EPC lineage, they lose CD133 but retain CD34 and VEGFR-2. Some circulating EPCs and, to a greater extent, relatively more differentiated EPCs express the endothelial lineage-specific markers vascular endothelial (VE)-cadherin or E-selectin. However, when immature EPCs commit to the hematopoietic lineage, they no longer express CD133 and VEGFR-2. Indeed, stem/progenitor cell markers are not expressed on differentiated hematopoietic cells.

In summary, CD133 is expressed on the surface of immature EPCs and primitive HSCs but not circulating relatively committed EPCs. Circulating committed EPCs may be isolated by selecting for their antigenicity to CD34 and VEGFR-2. In turn, hematopoietic stem/progenitor cells can be distinguished from committed EPCs by selecting for the former's antigenicity to VE-cadherin or E-selectin.

Interestingly, EPCs isolated from peripheral blood mononuclear cells have been shown to express CD14, MAC-1, and CD11c. The fact that these cell surface receptors are monocyte/macrophage markers suggests a possible monocyte/macrophage origin. It has also been shown that some CD34^{-} cells within the mononuclear peripheral cell population express CD14 and differentiate into endothelial cells.[11] Together, these findings raise the intriguing possibility that EPCs (CD34^{+}VEGFR-2^{+}CD133^{+}) are more plastic than originally thought, that a common precursor progenitor cell can pass through different developmental stages, and that there are surface markers yet to be discovered that may distinguish even more reliably between stem cell subtypes.

Table 1.1 Surface markers used to identify stem cells in bone marrow and blood

Cell surface marker	*Stem cell types*	*Significance*
BMPR	MSC, progenitor cell	■ Distinguishes committed mesenchymal cell types from mesenchymal and progenitor cells ■ Identifies early mesenchymal lineages (stem and progenitor cells)
CD4	WBC	■ Protein marker specific for mature T-lymphocyte (WBC) subtype
CD8	WBC	■ Protein marker specific for mature T-lymphocyte (WBC) subtype
CD34	HSC, EPC, satellite cell	■ Identifies bone marrow cells, especially HSCs and EPCs
CD38	Absent on HSC Present on WBC lineages	■ Cell-surface molecule that identifies WBC lineages. Selection of $CD34^{+}/CD38^{-}$ cells allows for purification of HSC populations
CD44	Mesenchymal cell	■ A type of cell-adhesion molecule used to identify specific types of mesenchymal cells
Lin	HSC, MSC	■ Cell adhesion molecule used to identify specific types of mesenchymal cells
Sca-1	HSC, MSC	■ Family of 13 or 14 cell surface proteins that are markers of mature blood cell lineages (*Note*: the presence of Lin^{-} cells assists in the purification of HSCs and hematopoietic progenitor cell populations)
Stro-1	Stromal (mesenchymal) precursor cell, hematopoietic cell	■ Antigen found on bone marrow cells that is used to identify HSCs and MSCs ■ Cell surface glycoprotein found on bone marrow stromal cells (*Note:* $Stro\text{-}1^{+}$ mesenchymal precursor cells can give rise to adipocytes, osteocytes, smooth myocytes, fibroblasts, chondrocytes, and blood cells)

BMPR, bone morphogenetic protein receptor; EPC, endothelial progenitor cell; HSC, hematopoietic stem cell; MSC, mesenchymal stem cell; WBC, white blood cell; Lin, lineage surface antigen; Sca-1, stem cell antigen 1; Stro-1, stromal cell antigen 1.

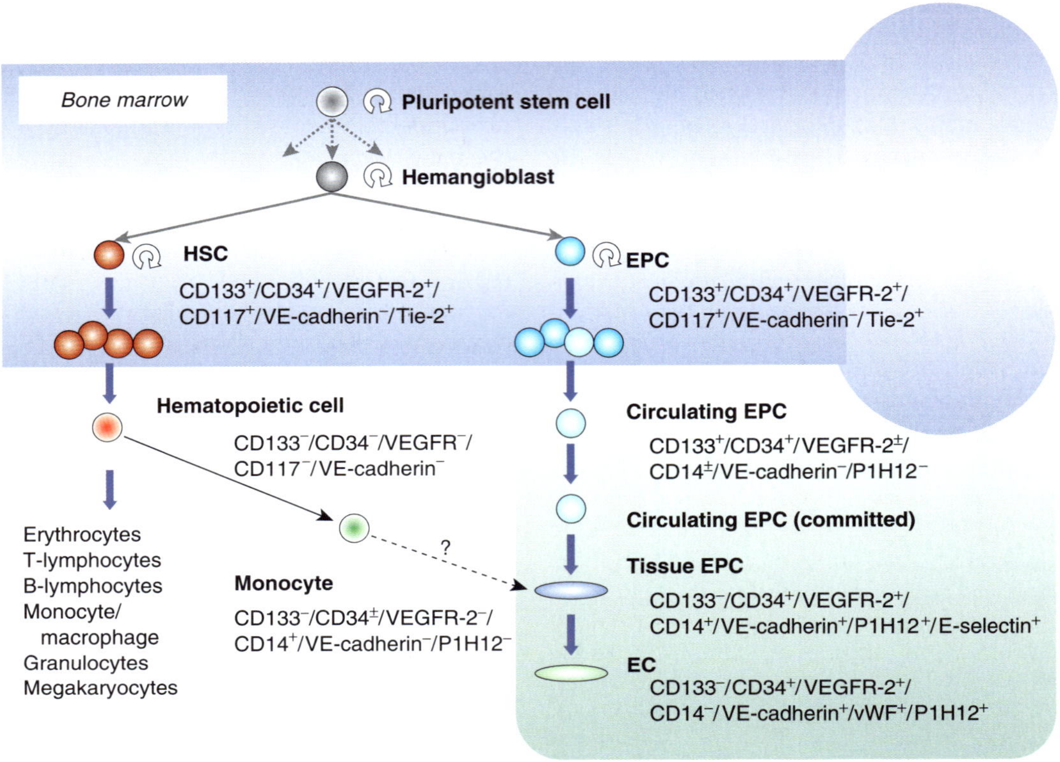

Figure 1.1 *Putative cascade and expressional profiles of human bone-marrow-derived endothelial progenitor cell differentiation. EC, endothelial cell; EPC, endothelial progenitor cell; HSC, hematopoietic stem cell; VE, vascular endothelial; VEGFR-2, vascular endothelial growth factor receptor 2 (KDR/FLK-1); vWF, von Willebrand factor. Reprinted from Iwami Y et al. J Cell Mol Med 2004;8:488–97 with permission.*

Despite their limitations, cell surface receptors remain the most popular and effective means of identifying stem cell subtypes for use in cardiac repair.

How Do Stem Cells Work?

Preclinical experiments have provided evidence for the efficacy of stem cell therapy. Further investigations are now underway to elucidate the mechanistic aspects of stem cell therapy at the molecular level. So far, the questions outnumber the answers. Numerous groups, using various methods in diverse experimental settings, have proposed widely differing mechanisms for the apparent transformation of stem cells into cells of other tissue types.[2] Some investigators attribute the transformation to the transdifferentiation potential of stem cells. Others attribute it to cell fusion.[2]

Initial experimental evidence indicated that autologous BMMNCs (ABMMNCs) can transdifferentiate into endothelial cells and cardiac myocytes. Recent studies in mice, however, have challenged this notion, generating enormous controversy.[21,22] Murry et al[22] detected no transdifferentiation of ABMMNCs into cardiomyocytes despite using sophisticated genetic techniques to follow cell fate and engraftment. Others have shown experimentally that ABMMNCs depend on external signals to trigger their secretory properties and differentiation.[23] The local environment of viable myocardial cells may provide the milieu necessary for inducing

ABMMNC myocyte differentiation.[23] Therefore, in recent studies of occlusion-induced myocardial infarctions in rats and depending on the injection site, few (if any) ABMMNCs might have been expected to differentiate and express specific cardiac myocyte proteins; however, the reverse was true.

In an attempt to resolve the controversy between transdifferentiation versus fusion, Zhang et al[24] performed an elegant study involving flow-cytometric analysis of cardiac cell isolates from mice that had received human $CD34^+$ cells. Human leukocyte antigen (HLA)-ABC antigen and cardiac troponin T (Tnt) or Nkx 2.5 were used to identify cardiomyocytes derived from the $CD34^+$ cells, and HLA-ABC and VE-cadherin were used to identify transformed endothelial cells. Cells positive for both sets of markers were evaluated for the expression of human and mouse X chromosomes. Surprisingly, 73.3% of nuclei derived from HLA^+ and Tnt^+ or Nkx 2.5^+ cardiomyocytes contained both human and mouse X chromosomes; 23.7% of nuclei contained only human X chromosomes. In contrast, the nuclei of HLA^- Tnt^- cells contained only mouse X chromosomes. Furthermore, 97.3% of endothelial cells derived from $CD34^+$ cells contained only human X chromosomes. On the basis of these data, Zhang et al concluded that (a) some human $CD34^+$ cells had both fused with and transdifferentiated into cardiomyocytes and (b) others had transdifferentiated into endothelial cells in this model.

The transdifferentiation of HSCs into endothelial cells in the heart[25] is less controversial. In animal models of stem cell therapy for ischemic heart disease, the evidence points toward increased neovascularization (with reduced myocardial ischemia) and consequent improvement in cardiac function.[26,27] The evidence also suggests that bone marrow stem cells may contribute directly to an increase in contractility or, more likely, passively limit infarct expansion and remodeling. Unfortunately, the limitations of the present animal models leave this particular question unanswered.

According to the current understanding of bone marrow stem cell engraftment, most therapeutic stem cells die within days after delivery. Arteriogenesis and vasculogenesis have long been known to be highly dependent on vascular growth factors. In another elegant study, Kinnaird et al[28,29] concluded that MSCs contribute to angiogenesis by means of paracrine mechanisms. This new understanding allows one to postulate that the paracrine effects of bone marrow stem cell therapy may help to recruit circulating progenitor cells, activate resident cardiac stem cells, or both, triggering a cascade of events resulting in cardiac repair. Meanwhile, details about the important role of resident cardiac stem cells in the process of cardiac repair continue to emerge.[30,31]

What Insights Have Been Gained into Vascular and Cardiac Repair Mechanisms?

The field of stem cell therapy has benefited greatly from the work of numerous researchers in both basic and clinical sciences. Their studies have greatly improved our understanding of the processes involved in cardiac repair and neovascularization.

The creation of new blood vessels (neovascularization) implies the formation of new mature endothelial cells. This process involves either the migration and proliferation of endothelial cells from existing vessels (angiogenesis) or the generation of new vessels from bone marrow-derived progenitor cells (vasculogenesis).[32] Asahara et al[33] were the first to describe a unique population of EPCs that are derived from bone marrow and are present in the peripheral circulation. These EPCs share similarities with bone marrow hematopoietic progenitor cells. Before EPCs were discovered, vasculogenesis was thought to occur only in the human embryonic phase. In animal models of ischemia, however, EPCs have been shown to participate in new vessel development, thus establishing a new paradigm of postnatal vasculogenesis.

The importance of postnatal vasculogenesis to stem cell therapy has been highlighted by several recent studies. Bone marrow-derived EPCs have been shown to contribute functionally to vasculogenesis after an AMI, during wound healing, and in limb ischemia.[11] These cells have also been implicated in the endothelialization of vascular grafts.[34] The number of circulating EPCs and their migratory capacity have been shown to correlate inversely with risk factors for CAD, such as smoking and hypercholesterolemia.[35] EPCs have also been implicated in the pathogenesis of allograft transplant vasculopathy and coronary restenosis after stent implantation. These cells are recruited by appropriate cytokines, growth factors, and hormones through autocrine, paracrine, and endocrine mechanisms.[11] EPC mobilization is a natural response to vascular trauma, as seen in patients who undergo coronary artery bypass graft surgery or suffer burns or an AMI.[11] Because EPCs play such an important and dynamic role in vascular repair, they are good candidates for use in cardiac stem cell therapy.

Adult tissue-specific stem cells are present in other organs that are capable of self-renewal, including the liver, pancreas, skeletal muscle, and skin. As mentioned at the outset, the heart was until very recently considered a terminally differentiated, postmitotic organ whose number of myocytes was finite and established at birth. This dogma has been challenged, however, by the observation that HSCs can transdifferentiate into cardiomyocytes[36] and that stem cells may reside in the heart. Such resident cardiac stem cells are thought to occupy niches in the atria and apex and have been observed in the border zones of myocardial infarcts.[37] These observations have in turn drastically changed our understanding of the cardiac repair process. It now appears that the injured heart may be repaired by means of resident cardiac stem cells and possibly by stem cells originating from bone marrow. Once adequate signaling has been established with cytokines and growth factors, bone marrow cells are mobilized.[11] This concept has been strengthened by evidence from animal studies showing that AMI repair involves bone marrow cells[38] and by evidence of chimerism in transplanted hearts.[39]

In biologic terms, a chimera is an organism formed from aggregates of genetically different groups of cells derived from the same or a different species. Human chimerism is a well-recognized phenomenon involving two-way migration of cells from a host to a transplanted organ and vice versa. The unequivocal discovery of Y chromosome-positive cells in female donor hearts transplanted into male recipients has led to the theory that host cells replace donor heart cells that are lost as a result of transplant-associated ischemia/reperfusion injury. Chimerism in sex-mismatched transplanted hearts indicates that host cells produce not only cardiac myocytes but also endothelial and smooth muscle cells in those hearts. The biologic and clinical importance of chimerism and the true source of these host cells (whether bone marrow or the remaining atria of the transplant recipient) remain to be determined. It is most intriguing, however, that a population of host cells expressing progenitor cell surface markers (c-Kit, MDR1, and Sca-1) has been found in both the atria and the ventricles of transplanted hearts.[39]

Further evidence for the existence of a dynamic cardiac renewal process throughout adulthood comes from the recent identification of a novel population of early tissue-committed stem cells in the circulating pool of mononuclear cells.[40] These tissue-committed stem cells may be part of a group of circulating progenitor cells involved in cardiac repair. The particularities and interactions of resident and circulating stem cells in this setting continue to be delineated.

Conclusions

In summary, the potential for stem cell therapy in medicine – more specifically, in cardiology – is enormous. Principles relating to regenerative medicine are beginning to be understood as we start to identify some of the players and their roles. Cells are being studied intensely at the molecular level to help provide mechanistic answers and build a construct of knowledge in a relatively unknown field. This knowledge is being applied successfully in preclinical protocols, with a defined strategy of translational research that aims toward clinical applications. The field is moving fast, and not all the science is completely (or even somewhat!) understood; this has generated controversy among researchers, who caution against clinical advancement without the development of fundamental knowledge.

On the other hand, the clinical application is too promising to be held back, especially in light of the initial safety demonstrated in limited clinical trials. Real-world patients can benefit from real-world therapy when they are faced with the grim reality of death. To understand and apply this new therapy, the clinician will need to become familiar with the concepts outlined in this chapter and be ready for a future shift in the cardiovascular therapy paradigm.

References

1. American Heart Association. Heart Disease and Stroke Statistics – 2004 Update. Dallas: American Heart Association, 2003.
2. Perin E, Silva GV. Stem cell therapy for cardiac diseases. Curr Opin Hematol 2004;11:399–403.
3. Honold J, Assmus B, Lehman R, Zeiher AM, Dimmeler S. Stem cell therapy of cardiac disease: an update. Nephrol Dial Transplant 2004;19: 1673–7.
4. Nadal-Ginard B. Generation of new cardiomyocytes in the adult heart: prospects of myocardial regeneration as an alternative to cardiac transplantation. Rev Esp Cardiol 2001;54:543–50.
5. Asahara T, Masuda H, Takahashi T et al. Bone marrow origin of endothelial progenitor cells responsible for postnatal vasculogenesis in physiological and pathological neovascularization. Circ Res 1999;85:221–8.
6. Deb A, Wang S, Skelding KA, et al. Bone marrow-derived cardiomyocytes are present in adult human heart. A study of gender-mismatched bone marrow transplantation patients. Circulation 2003;107:1247–9.
7. Weissman IL. Stem cells: units of development, units of regeneration, and units in evolution. Cell 2000;100:157–68.
8. Blau HM, Brazelton TR, Weimann JM. The evolving concept of a stem cell: entity or function? Cell 2001;105:829–41.
9. www.nih.org.
10. Korbling M, Estrov Z. Adult stem cells for tissue repair – a new therapeutic concept? N Engl J Med 2003;349:570–82.
11. Hristov M, Erl W, Weber PC. Endothelial progenitor cells: mobilization, differentiation, and homing. Arterioscler Thromb Vasc Biol 2003;23:1–6.
12. Bruder SP, Jaiswal N, Haynesworth SE. Growth kinetics, self-renewal, and the osteogenic potential of purified human mesenchymal stem cells during extensive subcultivation and following cryopreservation. J Cell Biochem 1997;64: 278–94.
13. Bruder SP, Kurth AA, Shea M, Hayes WC, Jaiswal N, Kadiyala S. Bone regeneration by implantation of purified, culture-expanded human mesenchymal stem cells. J Orthop Res 1998;16:155–62.
14. Kadiyala S, Young RG, Thiede MA, Bruder SP. Culture expanded canine mesenchymal stem cells possess osteochondrogenic potential in vivo and in vitro. Cell Transplant 1997;6:125–34.
15. Young RG, Butler DL, Weber W, Caplan AI, Gordon SL, Fink DJ. Use of mesenchymal stem cells in a collagen matrix for Achilles tendon repair. J Orthop Res 1998;16:406–13.
16. Awad HA, Butler DL, Boivin GP, et al. Autologous mesenchymal stem cell-mediated repair of tendon. Tissue Eng 1999;5:267–77.
17. Ferrari G, Cusella-De Angelis G, Coletta M, et al. Muscle regeneration by bone marrow-derived myogenic progenitors. Science 1998;279:1528–30.
18. Galmiche MC, Koteliansky VE, Briere J, Herve P, Charbord P. Stromal cells from human long-term marrow cultures are mesenchymal cells that differentiate following a vascular smooth muscle differentiation pathway. Blood 1993;82:66–76.
19. Dennis JE, Merriam A, Awadallah A, Yoo JU, Johnstone B, Caplan AI. A quadripotential mesenchymal progenitor cell isolated from the marrow of an adult mouse. J Bone Miner Res 1999;14:700–9.
20. Prockop DJ. Marrow stromal cells as stem cells for nonhematopoietic tissues. Science 1997;276:71–4.
21. Hocht-Zeisberger E, Kahnert H, Kaomei G. Cellular repopulation of myocardial infarction in patients with sex-mismatched heart transplantation. Eur Heart J 2004;25:749–58.
22. Murry CE, Soonpaa MH, Reinecke H, et al. Haematopoietic stem cells do not transdifferentiate into cardiac myocytes in myocardial infarcts. Nature 2004;428:664–8.
23. Losordo DW, Dimmeler S. Therapeutic angiogenesis and vasculogenesis for ischemic disease – Part II: Cell-based therapies. Circulation 2004;109: 2692–7.
24. Zhang S, Wang D, Estrov Z. Both cell fusion and transdifferentiation account for the transformation of human peripheral blood CD34-positive cells into cardiomyocytes in vivo. Circulation 2004;110:3803–7.
25. Forrester JS, Price MJ, Makkar RR. Stem cell repair of infarcted myocardium: an overview for clinicians. Circulation 2003;108:1139–45.
26. Tang YL, Zhao Q, Zhang YC, et al. Autologous mesenchymal stem cell transplantation induce VEGF and neovascularization in ischemic myocardium. Regul Pept 2004;117:3–10.
27. Duan HF, Wu CT, Wu DL, et al. Treatment of myocardial ischemia with bone marrow-derived mesenchymal stem cells overexpressing hepatocyte growth factor. Mol Ther 2003;3:467–74.

28. Kinnaird T, Stabile E, Burnett MS. Local delivery of marrow-derived stromal cells augments collateral perfusion through paracrine mechanisms. Circulation 2004;109:1543–9.
29. Kinnaird T, Stabile E, Burnett MS. Marrow-derived stromal cells express genes encoding a broad spectrum of arteriogenic cytokines and promote in vitro and in vivo arteriogenesis through paracrine mechanisms. Circ Res 2004;94:678–85.
30. Anversa P, Nadal-Ginard B. Myocyte renewal and ventricular remodeling. Nature 2002;415:240–3.
31. Anversa P, Sussman MA, Bolli R. Molecular genetic advances in cardiovascular medicine focus on the myocyte. Circulation 2004;109:2832–8.
32. Rumpold H, Wolf D, Koeck R, Gunsilius E. Endothelial progenitor cells: a source for therapeutic vasculogenesis? J Cell Mol Med 2004;8:509–18.
33. Asahara T, Murohara T, Sullivan A, et al. Isolation of putative progenitor endothelial cells for angiogenesis. Science 1997;275:964–7.
34. Bhattacharya V, McSweeney PA, Shi Q, et al. Enhanced endothelialization and microvessel formation in polyester grafts seeded with $CD34^+$ bone marrow cells. Blood 2000;95:581–5.
35. Vasa M, Fichtlscherer S, Aicher A, et al. Number and migratory activity of circulating endothelial progenitor cells inversely correlate with risk factors for coronary artery disease. Circ Res 2001; 89:E1–7.
36. Graf T. Differentiation plasticity of hematopoietic cells. Blood 2002;99:3089–101.
37. Oh H, Bradfute SB, Gallardo TD, et al. Cardiac progenitor cells from adult myocardium: homing, differentiation, and fusion after infarction. Proc Natl Acad Sci USA 2003;100:12313–18.
38. Orlic D, Kajstura J, Chimenti S, et al. Bone marrow cells regenerate infarcted myocardium. Nature 2001;410:701–5.
39. Quaini F, Urbanek K, Beltrami AP, et al. Chimerism of the transplanted heart. N Engl J Med 2002;346: 5–15.
40. Kucia M, Ratajczak J, Ratajczak MZ. Bone marrow as a source of circulating $CXCR4^+$ tissue-committed stem cells. Biol Cell 2005;97:133–46.

chapter 2

The Basics of Embryonic Stem Cells in Comparison to Adult Stem Cells

Yong-Jian Geng

Introduction

Recent advances in biotechnology have given us a better understanding of the molecular and cellular basis of stem cell survival, growth, and differentiation, and of the potential for using stem cells to treat various diseases, including heart disease. Clinicians and basic research scientists are working closely to seek new stem cell sources and to develop new methodologies for stem cell isolation, growth, and transplantation. They are primarily studying two kinds of animal and human stem cells: embryonic stem cells (ESCs) and adult stem cells. Each of these two types of stem cells plays a role in tissue morphogenesis and postinjury repair, albeit differing in metabolism, function, and morphology. Before transplanting stem cells into damaged or diseased organs or tissues, however, investigators need to address many issues. The source, quality, and availability of stem cells should be considered first. ESCs are the most potent stem cells and so hold great promise for the development of new therapy. However, ethical considerations, limited numbers of cell lines in the USA, limited resources, the difficulty of obtaining autologous stem cells, and the potential risk for tumorigenesis have restricted their clinical application. On the other hand, adult stem cells can be obtained from the patient's own tissues, and their application does not raise ethical considerations, but their potency is limited.

In this chapter, we will focus on several fundamental issues in stem cell biology and on the potential application of stem cells in cardiovascular disease.

Methods for Establishing Embryonic Stem Cell Lines

There are several ways to isolate and establish ESC lines for cardiovascular research. After an oocyte has been fertilized in vitro by a sperm cell, the following events occur according to a fairly predictable timeline. Day 1 ends 18–24 hours after fertilization of the oocyte. By day 2, the zygote (fertilized egg) has undergone its first cleavage, producing a 2-cell embryo. By the end of day 3 (72 hours), the embryo has reached the 8-cell stage and is called a morula. At this stage, the embryo's development starts being controlled by its own genome. This means that maternal influences – due to the presence of mRNA and proteins in the oocyte cytoplasm – are significantly reduced. On day 4, the cells of the embryo adhere tightly to each other in a process known as compaction, and on day 5, the cavity of the blastocyst is completed.[1]

ESCs are derived from the blastocyst stage. This is the stage before the embryo is implanted into the uterine wall. Human and mouse blastocysts consist of 200–250 and 150 cells, respectively. The blastocyst cells are organized into an outer

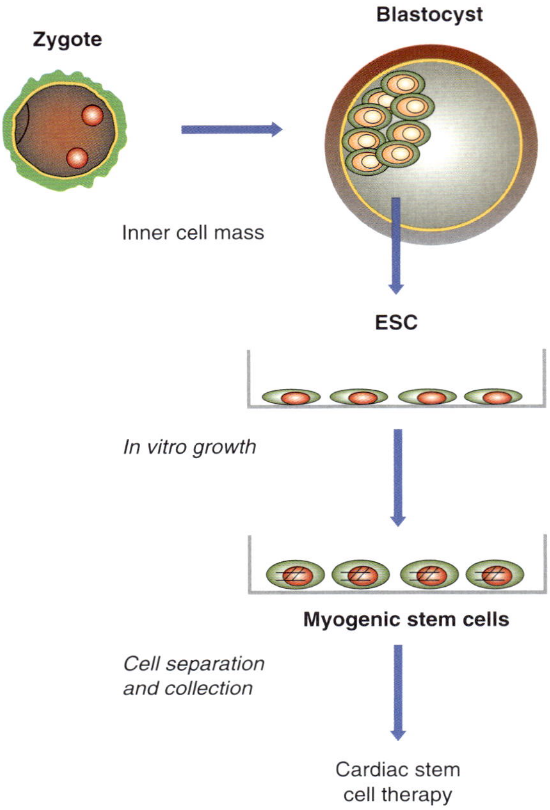

Figure 2.1 Embryonic stem cell (ESC) isolation and culture from the inner cell mass of the blastocyst.

layer (trophectoderm, which consists of most of the cells), a fluid-filled cavity (blastocele), and an inner cluster of cells (inner cell mass). The inner cell mass is the main source of ESCs (Figure 2.1). To derive ESC cultures, the trophectoderm is removed, either by microsurgery or immunosurgery (in which antibodies against the trophectoderm help break it down), thus freeing the inner cell mass. At this stage, the human inner cell mass is composed of only 30–34 cells. The in vitro conditions for growing a human embryo to the blastocyst stage vary. However, once the inner cell mass has been obtained from a mouse or human blastocyst, the techniques for growing ESCs are similar.[1]

ESCs can also be generated through somatic nucleus transfer or cloning technology. In theory, the nucleus of a differentiated mouse somatic cell can be reprogrammed by injecting it into an oocyte. The resultant pluripotent cell would be immunologically compatible with the donor because it would be genetically identical to the donor cell.[1]

Maintaining the pluripotency of ESCs was a major challenge to scientists. Establishment of ESC lines derived from mouse blastocysts became possible 20 years ago with the invention of techniques that allowed the cells to be grown but not differentiated in vitro.[1] The discovery of various growth factors (e.g., leukemia inhibitory factor, LIF) made the culture of ESCs possible. In the presence of LIF, stem cells stop differentiating and yet maintain their ability to proliferate.[2–4] However, stem cells from different species have different sensitivities to LIF. In humans, growth of ESCs requires additional factors, including fibroblast growth factors (FGFs) and colony-stimulating factors.

ESC lines may be derived from early embryos, in which case they closely resemble the cells of a preimplantation embryo, or from later embryos, in which case they are similar to cells derived from neonatal or adult tissues. Hence, stem cell lines may be heterogeneous. Nonetheless, all ESCs can proliferate extensively and differentiate into all adult cell types. When they are isolated and grown ex vivo (outside the organism), they continue to replicate and show the potential to differentiate. Although scientists are still debating how to define ESCs, some defining characteristics are presently accepted (Table 2.1).

The recent development of the somatic cell nucleus transfer (SCNT) technique has offered a new approach for establishing stem cells that immunologically and genetically match those of patients. In SCNT, a nucleus from one of the patient's own cells (e.g., a fibroblast) is injected into an oocyte that has had its nucleus removed. This procedure is also called therapeutic cloning. Because the stem cells derived from the oocyte carry almost the entire genomic material of the donor patient, therotically speaking, they carry the same immunogenic signals as the donor cells, and therefore do not provoke an immunorejection response, a major factor causing the failure of stem cell therapy.

Table 2.1 Biologic properties of embryonic stem cells (ESCs)[1]

- Derived from the inner cell mass of the blastocyst
- Capable of undergoing an unlimited number of symmetrical divisions without differentiating (long-term self-renewal)
- Exhibit and maintain a stable, full (diploid), normal complement of chromosomes (karyotype)
- Can give rise to differentiated cell types that are derived from all three primary germ layers of the embryo (endoderm, mesoderm, and ectoderm)
- Capable of differentiating into all fetal tissues during development (mouse ESCs maintained in culture for long periods can still generate any tissue when they are reintroduced into an embryo to generate a chimera)
- Capable of colonizing the germline and giving rise to oocytes or sperm cells
- Clonogenic (can give rise to a colony of genetically identical cells, or clones, that have the same properties as the original cell)
- Express the transcription factor Oct-4, which then activates or inhibits a host of target genes and maintains ESCs in a proliferative, nondifferentiating state
- Can be induced to continue proliferating or to differentiate
- Lack the G_1 checkpoint in the cell cycle. ESCs spend most of their time in the S phase of the cell cycle, during which they synthesize DNA. Unlike differentiated somatic cells, ESCs do not require an external stimulus to initiate DNA replication
- Do not show X inactivation. In every somatic cell of a female mammal, one of the two X chromosomes becomes permanently inactivated: this X inactivation does not occur in ESCs

SCNT was first explored by Hans Spemann in the 1920s for genetics research and is now explored for potential clinical application.[5] By definition, a somatic cell is any cell other than a sperm, an oocyte, or a cell that gives rise to a sperm or oocyte. SCNT requires two cells: a donor cell and an oocyte. The procedure of SCNT has multiple steps (Figure 2.2):

1. Isolate the donor nucleus from a somatic cell (e.g., a fibroblast or myofibroblast) of a mature donor. The donor cell is usually at the G_0 ("gap zero") phase of the cell cycle, a dormant phase, causing the cell to shut down but not die. In this state, the nucleus is ready to be accepted by the oocyte.
2. Remove the nucleus of the oocyte (containing its DNA). The recipient oocyte must be completely enucleated, which eliminates the majority of its genetic information.
3. Implant the somatic cell nucleus (and its DNA) in the nucleus-free oocyte. Either a fertilized or an unfertilized oocyte can be used, but the latter seems more likely to accept the donor nucleus as its own. The donor cell's nucleus can be placed inside the oocyte, through either cell fusion or transplantation. The egg cell is then prompted to begin forming an embryo. To harvest stem cells, the oocyte carrying the transferred nucleus is induced to divide until it reaches the blastocyst stage, at which time the cells of the inner cell mass are removed and cultured. These cells – ESCs – are pluripotent.

Although this technique shows great promise, it also has certain limitations. Ethical and biosafety issues remain major problems. In addition, because some genetic material from the mitochondria of the oocytes is still present, any defect or mutation in the mitochondrial DNA can pass down to the stem cells.

Methods for Testing Pluripotency

An ESC is characterized by its pluripotency. The following three kinds of experiments test whether a stem cell line (regardless of whether it originated from rodents or humans) is pluripotent and so determine whether it is an ESC.[1]

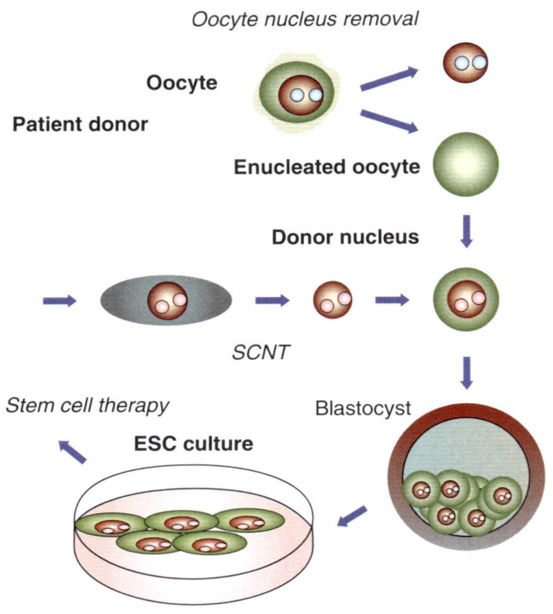

Figure 2.2 *Schematic presentation of the establishment of a patient-compatible embryonic stem cell (ESC) line for therapy by somatic cell nucleus transfer (SCNT).*

1. *Formation of chimeras*. This test is conducted by injecting ESCs derived from the inner cell mass of one blastocyst into the cavity of another blastocyst. The resulting combination embryos are then implanted in the uterus of a female mouse, and the progeny that result are known as chimeras. Chimeras are a mixture of tissues and organs derived from both the recipient blastocyst and donor ESCs. If the resulting chimeras are complete embryos, then the donor stem cells must have been pluripotent. Cultured ESCs can also replace the inner cell mass of a mouse blastocyst and produce a normal embryo, but the process is far less efficient than that of using cells taken directly from the inner cell mass. Whether mouse ESCs can generate a complete embryo depends on the number of times they have been passaged in vitro. A passage is the process of removing cells from one culture dish and replating them into fresh culture dishes. Whether the number of passages affects the differentiation potential of human ESCs remains to be determined.[1]
2. *Formation of mature tissues from transplants*. A second method for determining the pluripotency of mouse ESCs is to inject the cells into genetically identical or immune-deficient adult mice (under the skin or kidney capsule), so the tissue will not be rejected. If the injected cells are pluripotent, they develop into benign tumors called teratomas. These tumors contain cell types derived from all three primary germ layers of the embryo. Teratomas typically contain gut-like structures such as layers of epithelial cells and smooth muscle, skeletal or cardiac muscle (which may contract spontaneously), neural tissue, cartilage or bone, and sometimes hair. Even though mouse ESCs do not generate trophoblast tissues in vivo, ESCs that have been maintained for a long period in vitro can ultimately behave like pluripotent cells in vivo. In vitro, mouse ESCs can form an embryo by differentiating into any somatic cell type and can differentiate into a wide range of cell types in an adult.[1]
3. *In vitro differentiation*. A third technique for demonstrating pluripotency is to allow mouse ESCs to differentiate spontaneously in vitro or to direct their differentiation along specific pathways. The former is usually accomplished by removing feeder layers and adding LIF to the growth medium. Within a few days after changing the culture conditions, ESCs aggregate and may form embryoid bodies, which resemble teratomas. Embryoid bodies consist of a disorganized array of differentiated or partially differentiated cell types that are derived from the three primary germ layers of the embryo.[1]

Understanding how ESCs replicate for hundreds of population doublings without differentiating is a major task that has been pursued for decades.[1] To date, two major areas of investigation have provided some clues. One involves investigating the effects of secreted factors, such as LIF, on mouse ESCs in vitro. The second area of study involves investigating the effects of transcription factors, such as Oct-4. This is a protein expressed by mouse and human ESCs in vitro and by mouse inner cell mass cells in vivo. The cell cycle of the ESC also seems to play a role in preventing differentiation. Many factors must be balanced in a particular way for ESCs to remain in a self-renewing state. If the balance shifts, the stem cells begin to differentiate.

Directing Differentiation of Embryonic Stem Cells

Directing pluripotent stem cells, especially human ESCs, to tissue-specific development is a major challenge.[2] How genetic or environmental factors induce stem cells to develop into specialized cells is largely unknown.[6] The directed differentiation of ESCs is vital to their use in the development of new therapies. One of the most common approaches for directing tissue- or cell type-specific differentiation is to change the stem cell culture conditions. By adding growth factors to the culture medium or changing the chemical composition of the dish surface, the ESCs can be induced to grow in a direction favorable to a specific tissue. For example, the plastic culture dishes used to grow mouse and human stem cells can be treated with a variety of substances that allow the cells either to adhere to the surface of the dish or to avoid adhering and instead float in the culture medium. The floating of ESCs in the culture medium may help them differentiate into heart muscle cells. In general, an adherent substrate prevents ESCs from interacting and differentiating, whereas a nonadherent substrate allows them to aggregate and thereby interact with each other. Cell–cell interactions are critical to normal embryonic development, so allowing some of these in vivo interactions to occur in the culture dish is a fundamental strategy for inducing mouse or human stem cell differentiation in vitro. In addition, adding specific growth factors to the culture medium triggers the activation (or inactivation) of specific genes in stem cells. This initiates a series of molecular events that induces the cells to differentiate along a particular pathway. For example, overexpression of the GATA-4 transcription factor in ESCs may enhance cardiomyogenesis.[1,7]

Genetic manipulation may also help direct ESC differentiation. One can introduce foreign genes into the cells via transfection or other methods. The added foreign genes trigger the cells to differentiate along a particular pathway. This approach is a precise way of regulating ESC differentiation, but it will work only if it is possible to identify which gene must be active at which particular stage of differentiation. Then the gene must be inserted into the genome at the proper location and activated during the correct stage of differentiation. Gene-guided differentiation has several pitfalls, including the lack of specific target genes, potential toxicity to stem cells, and modification of stem cells by vectors themselves.

All of the techniques described are still highly experimental. Nevertheless, within the past several years, it has become possible to generate differentiated, functional cells by manipulating the growth conditions of mouse ESCs in vitro.[6,7] How the directed differentiation occurs has not been explained. It is not known how or when gene expression is changed, which signal transduction systems are triggered, or what cell–cell interactions must occur to convert ESCs into precursor cells and, finally, into differentiated cells that look and function like their in vivo counterparts.[1]

Directing Differentiation of Adult Stem Cells

Upon stimulation by extrinsic or intrinsic factors, the adult stem cell can renew itself and yield all cell types of the tissue from which it originated. In theory, adult stem cells are capable of self-renewal throughout an organism's lifetime. However, as the organism ages, the number of tissue-specific stem cells declines, impairing regeneration or repair in adult tissues and organs. Different tissues and organs have different abundances of stem cells. Theoretically, tissues and organs such as the heart and the brain, with highly specialized, long-living cells, have fewer adult stem cells than do fast-turnover

Table 2.2 Comparison of biologic properties between embryonic and adult stem cells

Characteristic	*Embryonic Stem Cells*	*Adult Stem Cells*
Origin	Inner mass of the blastocyst	Various tissues (e.g., bone marrow, heart, adipose tissue)
Growth	Unlimited, symmetrical divisions	Limited, often asymmetrical divisions
Differentiation potential	Higher	Lower
Stable cell lines	Exist	Do not exist
Immunogenicity	Lower	Higher
Tumorigenicity	Higher	Lower
Ethical issues	Yes	No

tissues and organs such as the bone marrow and skin.

Recent studies have shown that certain types of adult stem cells, including those from bone marrow, are capable of differentiating into specialized cells in somatic tissues, such as those of the skeletal muscle, liver, heart, and brain. This ability to transdifferentiate, or differentiate into a cell type of a tissue other than the originating tissue, is called *cytoplasticity*.

Thus, transplanting adult stem cells into an infarcted heart may help in myocardial tissue repair or regeneration. The adult heart contains limited numbers of adult stem cells, and its regenerative capacity is generally lower than that of other tissues such as the liver and bone marrow. Because adult stem cells can transdifferentiate, they can be transplanted into the heart from other tissues such as bone marrow. In our institution and elsewhere, clinical trials have shown some therapeutic benefits in selected groups of patients with ischemic heart failure or myocardiac infarction.[8–10]

However, adult stem cells have some disadvantages over ESCs in terms of potency in growth and differentiation (Table 2.2). Usually, it is very difficult to establish a stable adult stem cell line, and adult stem cells have limited passage capacity. Therefore, isolation and growth of a large number of adult stem cells constitutes a major challenge to clinical adult stem cell application. Adult stem cells appear to show stronger immunogenicity – i.e., allogeneic adult stem cells may provoke immune cells more frequently than allogeneic ESCs. Because of this, the SCNT approach to establishing a customized stem cell line with the patient's own nucleus has been explored very recently.[5]

Adult Stem Cells and Cardiac Repair

Researchers now know that under highly specific growth conditions in laboratory culture dishes, adult stem cells can transdifferentiate into new cardiomyocytes and vascular endothelial cells. To test the ability of these cells to restore cardiac function, investigators have used animal models of a heart attack.[11] In the experimental procedures, a ligature is placed around a major blood vessel serving the heart muscle, thereby depriving the cardiomyocytes of their oxygen and nutrient supplies and causing a heart attack. Over the past several years, researchers using such models have made several key discoveries that kindled interest in the application of adult stem cells to heart muscle repair.[1]

Orlic et al[12] reported an experimental application of hematopoietic stem cells for cardiac tissue regeneration. In this study, a heart attack was induced in mice by tying off a major blood vessel, the left main coronary artery. By identifying unique cellular surface markers, the investigators then isolated a select group of adult hematopoietic stem cells. When injected into the damaged wall of the ventricle, these cells led to the formation of new cardiomyocytes, vascular endothelial cells, and smooth muscle cells, thus generating de novo myocardium, including coronary arteries, arterioles, and capillaries. Nine days after the bone marrow cells were transplanted, the newly formed myocardium occupied 68% of the damaged portion of the ventricle, in effect replacing the dead myocardium with living, functioning tissue. The researchers found that mice that received the injected cells survived in greater numbers than mice that did not receive the mouse stem cells. Follow-up experiments are now being conducted to extend the post-transplantation analysis time to determine the longer-range effects of such therapy. The partial repair of the damaged heart muscle suggests that the injected mouse hematopoietic stem cells responded to signals in the environment near the injured myocardium and migrated to the damaged region of the ventricle, where they multiplied and became cardiomyocytes.[1]

Cardiac tissue can also be partially regenerated in the mouse heart attack model through the transplantation of adult stem cells from mouse bone marrow. Using this model, investigators purified a side population of hematopoietic stem cells from a genetically altered mouse strain.[13] These cells were then transplanted into the marrow of lethally irradiated mice. Ten weeks later, the recipient mice were subjected to a heart attack via the tying off of a different major cardiac blood vessel, the left anterior descending (LAD) coronary artery. Two to four weeks after the induced cardiac injury, the survival rate was 26%. As with the study by Orlic et al,[12] donor-derived cardiomyocytes and endothelial cells were found surrounding the damaged tissue in surviving mice. Thus, the mouse hematopoietic stem cells transplanted into the bone marrow had responded to signals in the injured heart, migrated to the border region of the damaged area, and differentiated into several types of tissue needed for cardiac repair. This study suggests that mouse hematopoietic stem cells can be delivered to the heart through bone marrow transplantation in addition to through direct injection.[1]

More evidence for the potential of stem cell-based therapies to treat heart disease is provided by a study that showed that human adult hematopoietic stem cells are capable of giving rise to vascular endothelial cells when transplanted into rats.[14] As in the previous study, these researchers induced a heart attack by tying off the LAD coronary artery. They took great care to identify a population of human hematopoietic stem cells that give rise to new blood vessels. These cytoplastic cells were used to form new blood vessels in the damaged area of the rats' hearts and to encourage proliferation of preexisting vasculature following the experimental heart attack.[1]

Under the appropriate culture conditions, human hematopoietic stem cells, like mouse hematopoietic stem cells, can be induced to transdifferentiate into numerous tissue types, including cardiac muscle. When injected into the bloodstream leading to the damaged rat heart, these cells have prevented the death of hypertrophied, or thickened but otherwise viable, myocardial cells and reduced progressive formation of collagen fibers and scars.[15] Furthermore, the hematopoietic cells could be identified on the basis of highly specific cell markers that differentiated them from cardiomyocyte precursor cells. This would enable the cells to be used alone or in conjunction with myocyte regeneration strategies or pharmacologic therapies.[1]

Embryonic Stem Cells and Cardiac Repair

Because of their ability to differentiate into any cell type in the adult body, ESCs are another possible source population for cardiac repair cells. The first step in this application was taken by Itskovitz-Eldor et al,[16] who demonstrated that human ESCs can reproducibly differentiate in vitro into embryoid bodies. Among the various cell types found in the embryoid bodies were cells that had the physical appearance of cardiomyocytes, showed cellular markers consistent with heart cells, and demonstrated contractile activity similar to that of cardiomyocytes.[1]

In a continuation of this early work, scientists found structural and functional properties of early-stage cardiomyocytes in the cells that developed from embryoid bodies. Using antibody markers, Kehat et al[17] identified the cells that spontaneously contracted as myosin heavy chain, α-actinin, desmin, antinatriuretic protein, and cardiac troponin – all proteins found in heart tissue. A genetic analysis of these cells showed that the transcription factor genes expressed were consistent with early-stage cardiomyocytes. Electrical recordings from these cells, changes in calcium ion movement within the cells, and the cells' contractile responsiveness to catecholamine hormone stimulation were similar to those seen in early cardiomyocytes observed during mammalian development.[1]

Min et al[18] induced heart attacks in rodents by ligating the LAD coronary artery, then transplanted ESCs from culture. Cardiac function improved. Using markers, the researchers found that cells in the recipient hearts, including the myocardium, were derived from the ESCs. This research shows that, like adult stem cells, ESCs can repair cardiac tissue in rodents.

Evaluation of the Use of Stem Cells in Cardiac Repair

These breakthrough discoveries in rodent models present new opportunities for using stem cells to repair damaged heart muscle. But the evidence is not complete. The mouse hematopoietic stem cell populations that give rise to cardiac replacement cells are not homogeneous. Rather, they are enriched for the cells of interest through specific and selective stimulating factors that promote cell growth. Thus, the originating cell population of these injected cells has not been identified, and the injected cells may originate from cell populations that could cause the recipient to reject the transplanted cells. This is a major issue for clinical applications, but it is not as relevant in the experimental models described here because the experimental rodents have been bred to be genetically similar. Another issue is the ability to produce a sufficient number of cells for clinical application: the repair of one damaged human heart would likely require millions of cells. Thus, the unique capacity of ESCs to replicate easily in culture may give them an advantage over adult stem cells.[1]

Although researchers know that adult stem cells and ESCs can repair damaged heart tissue, many questions need to be answered before any widespread clinical applications can be considered. For example, how long will the replacement cells continue to function? Do the rodent research models accurately reflect human heart conditions and transplantation responses? Do these replacement cardiomyocytes have the electrical signal conducting capabilities of native cardiac muscle cells?[1]

Stem cells may well serve as the foundation upon which a future form of cellular therapy is constructed. In current animal models, the time between injury to the heart and application of stem cells affects the degree to which regeneration takes place, and this has real implications for the patient who is rushed unprepared to the emergency room in the wake of a heart attack. In the future, could the patient's cells be harvested and expanded for use in an efficient manner? Alternatively, could at-risk patients donate their cells in advance, thus minimizing the preparation necessary for the cells' administration? Moreover, could stem cells be genetically programmed to migrate directly to the site of injury and immediately synthesize the heart proteins necessary for the regeneration process? Investigators are currently addressing these questions, thus providing a promising future for cardiac repair.[1]

Conclusions

Stem cells show great potential in regenerative medicine. Establishment of ESC lines and isolation of adult stem cells provide a great opportunity to develop a potentially novel therapy for treating many medical disorders, including several life-threatening cardiovascular conditions and diseases, such as myocardial infarction and heart failure. ESCs have a higher potency of replication and cell lineage differentiation than do adult stem cells. Both ESCs and adult stem cells can develop into cardiovascular cells, including cardiac myocytes, smooth muscle cells, and endothelial cells. And yet, it is largely unknown whether the two types of stem cells have the same potential for repopulating cardiomyocytes and improving heart function. Because of ethical and biosafety issues, ESCs have not been used for clinical application. The majority of information about the potential application of ESCs in regenerative cardiovascular medicine comes from laboratories and experimental animal models. However, studies involving an array of adult stem cell types have been done. Most recently, attention has shifted to the use of autologous bone marrow-derived stem cells, with encouraging results. Cardiac function has improved in selected patients who have undergone treatment with autologous bone marrow-derived stem cells delivered via a transendocardial or an intracoronary approach.

Acknowledgments

The work of the author is partially supported by grants from the National Institutes of Health, the Texas Higher Education Board ATP/ADP programs, and the DREAMS/T5 Research Program awarded by the US Department of Defense.

References

1. Report on stem cells. National Institutes of Health 2001. http://stemcells.nih.gov/info/scireport Accessed June 17, 2005.
2. Lebkowski JS, Gold J, Xu C, et al. Human embryonic stem cells: culture, differentiation, and genetic modification for regenerative medicine applications. Cancer J 2001;7(Suppl 2):S83–93.
3. Murray R, Lee F, Chiu CP. The genes for leukemia inhibitory factor and interleukin-6 are expressed in mouse blastocysts prior to the onset of hemopoiesis. Mol Cell Biol 1990;10:4953–6.
4. Nir SG, David R, Zaruba M, et al. Human embryonic stem cells for cardiovascular repair. Cardiovasc Res 2003;58:313–23.
5. Hwang WS, Roh SI, Lee BC, et al. Patient-specific embryonic stem cells derived from human SCNT blastocysts. Science 2005;308:1777–83.
6. Maltsev VA, Wobus AM, Rohwedel J, et al. Cardiomyocytes differentiated in vitro from embryonic stem cells developmentally express cardiac-specific genes and ionic currents. Circ Res 1994;75:233–44.
7. Grepin C, Nemer G, Nemer M. Enhanced cardiogenesis in embryonic stem cells overexpressing the GATA-4 transcription factor. Development 1997;124:2387–95.
8. Perin EC, Dohmann HF, Borojevic R, et al. Transendocardial, autologous bone marrow cell transplantation for severe, chronic ischemic heart failure. Circulation 2003;107:2294–302.
9. Perin EC, Dohmann HF, Borojevic R, et al. Improved exercise capacity and ischemia 6 and 12 months after transendocardial injection of autologous bone marrow mononuclear cells for ischemic cardiomyopathy. Circulation 2004; 110(11 Suppl 1): II213–18.
10. Silva GV, Perin EC, Dohmann HF, et al. Catheter-based transendocardial delivery of autologous bone-marrow-derived mononuclear cells in patients listed for heart transplantation. Tex Heart Inst J 2004;31:214–19.
11. Silva GV, Litovsky S, Assad JA, et al. Mesenchymal stem cells differentiate into an endothelial phenotype, enhance vascular density, and improve heart function in a canine chronic ischemia model. Circulation 2005;111:150–6.
12. Orlic D, Kajstura J, Chimenti S, et al. Bone marrow cells regenerate infarcted myocardium. Nature 2001;410:701–5.
13. Jackson KA, Majka SM, Wang H, et al. Regeneration of ischemic cardiac muscle and vascular endothelium by adult stem cells. J Clin Invest 2001;107: 1395–402.
14. Kocher AA, Schuster MD, Szabolcs MJ, et al. Neovascularization of ischemic myocardium by human bone-marrow-derived angioblasts prevents cardiomyocyte apoptosis, reduces remodeling and improves cardiac function. Nat Med 2001;7:430–6.
15. Pittenger MF, Mackay AM, Beck SC, et al. Multilineage potential of adult human mesenchymal stem cells. Science 1999;284:143–7.
16. Itskovitz-Eldor J, Schuldiner M, Karsenti D, et al. Differentiation of human embryonic stem cells into embryoid bodies compromising the three embryonic germ layers. Mol Med 2000;6:88–95.
17. Kehat I, Kenyagin-Karsenti D, Snir M, et al. Human embryonic stem cells can differentiate into myocytes with structural and functional properties of cardiomyocytes. J Clin Invest 2001;108:407–14.
18. Min JY, Yang Y, Converso KL, et al. Transplantation of embryonic stem cells improves cardiac function in postinfarcted rats. J Appl Physiol 2002;92:288–96.

chapter 3

The Basics of Mesenchymal Lineage Progenitor Cells

Silviu Itescu

Introduction

The mammalian bone marrow comprises two distinct stem cell populations that co-operate and are functionally interdependent, the hematopoietic and mesenchymal lineage progenitors. Traditionally, mesenchymal lineage progenitors within the bone marrow stroma have been viewed largely in terms of their well-documented role in supporting the proliferation, differentiation, and maturation of hematopoietic stem cells (HSCs). However, while hematopoietic lineage stem cells appear to be relatively restricted in their range of tissue differentiation to cells of hematopoietic and endothelial lineage, mesenchymal lineage progenitors have recently been shown to contain multipotent stem cells with the capacity to give rise to a variety of differentiated cell lineages, including bone, cartilage, adipose, smooth muscle, and even cardiac muscle tissue.

The increasing recognition of the multipotential properties of mesenchymal lineage progenitor cells, together with their apparent ease of manipulation in culture, has generated great interest in using these cells for diverse clinical applications. More intriguing recent data have focused on the ability of these cells to evade recognition by the immune cells of unrelated recipients, raising the possibility that they may potentially constitute a source of allogeneic cellular therapeutic products. This review will give an overview of the identity, nature, developmental origin and functional characteristics of mesenchymal lineage progenitor cells, their amenability to ex vivo culture manipulation, and their therapeutic potential, particularly for patients with cardiovascular disease.

Mammalian Marrow Contains Mesenchymal Lineage Progenitors That Have High Proliferative Capacity and Are Clonogenic in Vitro

Friedenstein et al[1] were the first to establish a reproducible biologic assay to identify the presence of cells in mammalian bone marrow capable of giving rise to multiple tissues of mesenchymal lineage, including bone, cartilage, and fat. Using gentle mechanical disruption of bone marrow tissue, these researchers were able to readily dissociate stromal and hematopoietic cells into a single-cell suspension. The bone marrow stromal cells rapidly adhere, can be easily separated from the nonadherent hematopoietic cells by repeated washing, and, under appropriate culture conditions, give rise to distinct colonies. The clonogenic stromal progenitor cells responsible for colony growth under these conditions are termed fibroblast colony-forming cells (CFU-Fs, for "colony-forming units – fibroblast") and are rapidly adherent, nonphagocytic, clonogenic cells capable of extended proliferation in vitro.

The degree of CFU-F proliferative activity in vitro is greatly dependent on the mitogenic factors present in the culture media. The most important of these include platelet-derived growth factor (PDGF), epidermal growth factor (EGF), basic fibroblast growth factor (bFGF), transforming growth factor β (TGF-β), and insulin-like growth factor I (IGF-I).[2,3] Under optimal conditions, cultured cells combined from multiple CFU-F colonies can undergo more than 50 cell doublings, or over 25 culture passages, demonstrating extensive self-replicative capacity.

Marrow Mesenchymal Lineage Progenitors Isolated on the Basis of Physical Properties Demonstrate Functional in Vitro Heterogeneity

Neither CFU-F outgrowth nor expression of osteogenic, chondrogenic, or adipogenic phenotypic markers in culture (detected either by mRNA expression or by histochemical techniques) necessarily constitutes multipotency of a given clone.[4] Typically, CFU-F outgrowth is heterogeneous and is characterized by a broad range of colony sizes and different cell morphologies, representing varying growth rates of different cell types, ranging from spindle-shaped cells to large flat cells. Moreover, different clones may spontaneously differentiate to different tissues under inductive conditions in vitro or following transplantation in vivo.[5,6]

Interestingly, the bone marrow stromal population from which mesenchymal lineage stem cells are derived shares properties with cells of fibroblast, myofibroblast, and endothelial cell lineage, expressing matrix proteins and α smooth muscle actin (α-SMA), as well as endoglin/CD105 and MUC-18/CD146. Despite attempts to use only those clones that have been distinctively characterized phenotypically following ex vivo culture and passage of cells initially isolated from bone marrow stroma by simple density gradient separation and plastic adherence, the resulting clones continue to display varying degrees of multipotentiality.[7] To date, no surface marker expressed by in vitro cultured mesenchymal lineage cells has consistently shown predictability of the biologic behavior of any given clone either in vitro or in vivo.

Prospective Immunoselection of Mesenchymal Lineage Precursor Cells Enhances Reproducible Functional Outgrowth

To generate mesenchymal lineage stem cells with sufficient functional reproducibility to enable clinical use, investigators have sought to develop more precise methods to identify and isolate the subset of marrow mesenchymal lineage precursors with the most extensive replication and differentiation potential. This requires prospective linkage between surface phenotype, genotype, and multipotency displayed in transplantation assays. By immunizing mice with human mesenchymal lineage precursors, several laboratories have developed monoclonal antibodies reactive with and suitable for isolation of highly purified mesenchymal precursor cell populations.[8–11] Use of a monoclonal antibody reactive with an antigen termed Stro-1 enables identification of a population of marrow stromal cells that are clonogenic (Stro-1^{bright})[12] and results in a 10- to 20-fold enrichment of CFU-Fs relative to their incidence in unseparated bone marrow.[13] Freshly isolated Stro-1^{bright} cells, containing multipotent stromal/mesenchymal lineage stem cells, have been extensively characterized for a long list of markers expressed by fibroblasts, myofibroblasts, endothelial cells, and hematopoietic cells in several different laboratories.[14–17] In these studies, combined use of monoclonal antibodies against Stro-1 and vascular cell adhesion molecule 1 (VCAM-1/CD106) results in up to 1000-fold enrichment of CFU-Fs relative to their incidence in unseparated bone marrow, with a CFU-F incidence of approximately 1 per 2 cells plated.[17] At a clonal level, Stro-1^{bright} VCAM-1^{+} cells are devoid of hematopoietic, fibroblast, or endothelial lineage cells, and demonstrate multipotential capability, differentiating to bone, cartilage, and adipose tissue. Thus, in order to maximize functional reproducibility, all efforts should be made to initiate mesenchymal lineage stem cell culture expansion with as pure and homogeneous a population of Stro-1^{bright} VCAM-1^{+} cells as possible.

Distinctive Anatomic Location of Mesenchymal Lineage Precursor Cells Suggests a Shared Identity with Vascular Pericytes

There are now cumulative data from a number of investigators that convincingly point toward the identity of clonogenic stromal/mesenchymal lineage stem cell precursors as being cells intimately associated with blood vessel walls – generally referred to as vascular smooth muscle cells or pericytes. By immunohistochemistry, Stro-1^{+} cells in human bone marrow, as well as at other sites (including abdominal fat, dental pulp, skin, and liver), are predominantly localized anatomically to perivascular and sinusoidal sites.[18] Here, they are found to coexpress markers typically associated with both vascular smooth muscle, such as α-SMA, and with endothelium, such as MUC-18/CD146.

Observations from cultured bone marrow-derived stromal cells support the interpretation that mesenchymal precursor cells are vascular pericytes in vivo. Cultured stromal cells/mesenchymal lineage stem cells coexpress α-SMA as well as other markers of pericytes/smooth muscle cells, such as caldesmon, metavinculin, calponin, and smooth muscle myosin heavy chains.[19] Moreover, cultured pericytes and marrow stromal cells synthesize very similar extracellular matrix proteins, including a variety of basal lamina and interstitial collagens.[20,21] In addition, marrow stromal cells respond exuberantly to culture with PDGF-BB[22] a cytokine whose interaction with its cognate receptor is involved in pericyte recruitment and viability.[23] Finally, vascular pericytes isolated from blood vessels or the retina fulfill criteria for being multipotential mesenchymal precursors, demonstrating capability for differentiation into a variety of cell types, including osteoblasts, adipocytes, chondrocytes, and fibroblasts.[24–29]

Formation of Vascular Structures During Embryogenesis: Inter-relationship Between Pericytes and Endothelial Precursors

In order to develop successful methods for inducing neovascularization of the adult heart, one needs to understand the process of definitive vascular network formation during embryogenesis. In the prenatal period, hemangioblasts derived from the human ventral aorta give rise to cellular elements involved in both vasculogenesis, or formation of the primitive capillary network, and hematopoiesis.[30,31] Under the regulatory influence of various transcriptional and differentiation factors, embryonic hemangioblasts mature, migrate, and differentiate to become endothelial lining cells and create the primitive vasculogenic network. Subsequent to capillary tube formation, the newly created vasculogenic vessels undergo sprouting, tapering, remodeling, and regression under the direction of vascular endothelial growth factor (VEGF), angiopoietins, and other factors – a process termed angiogenesis. The final component required for definitive vascular network formation to sustain embryonic organogenesis is an influx of mesenchymal lineage cells to form the vascular supporting mural cells such as vascular smooth muscle cells (vSMCs) and pericytes.

The embryologic origins of pericytes and vSMCs include mesenchymal cells surrounding the dorsal aorta,[32,33] neural crest cells in the forebrain and cardiac outflow tract,[34] and epicardial cells in heart coronary vessels.[35] In the mature vascular system, the endothelium is supported by mural cells, with the smallest capillaries partially covered by solitary pericytes and with arteries and veins surrounded by single or multiple layers of vSMCs. It has been suggested that pericytes and vSMCs represent a continuum of a common mural cell lineage and that pericytes may give rise to vSMCs during vessel enlargement or remodeling (arteriogenesis).[36] The vSMCs provide structural support to large vessels and are important regulators of arteriolar blood flow due to contractile characteristics. Whereas pericytes directly contact endothelial cells via N-cadherin- and β-catenin-based adherens junctions,[37] vSMCs are separated from the endothelium by a basement membrane, and in larger arteries by the intima.

Pericytes form intimate connections with endothelial cells, alterations in these interactions having significant consequences on microvasculature morphology and physiology. Injecting N-cadherin-neutralizing antibodies into the developing chick brain has profound effects on vascular integrity,[38] while injecting neutralizing PDGF receptor β (PDGFR-β) antibodies in newborn mice results in almost complete impairment of pericyte recruitment to the retinal microvasculature, with severe defects in vascular patterning.[39] Detailed analysis of the microvasculature in PDGF-B and PDGFR-β knockout mice demonstrates abnormal capillary diameters, rupturing microaneurysms, endothelial hyperplasia, defects in endothelial junction formation, and formation of numerous cytoplasmic folds at the luminal surface of the endothelium.[23] Together with physiological signs of hypoxia in these knockout animals, such as upregulation of VEGF-A expression,[23] these observations indicate that pericytes control endothelial differentiation in vivo, have a profound role in sprouting angiogenesis in the retina, and have a major effect on capillary blood flow in general.

Human Mesenchymal Precursor Cells as Progenitors of the Vascular Network

As with the development of other organs in the embryo, establishment of the primitive marrow stroma involves a complex series of events that require vascular invasion of primitive bone rudiments.[40] The relevance of the vascular system persists in the postnatal skeleton, with the medullary vascular network consisting of a continuous layer of endothelial cells and subendothelial pericytes and being shared by bone and bone marrow.[41,42] Under normal steady-state conditions, human bone marrow expression of α-SMA is limited to vSMCs in the media of arteries, pericytes lining capillaries, and occasional flattened cells on the endosteal surface of bone.[43] Strikingly, pericytes in the arterial and capillary sections of the medullary vascular network coexpress α-SMA and Stro-1, consistent with the identity and anatomic location of stromal/mesenchymal progenitors as vSMCs/pericytes.[18]

The perivascular in vivo location of human mesenchymal lineage precursors, together with their coexpression of markers of both endothelial and smooth muscle lineage cells and their multipotential capabilities, raises the intriguing possibility that mesenchymal lineage precursors may be true progenitors of the vascular tree. This possibility is supported by work with embryonic stem cells, where a common vascular endothelial growth factor receptor 2 (VEGFR-2, FLK-1/KDR)-positive precursor gives rise to cells of both endothelial and smooth muscle lineage, resulting in development of the embryonic vasculature.[44,45]

The intimate proximity of human perivascular mesenchymal lineage precursors to vascular endothelium suggests that each cell type influences the biology of the other. Migration of mesenchymal lineage precursors and formation of a pericyte coating in physical continuity with the nascent vascular network is dependent on production of EGF and PDGF-B by nascent endothelial tubes.[46] Conversely, maintenance of vessel integrity, stabilization, and prevention of vessel pruning are dependent on pericyte coating of the microvessel.[46]

During normal bone development, new bone formation occurs in a precise spatial and temporal sequence, best visualized in metaphyseal growth plates. Importantly, new bone cell growth accompanies endothelial cell growth, pericyte coverage, and active angiogenesis. Inhibition of angiogenesis results in blockade of both metaphyseal endochondral bone formation and related activities in the adjacent cartilage growth plates.[47] Together, these observations suggest that Stro-1$^+$ mesenchymal lineage precursors serve as important regulators of new blood vessel formation in the bone marrow, in growing bone, and, in view of their ubiquitous expression throughout the body, perhaps in various tissues during periods of growth, damage, or remodeling.

New Vascular Network Formation is a Prerequisite for Long-term Survival of Cardiomyocyte Precursors Implanted into Ischemic Myocardium

A major limitation to successful cellular therapy in animal models of myocardial damage has been the inability of the introduced donor cells to survive in their host environment, whether such transplants have been congenic (analogous to the autologous scenario in humans) or allogeneic. One major reason for the poor survival of transplanted cardiomyocytes or skeletal myoblasts is that viability and prolonged function of transplanted cells requires an augmented vascular supply. Recent studies have shown that development of thin-walled capillaries in ischemic myocardium following transplantation of hematopoietic lineage endothelial precursors enhances survival of endogenous cardiomyocytes.[48] Moreover, transplanting cultured cardiomyocytes that incorporate more vascular structures in vivo results in significantly greater cell survival and protection against apoptosis.[49] Finally, in situations where transplanted cardiomyocyte precursors contained an admixture of cells also giving rise to vascular structures, survival and function of the newly formed cardiomyocytes have been significantly augmented.[50]

As a corollary of the above, it is reasonable to anticipate that cellular therapies for the treatment of ischemic cardiomyopathy will need to address two interdependent processes: (a) a renewable source of proliferating, functional cardiomyocytes, and (b) development of a network of capillaries and larger blood vessels for supply of oxygen and nutrients both to the chronically ischemic, endogenous myocardium and to the newly implanted cardiomyocytes. To achieve these endpoints, a common cellular source for regenerating cardiomyocytes, vascular structures, and supporting cells such as pericytes and smooth muscle cells would be ideal. The mesenchymal lineage precursor cell would appear to be just such a cellular source.

Mesenchymal Precursor Cells as Cardiomyocyte Progenitors

Over the past several years, a number of studies have suggested that stromal or mesenchymal lineage stem cells can be used to generate cardiomyocytes ex vivo for potential use in a range of cardiovascular diseases.[51–54] The newly generated cardiomyocytes appear to resemble normal cardiomyocytes in terms of phenotypic properties, such as expression of actinin, desmin, and troponin I, and function, including positive and negative chronotropic regulation of contractility by pharmacological agents and production of vasoactive factors such as atrial and brain natriuretic peptides.[51,52] Moreover, in vivo transplantation of bone marrow-derived mesenchymal lineage stem cells has resulted in incorporation within endogenous heart tissue[53] and in cardiac muscle differentiation.[54]

However, significant and sustained functional cardiac improvement following in vivo transplantation of stromal/mesenchymal lineage stem cell-derived cardiomyocytes has been exceedingly difficult to show to date. In part, this may be because the signals required for cardiomyocyte differentiation and functional regulation are complex and poorly understood. For example, phenotypic and functional differentiation of mesenchymal stem cells to cardiomyocyte lineage cells in vitro requires culture with exogenously added 5-azacytidine.[55] An alternative explanation is that xenogeneic components of the culture media, such as bovine calf serum, result in immunogenic modification of the cells during the ex vivo culture process, as has been shown for myocardial implantation of skeletal muscle. In the absence of tissue culture, skeletal myoblast implantation does not induce any adverse immune response and results in grafts showing excellent survival for up to 1 year, whereas injection of cultured isolated (congenic) myoblasts results in massive and rapid necrosis of donor myoblasts, with over 90% dead within the first hour after injection.[56–58] Rejection of the cells modified by tissue culture conditions is mediated by host natural killer (NK) cells that recognize foreign proteins on the surface of the modified autologous or congenic cells. Other possible reasons for lack of sufficient engraftment and long-term survival of these cells include the lack of appropriate survival signals present in the ischemic myocardium or within the matrix/scaffolds in which the cells are delivered. Methods to increase endogenous expression of cell survival signals, such as by Akt genetic modification of stromal/mesenchymal lineage cells, can result in prolonged cellular survival in vivo and functional cardiac recovery.[59]

Potential for Allogeneic Use of Mesenchymal Lineage Precursor Cells

Some of the most exciting data that have been generated recently relate to the ability of mesenchymal lineage stem cells to evade recognition by the immune cells of unrelated recipients, raising the possibility that they may potentially constitute a source of allogeneic cellular therapeutic products. Despite the expression of human leukocyte antigen (HLA) molecules on their surface, these cells do not induce allogeneic mixed lymphocyte responses, even after being differentiated to bone, cartilage, or adipocytes.[60,61] Moreover, they suppress third-party mixed lymphocyte responses in vitro in a dose-dependent manner[62] and can suppress an ongoing immune response in vivo, as demonstrated in a recent study where haploidentical mesenchymal stem cells inhibited a potentially fatal graft-versus-host response in a bone marrow transplant recipient.[63]

Allogeneic mesenchymal stem cells loaded on hydroxyapatite–tricalcium phosphate implants enhanced the repair of a critical-sized segmental defect in the canine femur without the use of immunosuppressive therapy, with no adverse immune responses detected for up to 4 months of follow-up.[64] These are the first animal studies to support the feasibility of using allogeneic mesenchymal lineage cells for tissue regeneration. If similar studies can be extended to large animal models of cardiovascular disease, this will open the exciting prospect of using well-regulated, centrally manufactured, allogeneic mesenchymal lineage cell therapy in patients with heart disease.

Conclusions

Adult bone marrow stromal or mesenchymal lineage precursors can be isolated with great purity by physical and immunologic techniques, expanded easily by ex vivo culture techniques, and used to generate both vascular networks and new heart muscle when implanted into ischemic myocardium. However, challenges remain in optimizing the culture expansion protocols and techniques for delivery of these cells before they can be considered ready for in vivo human transplantation. Specifically, their capacity for vascular network formation needs to be harnessed, conditions to direct their differentiation to cardiomyocytes need to be defined, immunogenic factors in the culture media need to be eliminated, and biologic matrices/scaffolds in which the cells are delivered in vivo need to be optimized to provide adequate cell survival signals.

References

1. Friedenstein AJ, Chailakhyan RK, Lalykina KS. The development of fibroblast colonies in monolayer cultures of guinea pig bone marrow and spleen cells. Cell Tissue Kinet 1970;3:393–402.
2. Gronthos S, Simmons PJ. The growth factor requirements of STRO-1-positive human bone marrow stromal precursors under serum-deprived conditions in vitro. Blood 1995;85:929–40.
3. Kuznetsov SA, Krebsbach PH, Satomura K, et al. Single-colony derived strains of human marrow stromal fibroblasts form bone after transplantation in vivo. J Bone Miner Res 1997;12:1335–47.

4. Satomura K, Krebsbach P, Bianco P, et al. Osteogenic imprinting upstream of marrow stromal cell differentiation. J Cell Biochem 2000;78: 391–403.
5. Friedenstein AJ, Latzinik NW, Grosheva AG, et al. Marrow microenvironment transfer by heterotopic transplantation of freshly isolated and cultured cells in porous sponges. Exp Hematol 1982;10: 217–27.
6. Ashton BA, Allen TD, Howlett CR, et al. Formation of bone and cartilage by marrow stromal cells in diffusion chambers in vivo. Clin Orthop 1980; 151:294–307.
7. Pittenger MF, Mackay AM, Beck SC, et al. Multilineage potential of adult human mesenchymal stem cells. Science 1999;284:143–7.
8. Simmons PJ, Torok-Storb B. Identification of stromal cell precursors in human bone marrow by a novel monoclonal antibody, STRO-1. Blood 1991;78:55–62.
9. Haynesworth SE, Baber MA, Caplan AI. Cell surface antigens on human marrow-derived mesenchymal cells are detected by monoclonal antibodies. Bone 1992;13:69–80.
10. Joyner CJ, Bennett A, Triffitt JT. Identification and enrichment of human osteoprogenitor cells by using differentiation stage-specific monoclonal antibodies. Bone 1997;21:1–6.
11. Gronthos S, Graves SE, Ohta S, et al. The STRO-1$^+$ fraction of adult human bone marrow contains the osteogenic precursors. Blood 1994;84:4164–73.
12. Simmons PJ, Torok-Storb B. Identification of stromal cell precursors in human bone marrow by a novel monoclonal antibody, STRO-1. Blood 1991; 78:55–62.
13. Gronthos S, Simmons PJ. The biology and application of human bone marrow stromal cell precursors. J Hematother 1996;5:15–23.
14. Simmons PJ, Gronthos S, Zannettino A, et al. Isolation, characterization and functional activity of human marrow stromal progenitors in hemopoiesis. Prog Clin Biol Res 1994;389:271–80.
15. Filshie RJ, Zannettino AC, Makrynikola V, et al. MUC18, a member of the immunoglobulin superfamily, is expressed on bone marrow fibroblasts and a subset of hematological malignancies. Leukemia 1998;12:414–21.
16. Gronthos S, Mankani M, Brahim J, et al. Postnatal human dental pulp stem cells (DPSCs) in vitro and in vivo. Proc Natl Acad Sci USA 2000;97:13625–30.
17. Gronthos S, Zannettino AC, Hay SJ, et al. Molecular and cellular characterisation of highly purified stromal stems derived from human bone marrow. J Cell Sci 2003;116:1827–35.
18. Shi S, Gronthos S. Perivascular niche of postnatal mesenchymal stem cells in human bone marrow and dental pulp. J Bone Miner Res 2003;18:696–704.
19. Galmiche MC, Koteliansky VE, Briere J, Herve P, Charbord P. Stromal cells from human long-term marrow cultures are mesenchymal cells that differentiate following a vascular smooth muscle differentiation pathway. Blood 1993;82:66–76.
20. Schor AM, Canfield AE. Osteogenic potential of vascular pericytes. In: Beresford JN, Owen ME (eds). Marrow Stromal Cell Culture. Cambridge: Cambridge University Press, 1998:128–48.
21. Zuckerman KS, Wicha MS. Extracellular matrix production by the adherent cells of long-term murine bone marrow cultures. Blood 1983; 61:540–7.
22. Gronthos S, Simmons PJ. The growth factor requirements of STRO-1$^+$ human bone marrow stromal precursors under serum-deprived conditions. Blood 1995;85:929–40.
23. Hellstrom M, Kalen M, Lindahl P, Abramsson A, Betsholtz C. Role of PDGF-B and PDGFR-beta in recruitment of vascular smooth muscle cells and pericytes during embryonic blood vessel formation in the mouse. Development 1999;126: 3047–55.
24. Schor AM, Canfield AE, Sutton AB, Arciniegas E, Allen TD. Pericyte differentiation. Clin Orthop 1995;313:81–91.
25. Sims DE. The pericyte – a review. Tissue Cell 1986; 18:153–74.
26. Diaz-Flores L, Gutiérrez R, Gonzales P, Varela H. Inducible perivascular cells contribute to the neochondrogenesis in grafted perichondrium. Anat Rec 1991;229:1–8.
27. Doherty MJ, Ashton BA, Walsh S, Beresford JN, Grant ME, Canfield AE. Vascular pericytes express osteogenic potential in vitro and in vivo. J Bone Miner Res 1998;13:828–38.
28. Doherty MJ, Canfield AE. Gene expression during vascular pericyte differentiation. Crit Rev Eukaryot Gene Exp 1999;9:1–17.
29. Brighton CT, Lorich DG, Kupcha R, Reilly TM, Jones AR, Woodbury RA 2nd. The pericyte as a possible osteoblast progenitor cell. Clin Orthop 1992;275:287–99.
30. Tavian M, Coulombel L, Luton D, San Clemente H, Dieterlen-Lievre F, Peault B. Aorta-associated CD34 hematopoietic cells in the early human embryo. Blood 1996;87:67–72.
31. Jaffredo T, Gautier R, Eichmann A, Dieterlen-Lievre F. Intraaortic hemopoietic cells are derived from endothelial cells during ontogeny. Development 1998;125:4575–83.
32. Drake CJ, Hungerford JE, Little CD. Morphogenesis of the first blood vessels. Ann NY Acad Sci 1998;857:155–79.
33. Hungerford JE, Little CD. Developmental biology of the vascular smooth muscle cell: building a multilayered vessel wall. J Vasc Res 1999;36:2–27.

34. Bergwerff M, Verberne ME, DeRuiter MC, Poelmann RE, Gittenberger de Groot AC. Neural crest cell contribution to the developing circulatory system: implications for vascular morphology? Circ Res 1998;82:221–31.
35. Etchevers HC, Couly GF, Le Douarin NM. Morphogenesis of the branchial vascular sector. Trends Cardiovasc Med 2002;12:299–304.
36. Vrancken Peeters MP, Gittenberger-de Groot AC, Mentink MM, Poelmann RE. Smooth muscle cells and fibroblasts of the coronary arteries derive from the epithelial-mesenchymal transformation of the epicardium. Anat Embryol (Berl) 1999;199: 367–78.
37. D'Amore PA. Capillary growth: a two-cell system. Semin Cancer Biol 1997;3:49–56.
38. Gerhardt H, Wolburg H, Redies C. N-cadherin mediates pericytic endothelial interaction during brain angiogenesis in the chicken. Dev Dyn 2000; 218:472–9.
39. Uemura A, Ogawa M, Hirashima M, et al. Recombinant angiopoietin-1 restores higher-order architecture of growing blood vessels in mice in the absence of mural cells. J Clin Invest 2002;110: 1619–28.
40. Bianco P, Riminucci M. The bone marrow stroma in vivo: ontogeny, structure, cellular composition and changes in disease. In: Beresford JN, Owen M (eds). Marrow Stromal Cell Culture. Cambridge: Cambridge University Press, 1998:10–25.
41. Ascenzi A. Physiological relationship and pathological interferences between bone tissue and marrow. In: Bourne GH (ed). The Biochemistry and Physiology of Bone. New York: Academic Press, 1976:403–45.
42. Andreeva ER, Pugach IM, Gordon D, et al. Continuous subendothelial network formed by pericyte-like cells in human vascular bed. Tissue Cell 1998;30:127–35.
43. Bianco P, Riminucci M, Gronthos S, Robey PG. Bone marrow stromal stem cells: nature, biology, and potential applications. Stem Cells 2001;19: 180–92.
44. Ema M, Faloon P, Zhang WJ, et al. Combinatorial effects of Flk1 and Tal1 on vascular and hematopoietic development in the mouse. Genes Dev 2003;17:380–93.
45. Yamashita J, Itoh H, Hirashima M, et al. Flk1-positive cells derived from embryonic stem cells serve as vascular progenitors. Nature 2000;408: 92–6.
46. Benjamin LE, Hemo I, Keshet E. A plasticity window for blood vessel remodelling is defined by pericyte coverage of the preformed endothelial network and is regulated by PDGF-B and VEGF. Development 1998;125:1591–8.
47. Gerber HP, Vu TH, Ryan AM, et al. VEGF couples hypertrophic cartilage remodeling, ossification and angiogenesis during endochondral bone formation. Nat Med 1999;5:623–8.
48. Kocher AA, Schuster MD, Szabolcs MJ, et al. Neovascularization of ischemic myocardium by human bone-marrow-derived angioblasts prevents cardiomyocyte apoptosis, reduces remodeling and improves cardiac function. Nat Med 2001;7: 430–6.
49. Klug MG, Soonpaa MH, Koh GY, Field LJ. Genetically selected cardiomyocytes from differentiating embryonic stem cells form stable intracardiac grafts. J Clin Invest 1996;98:216–24.
50. Hescheler J, Fleischmann BK, Wartenberg M, et al. Establishment of ionic channels and signalling cascades in the embryonic stem cell-derived primitive endoderm and cardiovascular system. Cells Tissues Organs 1999;165:153–64.
51. Makino S, Fukuda K, Miyoshi S, et al. Cardiomyocytes can be generated from marrow stromal cells in vitro. J Clin Invest 1999;103:697–705.
52. Tomita S, Li R-K, Weisel RD, et al. Autologous transplantation of bone marrow cells improves damaged heart function. Circulation 1999;100:II-247.
53. Liechty KW, MacKenzie TC, Shaaban AF, et al. Human mesenchymal stem cells engraft and demonstrate site-specific differentiation after in utero transplantation in sheep. Nat Med 2000;6: 1282–6.
54. Toma C, Pittenger MF, Cahill KS, Byrne BJ, Kessler, D. Human mesenchymal stem cells differentiate to a cardiomyocyte phenotype in the adult murine heart. Circulation 2003;105:93–6.
55. Beauchamp JR, Morgan JE, Pagel CN, Partridge TA. Dynamics of myoblast transplantation reveal a discrete minority of precursors with stem cell-like properties as the myogenic source. J Cell Biol 1999;144:1113–22.
56. Smythe GM, Grounds MD. Exposure to tissue culture conditions can adversely affect myoblast behaviour in vivo in whole muscle grafts: implications for myoblast transfer therapy. Cell Transplant 2000;9:379–93.
57. Smythe GM, Hodgetts SI, Grounds MD. Problems and solutions in myoblast transfer therapy. J Cell Mol Med 2001;5:33–47.
58. Hodgetts SI, Beilharz MW, Scalzo T, Grounds MD. Why do cultured transplanted myoblasts die in vivo? DNA quantification shows enhanced survival of donor male myoblasts in host mice depleted of $CD4^+$ and $CD8^+$ or $NK1.1^+$ cells. Cell Transplant 2000;9:489–502.
59. Mangi AA, Noiseux N, Kong D, et al. Mesenchymal stem cells modified with Akt prevent remodeling and restore performance of infarcted hearts. Nat Med 2003;9:1195–201.
60. Di Nicola M, Carlo-Stella C, Magni M, et al. Human bone marrow stromal cells suppress T-lymphocyte proliferation induced by cellular or

nonspecific mitogenic stimuli. Blood 2002;99: 3838–43.

61. Le Blanc K, Tammik C, Rosendahl K, Zetterberg E, Ringdén O. HLA expression and immunologic properties of differentiated and undifferentiated mesenchymal stem cells. Exp Hematol 2003;31: 890–6.
62. Tse WT, Pendleton JD, Beyer WM, Egalka MC, Guinan E. Suppression of allogeneic T-cell proliferation by human marrow stromal cells: implications in transplantation. Transplantation 2003;75: 389–97.
63. Le Blanc K, Rasmusson I, Sundberg B, et al. Treatment of severe acute graft-versus-host disease with third party haploidentical mesenchymal stem cells. Lancet 2004;363:1439–41.
64. Arinzeh TL, Peter SJ, Archambault MP, et al. Allogeneic mesenchymal stem cells regenerate bone in a critical-sized canine segmental defect. J Bone Joint Surg Am 2003;85-A:1927–35.

chapter 4

The Basics of Therapeutic Potential of Endothelial Progenitor Cells

Carmen Urbich and Stefanie Dimmeler

Introduction

Ischemia-induced death of cardiac myocytes results in scar formation and reduced contractility of the ventricle. Various experimental studies have provided evidence that the infusion of stem or progenitor cells may reduce scar formation and fibrosis. Moreover, predominantly bone marrow-derived cells have been shown to augment blood flow, thereby providing a novel therapeutic option for the prevention and/or treatment of ischemic heart failure. In animal models, several stem and progenitor cells have exhibited the capacity to improve neovascularization and cardiac regeneration (Tables 4.1 and 4.2). The best established source is bone marrow, which contains hematopoietic stem cells and "side population" (SP) cells, which are identified by their capacity to exclude Hoechst dye.[1] Mesenchymal stem cells (MSCs) and multipotent adult progenitor cells (MAPCs) can also be isolated from bone marrow.[2,3] In addition, Asahara et al[4] and Shi et al[5] have defined a subset of bone marrow-derived hematopoietic progenitor cells: endothelial progenitor cells (EPCs). These cells can give rise to endothelial cells and contribute to endothelial recovery and new capillary formation after ischemia. EPCs have subsequently been defined as cells expressing hematopoietic stem cell markers such as CD34 and CD133 and the endothelial marker protein VEGFR-2 (see the following section). Stimulated by these pioneering results, ongoing studies have identified additional sources that can give rise to endothelial cells. Thus, bone marrow-derived non-hematopoietic stem well as tissue-derived progenitor cells have been shown to differentiate to endothelial cells in vitro and in vivo. The different sources of EPCs and their potential therapeutic applications are discussed in the following section.

Sources of EPCs

Bone marrow-derived EPCs

The first studies supporting the concept that hematopoietic stem cells (HSCs) can give rise to endothelial cells were performed using isolated cells expressing the classical HSC marker protein CD34 or the more immature HSC marker protein CD133 (also known as AC133 or prominin). Both cell populations differentiated to endothelial cells in vitro under appropriate endothelial conditions that promoted differentiation.[4,6] Most importantly, injection of $CD34^+$ or $CD133^+$ cells enhanced neovascularization in animal models after ischemia.[4,7] In accordance with the initial discovery, EPCs were defined as cells positive for both hematopoietic stem cell markers such as CD34 or CD133 and an endothelial marker protein such as vascular endothelial growth factor

Table 4.1 Neovascularization by infusion of bone marrow-derived progenitor cells (selected studies)

Cells	*Surface markers*	*Improvement*	*Incorporation rate*	*Ref*
Freshly isolated cells				
$CD34^+$ cells	$CD34^+$, $CD45^+$, VEGFR-2^+		13.4 ± 5.7% (mouse) or 9.7 ± 4.5% (rabbit) Dil-Ac-LDL^+EPCs in $CD31^+$ capillaries	4
	Tie-2^+, Dil-Ac-LDL^+	Hind-limb ischemia	Frequently detected (not quantified)	48
Sca-1^+ BM-MNCs	Sca-1^+	Hind-limb ischemia	Detected (not quantified)	49
PBMCs	T and B lymphocytes and monocyte-depleted MNCs	Hind-limb ischemia		49
Ex vivo-expanded cells				
Ex vivo expanded EPCs	Dil-Ac-LDL^+, $lectin^+$, VEGFR-2^+, VE-$cadherin^+$, $CD31^+$, $CD14^+$, $CD34^+$	Hind-limb ischemia	2.1 ± 0.4 EPCs into vessels in a ×10 field 241 ± 25 cells/mm^2 (day 3) 355 ± 30 cells/mm^2 (day 7)	13,50
	Dil-Ac-LDL^+, NO^+, VEGFR-2^+, VE-$cadherin^+$, $CD31^+$, vWF^+, $CD45^-$	Hind-limb ischemia	Frequently detected (not quantified)	29
	$CD31^+$, vWF^+, Dil-Ac-LDL^+, VEGFR-2^+, Tie-2^+	Vascular graft survival, neovessel remodeling	80% of graft lumen at day 15	51
	Dil-Ac-LDL^+, $lectin^+$, VEGFR-2^+, $CD105^+$, vWF^+, $CD45^+$	Hind-limb ischemia	19.8 ± 8% $CD146^+$HLA-DR^+ cells containing vessels	10

(Continued)

Table 4.1 (Continued)

Cells	*Surface markers*	*Improvement*	*Incorporation rate*	*Ref*
	Early EPCs: Dil-Ac-LDL$^+$, lectin$^+$ VEGFR-2$^+$, CD31$^+$, Tie-2$^+$, VE-cadherin$^-$, eNOS$^-$, CD14$^+$ *Outgrowing ECs:* VEGFR-2$^+$, CD31$^+$, Tie-2$^+$, VE-cadherin$^+$, eNOS$^+$, CD14$^-$	Matrigel capillaries: outgrowing ECs exhibited a greater capacity for capillary morphogenesis in in vitro and in vivo matrigel models	Not determined	52
	Early EPCs: weak VEGFR-1, eNOS, vWF, VE-cadherin, VEGFR-2; spindle shape *Late EPCs*: strong VE-cadherin, VEGFR-1, VEGFR-2, eNOS, vWF; cobblestone morphology	*In vitro:* late EPCs showed better incorporation and tube formation; early EPCs showed higher release of growth factors *In vivo:* comparable vasculogenic potential of early and late EPCs (limb perfusion, capillary density)	Detected (not quantified)	14
MAPC-derived ECs	*Copurified MAPCs:* CD34$^-$, VE-cadherin$^-$, CD133$^+$, VEGFR-2$^+$ *Angioblasts:* CD34$^+$, VE-cadherin$^+$, CD133$^-$, VEGFR-2$^+$	Tumor growth/angiogenesis	*MAPC-derived ECs* 35% tumor angiogenesis, 30–45% wound healing angiogenesis *Undifferentiated MAPCs*: 12%	15

BM-MNC, bone marrow mononuclear cell; EC, endothelial cell; eNOS, endothelial nitric oxide synthase; EPC endothelial progenitor cell; HLA, human leukocyte antigen; MAPC, multipotent adult progenitor cell; NO, nitric oxide; PBMC, peripheral blood mononuclear cell; VEGFR, vascular endothelial growth factor receptor; vWF, von Willebrand factor.

Table 4.2 Cardiac regeneration by infusion of bone marrow-derived progenitor cells (selected studies)

Cells	*Surface markers*	*Improvement*	*Incorporation rate*	*Ref*
Freshly isolated cells				
Side population (SP)	c-Kit$^+$, Sca-1$^+$ CD34$^{-/low}$	Regeneration of ischemic cardiac muscle and vascular endothelium	0.02% donor-derived cardiomyocytes 3.3% donor-derived endothelial cells	1
Angioblasts (mobilized CD34$^+$ cells)	CD117^{bright}, GATA-2$^+$/VEGFR-2$^+$, Tie-2$^+$, CD133$^+$	Improvement of myocardial function; inhibition of myocyte apoptosis and late myocardial remodeling	20–25% of total myocardial capillary vasculature	7
Bone marrow Lin$^-$c-Kit$^+$ cells	Lin$^-$, c-Kit$^+$	Contribution to newly formed myocytes, endothelial cells, and smooth muscle cells; improvement of LV hemodynamics	Detected	34
Ex vivo-expanded cells				
Bone marrow cells treated ex vivo with 5′-azacytidine		Improvement of neovascularization and systolic blood pressure	Detected (cardiomyocyte differentiation)	53
Bone marrow cells treated ex vivo with 5′-azacytidine		Improvement of LV hemodynamics	Detected (cardiomyocyte differentiation)	54
EPC	Dil-Ac-LDL$^+$/lectin$^+$ VEGFR-2$^+$, VE-cadherin$^+$, CD31$^+$, CD14$^+$, CD34$^+$	Improvement of myocardial neovascularization and preservation of LV function	Detected (endothelial differentiation)	31
Nonadhesive CD31$^+$ MNCs and CD34$^+$ MNCs, respectively	CD31$^+$ and CD34$^+$, respectively	Improvement of neovascularization and LV function	Detected (endothelial differentiation)	55

EPC, endothelial progenitor cell; LV, left ventricular; MNC, mononuclear cell; VEGFR, vascular endothelial growth factor receptor.

receptor 2 (VEGFR-2; also known as KDR/FLK-1). However, CD34 is not exclusively expressed on hematopoietic stem cells – it is also expressed on mature endothelial cells. Therefore, follow-up studies used the more immature hematopoietic stem cell marker CD133 to better discriminate between EPCs and mature endothelial cells.[8] Recent studies suggest that myeloid cells can differentiate into endothelial cells. In particular, $CD14^{+}CD34^{-}$ myeloid cells coexpress endothelial and macrophagocytic lineage markers and form tube-like structures under angiogenic conditions in vitro.[9] In addition, ex vivo cultivation of purified $CD14^{+}$ mononuclear cells under endothelial cell-specific conditions yielded cells with an endothelial phenotype, which incorporated in newly formed blood vessels in vivo and improved neovascularization after induction of ischemia.[10] Moreover, a subset of human peripheral blood monocytes act as pluripotent stem cells.[11] In summary, these studies indicate that myeloid cells within peripheral blood can differentiate (or transdifferentiate) to the endothelial lineage. A recent study has suggested that monocyte-derived EPCs appear to have a lower proliferative capacity compared with HSCs or cord blood-derived EPCs.[12] However, the different cell types have a similar capacity to augment neovascularization in experimental models,[10,13,14] suggesting either that the proliferative capacity is not of major importance in vivo or that the monocyte-derived cells may compensate for the reduced proliferation by additional mechanisms (e.g., an increased release of growth factors to augment neovascularization). Additional studies are essential to determine the differences in incorporation and particularly the long-term fate of HSC- versus monocyte-derived cells. However, since HSCs also give rise to monocytes, it is a challenging task to discriminate clearly between these different cell populations.

MAPCs, which copurify with MSCs, can also be isolated from postnatal human bone marrow. They have been shown to differentiate into cells with phenotypic and functional characteristics of endothelial cells in vitro and contribute to tumor and wound healing angiogenesis in vivo.[15] Likewise, MSCs differentiate to endothelial cells[16] and have been shown to improve neovascularization and heart function in vivo.[17,18]

The contribution of bone marrow-derived progenitor cells to improvement of neovascularization has been further documented by using bone marrow transplantation with genetically tagged cells to replenish bone marrow-derived HSCs after irradiation. Various experimental studies have shown that genetically tagged bone marrow-derived cells can be found in the ischemic tissue and contribute to neoangiogenesis after ischemia or in tumors.[1,19–22] The reported level of incorporation of bone marrow-derived cells in the endothelium of capillaries and vessels varies from 0% to 50%, the highest levels being detected in tumors.[19,23] Despite different levels and locations (endothelial versus perivascular) of incorporation, the infusion of different subsets of EPCs has been shown to enhance functional recovery in various animal models. The discrepancy between the functional improvement and the numbers of incorporated cells may be partially explained by the use of different techniques to detect the incorporated cells. However, the difference in incorporation in the animal models has also provoked questions regarding the different molecular mechanisms by which EPCs contribute to improvement of neovascularization (see below).

Non bone marrow-derived EPCs

Tissue-residing cells have attracted increasing interest during the last few years. Various tissues, including adipose tissue, neuronal tissue, and the heart itself, contain cells that are capable of differentiating to the endothelial lineage. Tissue-specific stem cells reside in certain adult tissues, yet their specific properties are often hard to assess because of their heterogeneity and technical difficulties in identifying them and tracing their progeny. Neural stem cells differentiate to the endothelial lineage in vitro and in vivo, independently of cell fusion,[24] supporting the concept of stem cell plasticity. Moreover, tissue-resident c-Kit^{+} stem cells that are capable of differentiating to the endothelial lineage have been isolated from the heart.[25] Although, it is not completely clear at present whether these cells derive entirely from repopulated bone marrow-derived (hematopoietic) stem cells or are tissue-residing remnants from embryonic development, it is of major scientific and possible therapeutic interest to determine whether these tissue-derived cells might have superior capacities compared with bone marrow-derived or peripheral blood-derived cells.

Another source of adult stem cells for autologous cell therapy is adipose tissue. Using this tissue, cells can easily be isolated in large amounts with minimal discomfort to patients. Human lipoaspirate contains multipotent cells that can differentiate in different lineages.[26] Additionally, adipose tissue-derived cultured stromal–vascular fractions have been isolated that lack the HSC marker CD34 and the endothelial marker CD31 (and thus resemble MSCs/stromal cells) and that differentiate to endothelial cells and promote angiogenesis.[27] Stromal–vascular fractions obtained from adipose tissue also contain cells that express the hematopoietic marker CD34 but are negative for the endothelial marker CD31. These $CD34^{+}CD31^{-}$ cells are also capable of differentiating to endothelial cells and are potent promoters of neovascularization.[28]

Cord blood

Cord blood is a rich source of EPCs. It contains higher numbers of $CD133^{+}$ and $CD34^{+}$ HSCs compared with peripheral blood from adults.[12] $CD133^{+}$ and $CD34^{+}$ cells isolated from cord blood have been cultivated ex vivo and have differentiated to endothelial cells.[29] Cord blood-derived EPCs show a higher proliferative capacity and express telomerase, a functional characteristic of stem cells that is very low or absent in other progenitor cell populations.[12] Interestingly, Hildbrand et al[30] described a subset of $CD34^{+}$ cells that express the myeloid marker CD11b and are most effective in differentiating to the endothelial lineage. These results may indicate that a myeloid subset of HSCs is indeed involved in endothelial lineage commitment. However, further studies are necessary to confirm this hypothesis.

Mechanism of Functional Improvement Mediated by EPCs

Infusion of HSCs or EPCs after myocardial infarction leads to engraftment of these cells in the border zone of the infarct.[1,7] After homing, stem or progenitor cells may contribute in several possible ways to neovascularization and cardiac regeneration (Figure 4.1). These include differentiation to other cell types as well as paracrine mechanisms of action. Whereas the capacity of adult stem cells to differentiate to cardiac myocytes in a reasonable number is still debated, it has been shown by various groups that stem/progenitor cells can differentiate to endothelial cells and that infusion of different subsets of EPCs increases the formation of new capillaries and stimulates functional recovery after ischemia. Infusion of these ex vivo-expanded EPCs augmented blood flow and heart function in animal models after hind-limb ischemia or myocardial infarction.[10,13,31] Similar results were achieved when HSCs were used.[7] The therapeutic implication is further underscored by the finding that wild-type stem cell infusion is capable of rescuing dysfunctional neovascularization as seen in endothelial nitric oxide synthase (eNOS)-deficient animals.[32] Likewise, young adult bone marrow-derived progenitor cells have been shown to improve aging-impaired cardiac angiogenic function.[33]

When dyes or genetic markers were used to track cells after engraftment, some of the injected cells expressed cardiac marker proteins.[1,7,34,35] These initial results suggested that the cells differentiate to the cardiac lineage and may thereby contribute to cardiac regeneration. Moreover, cocultivation of umbilical venous endothelial cells, EPCs, or $CD34^{+}$ cells with cardiac myocytes induced differentiation of human endothelial cells to a cardiomyogenic phenotype.[36–38] However, this concept has recently been challenged by two negative reports.[39,40] Several other studies suggest that the expression of cardiac marker proteins is not the result of a differentiation process but rather reflects cell–cell fusion. Such events were initially reported for embryonic

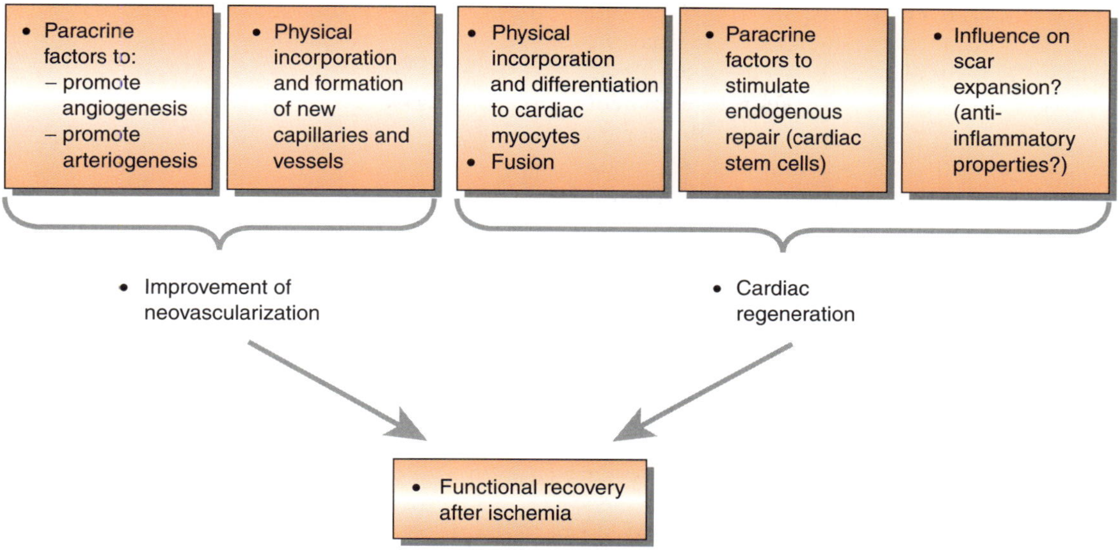

Figure 4.1 *Mechanisms of progenitor cell function: scheme depicting the potential mechanisms that might be involved in progenitor cell-mediated improvement of neovascularization and cardiac function after ischemia.*

stem cells and now have been confirmed with HSCs.[41] Interestingly, recent studies have shown that murine cardiac stem cells can fuse and differentiate to a similar extent when injected after a myocardial infarction.[42,43] The relative contributions of differentiation and fusion to cardiac regeneration by the different human cell types investigated thus far are unclear. Moreover, other mechanisms may account for the functional improvement, since, even in the study showing no differentiation of HSCs to cardiomyocytes, functional improvement was observed after cell infusion.[39]

The selective homing of HSCs and EPCs to sites of injury may also allow the local release of factors acting in a paracrine manner on the surrounding ischemic tissue and the vasculature. Bone marrow-derived mononuclear cells release angiogenic growth factors such as vascular endothelial growth factor (VEGF), basic fibroblast growth factor (bFGF), and angiopoietins, thereby enhancing the local angiogenic response.[44] Similarly, the reduction of postinfarction left ventricular dysfunction after injection of mesoangioblasts is likely mediated by the release of anti-apoptotic and angiogenic factors.[45] Moreover, isolated human EPCs also express various growth factors[46] that can promote cardiac myocyte survival and improve angiogenesis. Locally released paracrine factors may additionally act by promoting arteriogenesis.

Interestingly, a conditioned medium of cultivated EPCs can also stimulate the migration of cardiac progenitor cells in vitro.[46] These findings suggest that the release of paracrine factors may augment endogenous vascularization and cardiac regeneration. Moreover, the release of immunomodulatory cytokines by the infused cells may also change the environment and potentially limit scar expansion and inflammation. In particular, MSCs have recently been shown to reduce inflammation.[47] Future studies have to define the extent to which paracrine factors versus physical incorporation are involved. One may speculate that different progenitor cell types may be associated with different mechanisms.

References

1. Jackson KA, Majka SM, Wang H, et al. Regeneration of ischemic cardiac muscle and vascular endothelium by adult stem cells. J Clin Invest 2001;107:1395–402.
2. Pittenger MF, Mackay AM, Beck SC, et al. Multilineage potential of adult human mesenchymal stem cells. Science 1999;284:143–7.
3. Jiang Y, Vaessen B, Lenvik T, Blackstad M, Reyes M, Verfaillie CM. Multipotent progenitor cells can be isolated from postnatal murine bone marrow, muscle, and brain. Exp Hematol 2002;30:896–904.
4. Asahara T, Murohara T, Sullivan A, et al. Isolation of putative progenitor endothelial cells for angiogenesis. Science 1997;275:964–7.
5. Shi Q, Rafii S, Wu MH, et al. Evidence for circulating bone marrow-derived endothelial cells. Blood 1998;92:362–7.
6. Gehling UM, Ergun S, Schumacher U, et al. In vitro differentiation of endothelial cells from AC133-positive progenitor cells. Blood 2000;95:3106–12.
7. Kocher AA, Schuster MD, Szabolcs MJ, et al. Neovascularization of ischemic myocardium by human bone-marrow-derived angioblasts prevents cardiomyocyte apoptosis, reduces remodeling and improves cardiac function. Nat Med 2001;7:430–6.
8. Peichev M, Naiyer AJ, Pereira D, et al. Expression of VEGFR-2 and AC133 by circulating human $CD34^+$ cells identifies a population of functional endothelial precursors. Blood 2000;95:952–8.
9. Schmeisser A, Garlichs CD, Zhang H, et al. Monocytes coexpress endothelial and macrophagocytic lineage markers and form cord-like structures in Matrigel under angiogenic conditions. Cardiovasc Res 2001;49:671–80.
10. Urbich C, Heeschen C, Aicher A, Dernbach E, Zeiher AM, Dimmeler S. Relevance of monocytic features for neovascularization capacity of circulating endothelial progenitor cells. Circulation 2003;108:2511–16.
11. Zhao Y, Glesne D, Huberman E. A human peripheral blood monocyte-derived subset acts as pluripotent stem cells. Proc Natl Acad Sci USA 2003;100:2426–31.
12. Ingram DA, Mead LE, Tanaka H, et al. Identification of a novel hierarchy of endothelial progenitor cells utilizing human peripheral and umbilical cord blood. Blood 2004;29:29.
13. Kalka C, Masuda H, Takahashi T, et al. Transplantation of ex vivo expanded endothelial progenitor cells for therapeutic neovascularization. Proc Natl Acad Sci USA 2000;97:3422–7.
14. Hur J, Yoon CH, Kim HS, et al. Characterization of two types of endothelial progenitor cells and their different contributions to neovasculogenesis. Arterioscler Thromb Vasc Biol 2004;24:288–93.
15. Reyes M, Dudek A, Jahagirdar B, Koodie L, Marker PH, Verfaillie CM. Origin of endothelial progenitors in human postnatal bone marrow. J Clin Invest 2002;109:337–46.
16. Oswald J, Boxberger S, Jorgensen B, et al. Mesenchymal stem cells can be differentiated into endothelial cells in vitro. Stem Cells 2004;22:377–84.
17. Al-Khaldi A, Eliopoulos N, Martineau D, Lejeune L, Lachapelle K, Galipeau J. Postnatal bone marrow stromal cells elicit a potent VEGF-dependent neoangiogenic response in vivo. Gene Ther 2003;10:621–9.
18. Silva GV, Litovsky S, Assad JA, et al. Mesenchymal stem cells differentiate into an endothelial phenotype, enhance vascular density, and improve heart function in a canine chronic ischemia model. Circulation 2005;111:150–6.
19. Crosby JR, Kaminski WE, Schatteman G, et al. Endothelial cells of hematopoietic origin make a significant contribution to adult blood vessel formation. Circ Res 2000;87:728–30.
20. Llevadot J, Murasawa S, Kureishi Y, et al. HMG-CoA reductase inhibitor mobilizes bone marrow-derived endothelial progenitor cells. J Clin Invest 2001;108:399–405.
21. Murayama T, Tepper OM, Silver M, et al. Determination of bone marrow-derived endothelial progenitor cell significance in angiogenic growth factor-induced neovascularization in vivo. Exp Hematol 2002;30:967–72.
22. Garcia-Barros M, Paris F, Cordon-Cardo C, et al. Tumor response to radiotherapy regulated by endothelial cell apoptosis. Science 2003;300:1155–9.
23. Lyden D, Hattori K, Dias S, et al. Impaired recruitment of bone-marrow-derived endothelial and hematopoietic precursor cells blocks tumor angiogenesis and growth. Nat Med 2001;7:1194–201.
24. Wurmser AE, Nakashima K, Summers RG, et al. Cell fusion-independent differentiation of neural stem cells to the endothelial lineage. Nature 2004;430:350–6.
25. Beltrami AP, Barlucchi L, Torella D, et al. Adult cardiac stem cells are multipotent and support myocardial regeneration. Cell 2003;114:763–76.
26. Zuk PA, Zhu M, Mizuno H, et al. Multilineage cells from human adipose tissue: implications for cell-based therapies. Tissue Eng 2001;7:211–28.
27. Planat-Benard V, Silvestre JS, Cousin B, et al. Plasticity of human adipose lineage cells toward endothelial cells: physiological and therapeutic perspectives. Circulation 2004;109:656–63.
28. Miranville A, Heeschen C, Sengenes C, Curat CA, Busse R, Bouloumie A. Improvement of postnatal neovascularization by human adipose tissue-derived stem cells. Circulation 2004;110:349–55.
29. Murohara T, Ikeda H, Duan J, et al. Transplanted cord blood-derived endothelial precursor cells

augment postnatal neovascularization. J Clin Invest 2000;105:1527–36.
30. Hildbrand P, Cirulli V, Prinsen RC, et al. The role of angiopoietins in the development of endothelial cells from cord blood CD34+ progenitors. Blood 2004;104:2010–19.
31. Kawamoto A, Gwon HC, Iwaguro H, et al. Therapeutic potential of ex vivo expanded endothelial progenitor cells for myocardial ischemia. Circulation 2001;103:634–7.
32. Aicher A, Heeschen C, Mildner-Rihm C, et al. Essential role of endothelial nitric oxide synthase for mobilization of stem and progenitor cells. Nat Med 2003;9:1370–6.
33. Edelberg JM, Tang L, Hattori K, Lyden D, Rafii S. Young adult bone marrow-derived endothelial precursor cells restore aging-impaired cardiac angiogenic function. Circ Res 2002;90:E89–93.
34. Orlic D, Kajstura J, Chimenti S, et al. Bone marrow cells regenerate infarcted myocardium. Nature 2001;410:701–5.
35. Toma C, Pittenger MF, Cahill KS, Byrne BJ, Kessler PD. Human mesenchymal stem cells differentiate to a cardiomyocyte phenotype in the adult murine heart. Circulation 2002;105:93–8.
36. Condorelli G, Borello U, De Angelis L, et al. Cardiomyocytes induce endothelial cells to transdifferentiate into cardiac muscle: implications for myocardium regeneration. Proc Natl Acad Sci USA 2001;98:10733–8.
37. Badorff C, Brandes RP, Popp R, et al. Transdifferentiation of blood-derived human adult endothelial progenitor cells into functionally active cardiomyocytes. Circulation 2003;107:1024–32.
38. Yeh ET, Zhang S, Wu HD, Korbling M, Willerson JT, Estrov Z. Transdifferentiation of human peripheral blood CD34+-enriched cell population into cardiomyocytes, endothelial cells, and smooth muscle cells in vivo. Circulation 2003;108:2070–3.
39. Balsam LB, Wagers AJ, Christensen JL, Kofidis T, Weissman IL, Robbins RC. Haematopoietic stem cells adopt mature haematopoietic fates in ischaemic myocardium. Nature 2004;428:668–73.
40. Murry CE, Soonpaa MH, Reinecke H, et al. Haematopoietic stem cells do not transdifferentiate into cardiac myocytes in myocardial infarcts. Nature 2004;428:664–8.
41. Medvinsky A, Smith A. Stem cells: fusion brings down barriers. Nature 2003;422:823–5.
42. Oh H, Bradfute SB, Gallardo TD, et al. Cardiac progenitor cells from adult myocardium: homing, differentiation, and fusion after infarction. Proc Natl Acad Sci USA 2003;100:12313–18.
43. Zhang S, Wang D, Estrov Z, Raj S, Willerson JT, Yeh ET. Both cell fusion and transdifferentiation account for the transformation of human peripheral blood CD34-positive cells into cardiomyocytes in vivo. Circulation 2004;110:3803–7.
44. Kamihata H, Matsubara H, Nishiue T, et al. Implantation of bone marrow mononuclear cells into ischemic myocardium enhances collateral perfusion and regional function via side supply of angioblasts, angiogenic ligands, and cytokines. Circulation 2001;104:1046–52.
45. Galli D, Innocenzi A, Staszewsky L, et al. Mesoangioblasts, vessel-associated multipotent stem cells, repair the infarcted heart by multiple cellular mechanisms. A comparison with bone marrow progenitors, fibroblasts, and endothelial cells. Arterioscler Thromb Vasc Biol 2005;25: 692–7.
46. Urbich C, Aicher A, Heeschen C, et al. Soluble factors released by endothelial progenitor cells promote migration of endothelial cells and cardiac resident progenitor cells. J Mol Cell Cardiol 2005; 39:733–42.
47. Tse WT, Pendleton JD, Beyer WM, Egalka MC, Guinan EC. Suppression of allogeneic T-cell proliferation by human marrow stromal cells: implications in transplantation. Transplantation 2003;75: 389–97.
48. Schatteman GC, Hanlon HD, Jiao C, Dodds SG, Christy BA. Blood-derived angioblasts accelerate blood-flow restoration in diabetic mice. J Clin Invest 2000;106:571–8.
49. Takahashi T, Kalka C, Masuda H, et al. Ischemia- and cytokine-induced mobilization of bone marrow-derived endothelial progenitor cells for neovascularization. Nat Med 1999;5:434–8.
50. Yamaguchi J, Kusano KF, Masuo O, et al. Stromal cell-derived factor-1 effects on ex vivo expanded endothelial progenitor cell recruitment for ischemic neovascularization. Circulation 2003; 107:1322–8.
51. Kaushal S, Amiel GE, Guleserian KJ, et al. Functional small-diameter neovessels created using endothelial progenitor cells expanded ex vivo. Nat Med 2001;7:1035–40.
52. Gulati R, Jevremovic D, Peterson TE, et al. Diverse origin and function of cells with endothelial phenotype obtained from adult human blood. Circ Res 2003;93:1023–5.
53. Tomita S, Li RK, Weisel RD, et al. Autologous transplantation of bone marrow cells improves damaged heart function. Circulation 1999;100: II247–56.
54. Tomita S, Mickle DA, Weisel RD, et al. Improved heart function with myogenesis and angiogenesis after autologous porcine bone marrow stromal cell transplantation. J Thorac Cardiovasc Surg 2002; 123:1132–40.
55. Kawamoto A, Tkebuchava T, Yamaguchi J, et al. Intramyocardial transplantation of autologous endothelial progenitor cells for therapeutic neovascularization of myocardial ischemia. Circulation 2003;107:461–8.

chapter 5

Mechanistic Insights into Cardiac Stem Cell Therapy from a Histopathologic Perspective

Renu Virmani, Frank D Kolodgie, and Elena Ladich

Introduction

Of patients with ST-segment elevation myocardial infarction (STEMI), one-third will die, half of these deaths occurring within 1 hour. Over 36% of patients with a myocardial infarction will show a reduction of myocardial contractile function and develop heart failure.[1] Patients undergoing reperfusion therapy have a lower risk of post-infarction heart failure. Nevertheless, if further advances are to be made, new therapies will need to be developed. One such therapy for which promising results have been claimed is stem cell therapy. In this chapter, we will discuss the histologic changes in reperfused versus nonreperfused myocardial infarcts and the healing mechanisms that provide a means to determine whether stem cell therapy is effective in reducing myocardial ischemia and infarction while improving myocardial function. We will also discuss the use of various markers to identify the different cell types that have been proposed for myocardial salvage following myocardial infarction in animals and eventually in humans.

Normal Myocardium

During embryogenesis, growth of the heart occurs primarily through proliferation of cardiac myocytes. Prior to embryonic day 9.5 in the mouse, the heart tube is a thin-walled structure with atrial and ventricular chambers that are molecularly specified but morphologically indistinct. Growth of the heart from here on involves proliferation of cardiac myocytes along the wall of the heart tube and in the ventricular septum. Most of the proliferation occurs along the outer surface of the heart, which is a compact region. As the ventricles thicken, the myocytes along the inner wall become organized into fingerlike projections called trabeculae. It has been shown that retinoic acid produced by the epicardium is a critical regulator of cardiac growth. At birth, the myocardium is only a fraction of the thickness it will become during adulthood. Myocardial thickness increases at least fourfold in postnatal life due to myocyte hypertrophy rather than to myocyte division.

Healing and Repair of Myocardial Infarction (Figures 5.1 and 5.2)

Without a basic understanding of how the heart heals following a myocardial infarction, it is impossible to know whether cell therapy is effective. The cells within the myocardium and from the circulating blood are responsible for repair

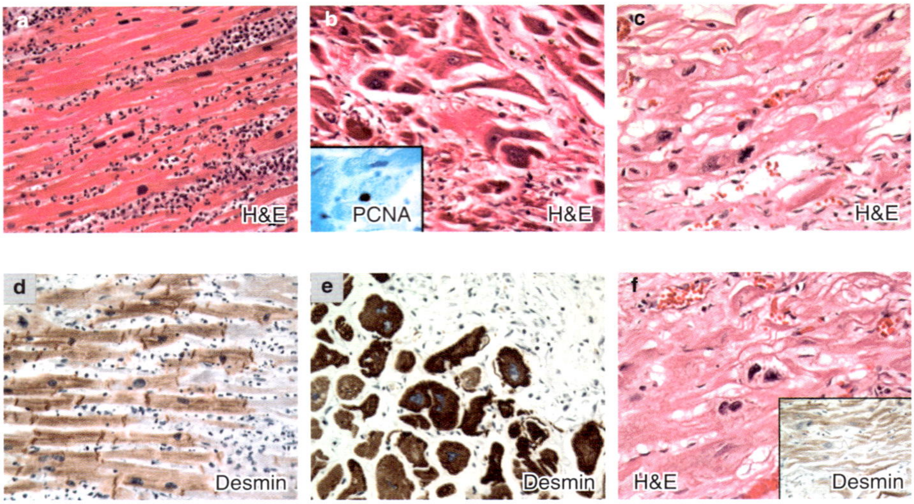

Figure 5.1 Morphologic changes at 3 days, 7–10 days, and 2–3 weeks following a myocardial infarction in a human. (a–c) Hematoxylin–eosin (H&E)-stained sections with marked acute inflammatory infiltrate (a), early granulation tissue and adjoining bizarre and multinucleate but viable myocytes (b), and a border area with multinucleated cells at 2–3 weeks (c). The myocytes in (b) are proliferating cell nuclear antigen (PCNA)-positive (insert in b). (d) and (e) are adjoining sections to (a) and (b) and are stained with anti-desmin antibodies; viable myocytes are stained by 3,3′-diaminobenzidine (brown). Being a different area than (c), (f) shows multinucleated myocytes, which stain positive with anti-desmin antibodies.

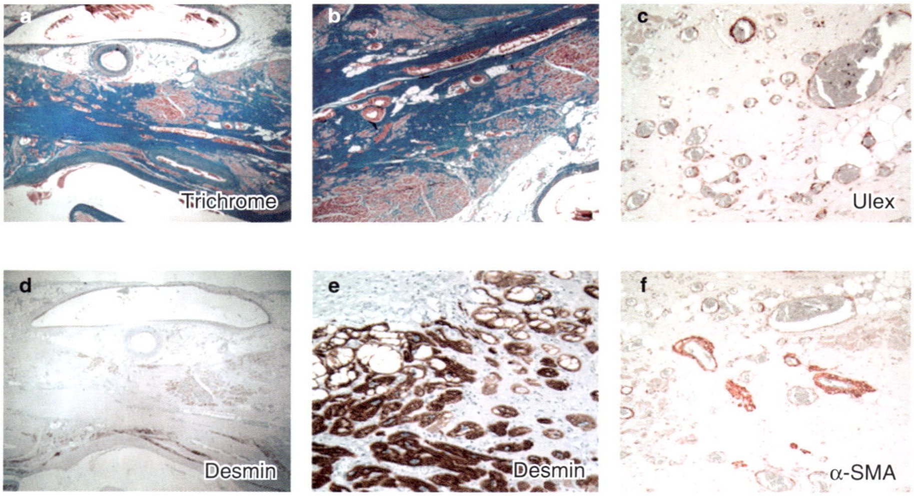

Figure 5.2 Images from a >2-month-old healed myocardial infarct. (a, b) Sections stained by Masson's trichrome show the area of healed myocardial infarction; note that the collagenized areas of the scar are blue, while the viable myocytes are red. (c) The scarred area is stained with Ulex europaeus lectin to identify capillaries, arterioles, muscular arteries, and venules. (d, e) Anti-desmin antibody-stained sections showing focal positivity, with only focal collections of viable myocytes (brown stain). The myocytes close to the endocardium in (e) are vacuolated but still viable. (f) Myocardial section stained with an antibody against α-smooth muscle actin (α-SMA) showing smooth muscle cells around established vessels.

mechanisms. The time and rate of their appearance and their relationship to one another are important parameters that need to be understood prior to determining strategies that may alter these mechanisms. The various processes that govern the mechanisms of repair after myocardial infarction, with and without reperfusion, as well as remodeling, are known to contribute to congestive heart failure. The rate of infarct healing is a function of the ratio of surface to volume. As infarct size increases, the surface/volume ratio decreases, and therefore large infarcts heal more slowly than small ones.[2–4] Nonreperfused myocardial infarcts in humans and animals heal more slowly than reperfused infarcts. The early phases of myocardial infarction are characterized by myocyte necrosis and acute inflammation, which in nonreperfused infarcts occurs only in the border areas, whereas in reperfused infarcts inflammatory cells are scattered throughout the infarcted myocardium. This is followed by macrophage and later fibroblast infiltration, both of which are accompanied by neoangiogenesis. Macrophages begin to appear by day 4 and granulation tissue by day 7, while neutrophils begin to disappear. This phase of healing is again accelerated in reperfused infarcts and is diffuse in nature; in nonreperfused infarcts, depending upon the infarct size, it is limited to the border areas. The necrotic myocardium begins to disintegrate at about day 8, soon after macrophages appear, and with the ingrowth of angiogenesis this eventually leads to removal of the necrotic tissue, which is complete by 4–6 weeks, depending upon infarct size. By 6 weeks, the infarcted areas become rich in collagen with interspersed intact myocytes. The islands of myocytes are far greater in number in reperfused than nonreperfused myocardium. Also, reperfused infarcts have hemorrhagic areas interspersed within the zone of necrosis, and the irreversibly injured myocytes show contraction band necrosis. The areas of viable myocytes in the border regions are greater in reperfused infarcts and are dependent upon the length of time for which the coronary artery has been occluded.

Angiogenesis in the Postinfarcted Myocardium

At day 8, the developing heart in the mouse has the form of a heart tube and is an avascular structure consisting of a few layers of myocytes and receiving oxygen through diffusion. As the heart grows, the trabeculations progressively increase in size, still allowing diffusion of oxygen. As the heart begins to contract at around day 9, a primitive vascular plexus starts to develop and a proepicardial organ attaches to the heart, which migrates within the subepicardial matrix. Eventually, these precursors differentiate into endothelial cells and form a primitive capillary network that will expand in an epi-to-endocardial direction and towards the base of the heart by endothelial sprouting, which eventually connects to the aorta. The myocardial capillaries become remodeled into larger vessels ramifying into smaller branches, and the larger vessels become surrounded by smooth muscle cells, with pericytes surrounding the smaller vessels.[5] In the mouse, after birth, the capillary density increases three- to fourfold, and the smooth muscle cell-covered coronary arteries increase tenfold during the first 3 weeks.[6] However, recent work suggests that the bone marrow-derived endothelial precursor cells contribute to neovascularization of the heart and liver during the postnatal period.[7]

The normal myocardium is rich in capillaries, differences being seen between the endocardial and epicardial myocardium. The epicardial capillary density has been reported to be 2439 capillaries/mm^2, which is 21% greater than the endocardial capillary density of 2014 capillaries/mm^2.[8] The endocardial myocytes (617 μm^2) have a greater cross-sectional area than the epicardial myocytes (403 μm^2). Thus, the ratio of myocyte to capillary density in the epicardium is different from that in the endocardium. We have observed that for every myocyte there are at least four or five capillaries. From our morphologic assessment in normal hearts, the number of capillaries per square millimeter is very similar to that reported by Stoker et al;[8] our study showed 2098 capillaries/mm^2, and the percentage area

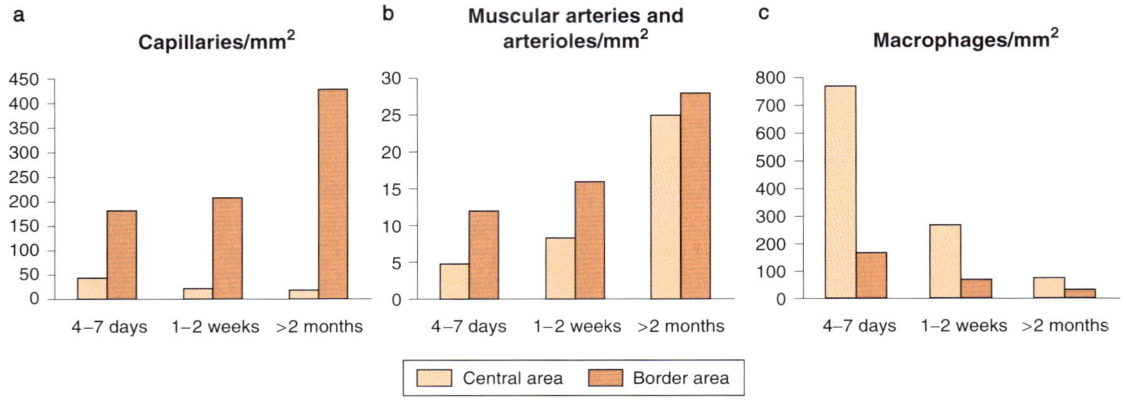

Figure 5.3 *Bar graphs showing the number of capillaries (a), muscular arteries and arterioles (b), and macrophage infiltrates (c) in the border and central regions of human infarcts aged 4–7 days, 1–2 weeks, and >2 months.*

occupied by the capillaries is fairly small (1.98%). We have also assessed the number of capillaries present in the area of the healed myocardial infarcts: only 36 capillaries/mm^2; however, the percentage area occupied by vessels is significantly greater in the healed infarcts than in normal myocardium (7.95%; $p=0.05$) (Figure 5.3).

Most quantitative work about changes in healing infarcts has been reported for the dog and mouse models.[4,9] Myocardial infarcts in humans take at least 8 weeks to heal.[10] Myocardial infarcts in dogs show complete healing by 6 weeks. In rats, infarct healing is essentially complete by 3 weeks. Virag and Murry[4] have shown that 4 days after permanent coronary occlusion in mice, fibroblast proliferation was more rapid than endothelial proliferation ($15.4\pm1.1\%$ and $2.9\pm0.5\%$, respectively). By 1 week, fibroblast and endothelial proliferation declined to $4.1\pm0.6\%$ and $0.7\pm0.1\%$, respectively, and at 2 weeks proliferation was $<0.5\%$. Vascular density declined from $3643\pm82/mm^2$ in control hearts to $2716\pm197/mm^2$ at 1 week and $1010\pm47/mm^2$ at 4 weeks post infarction; but the average percentage area occupied by the vessels increased, as we have seen in humans, although the proportions were quite different (Figure 5.3). In mice, the vessel area increased from $14.1\pm0.3\,mm^2$ in control hearts to $16.9\pm1.9\,mm^2$ at 1 week and to $38.7\pm7.9\,mm^2$ at 4 weeks.[4] Further data of this kind are needed before strategies are developed to alter wound healing of the infarcted myocardium.

Ventricular Remodeling after a Myocardial Infarction

Another possible strategy to improve ventricular function would be to prevent left ventricular remodeling after a myocardial infarction, as this contributes significantly to left ventricular dilatation and dysfunction.[11] It appears that currently used antiremodeling therapies do not prevent ventricular enlargement, and morbidity and mortality are still significant. It is clear that extracellular matrix proteins play an important role in remodeling and that targeting the extracellular matrix (with antifibrotic agents) may be beneficial in selected patients. Of the many collagen types, the major fibrillar collagens are types I and III, which are the main contributors to the healed infarcts. About 85% of total collagen is type I, and this is mainly in the form of thick fibers that contribute to the tensile strength of the infarct and resist stretch and deformation. Type III, a thin collagen, contributes only about 11% of the total collagen and confers resilience.[12,13] Other collagens also mediate important functions; these include elastin, glycosaminoglycans, integrins, fibronectin, and laminin. Degradation of the extracellular matrix by collagenases, gelatinases, stromelysins, and other proteolytic enzymes is an essential component of remodeling. This process is inhibited by tissue inhibitors of metalloproteinases, so these mechanisms must be balanced to prevent continued deterioration in a patient with a large myocardial infarction.[11]

Cell Types for the Treatment of Myocardial Infarction

A number of cell types have been advocated for the treatment of myocardial infarction, ranging from cardiomyoblasts to skeletal myoblasts and others from the stem cell family, including embryonic and adult stem cells. Within these categories, stem cells can be further divided according to the number of differentiated cell types they can produce, i.e., into totipotent and pluripotent cells. The latter may be multipotent or unipotent, depending upon the range of differentiated cell lineages.[14] We will not address all of these issues, as they are considered elsewhere in this book. However, each cell type has specific markers – transcription factors and other proteins expressed by the cell – so it is important to recognize these markers in order to enable identification of the cells in the target organ over time.

Cardiomyocytes

Cell proliferation and cell death are strictly regulated by developmental control mechanisms, and some cells withdraw from the cell cycle during the perinatal period and become postmitotic. In humans, brain and heart cells are of this type – the cells cannot divide, and in the case of the heart, postnatal needs are met through cellular enlargement (i.e., myocyte hypertrophy). Some investigators have questioned this concept and have shown myocyte replication (Ki-67$^+$ cells) in patients dying of a myocardial infarction at 4–12 days. However, the number of dividing cells has been very low: 0.08% in the zone adjacent to the infarct and 0.03% at sites away from it. The absence of myocyte division in humans may be explained by three observations, as pointed out by von Harsdorf et al.[15] Firstly, primary tumors of the heart (myxomas) are extremely rare, and an origin from cardiomyocytes has not been shown. Secondly, significant regeneration of myocytes has never been shown in humans, and if present is at an extremely low level (see above), although in MRL mice and amphibians the mitotic index is much higher (10–20% and 15–20%, respectively).[15] Thirdly, there is no experimental evidence to support the existence of significant cardiomyocyte replication in terminally differentiated myocytes. Therefore, the heart is encoded with a program that protects against uncontrolled replication of myocytes, as the myocytes lack expression of cell cycle-promoting factors and in fact have factors with inhibitory effects on cell cycle activity.[15]

Following intramyocardial injection of fetal or neonatal cardiomyocytes into infarcted or noninfarcted myocardium in mice, Muller-Ehmsen et al[16] have shown viable grafted cells at 6 months, with as many as 60% of the initial injected cells present at that time. The reasons for the better survival in the infarcted than the noninfarcted model are not clear. It may be related to less washout of cells from the infarct and to lack of contraction in the scar areas.

Cell-based Therapy as an Alternative Source for Cardiogenesis or Angiogenesis

Recognition of potential donor cells for regenerative biology

Identification and tracking of stem cells can be achieved by immune phenotyping of marker proteins using immunohistochemistry, flow cytometry, or emerging new genomic or proteomic approaches.[17–20] Expression of tissue-specific markers is not conclusive evidence that these cells will actually transform into the cardiac lineage. Careful documentation of cardiomyocyte differentiation must be performed to confirm the validity of stem cell therapy. Moreover, the benefits of cell grafting may not be exclusive or even related to the formation of new myocardium but may arise from secondary effects associated with postinfarct remodeling or increased angiogenesis.

Endothelial progenitor cells

An alternative strategy for neovascularization of the ischemic heart involves the utility of blood-borne endothelial progenitor cells (EPCs) that are thought to arise from a common hemangioblast precursor in adult bone marrow.[21,22] These cells express endothelial cell lineage markers, including CD34, Flk-1, VE-cadherin, platelet–endothelial cell adhesion molecule 1 (PECAM-1), von Willebrand factor (vWF), endothelial nitric oxide synthase (eNOS), and E-selectin. Transdifferentiation of CD34$^+$-enriched cells into cardiomyocytes and smooth muscle cells has been demonstrated in vivo.[23] There are, however, limitations on the therapeutic use of autologous EPCs for the treatment of tissue ischemia. The ability to expand these cells is limited by their scarcity in peripheral blood.[24,25] Further, functional impairment of EPCs has been observed in several pathologic conditions, and an inverse correlation has been reported between the number of circulating EPCs and the risk for cardiovascular events,[26] although increased circulating hematopoietic and endothelial progenitor cells have been found in patients in the early phase of acute myocardial infarction.[27] Risk factors for coronary artery disease such as age and diabetes reduce the number and functional activity of EPCs, limiting the therapeutic usefulness of autologous EPC transplantation in these patients.[28] Potential technical improvements to overcome these limitations may include isolation and expansion of EPCs from alternative sources, such as bone marrow, or the use of allogeneic EPCs from chord blood.

CD133$^+$ cells

Initially EPCs were defined as cell populations positive for both hematopoietic stem cell markers such as CD34 and an endothelial marker protein such as vascular endothelial growth factor receptor 2 (VEGFR-2, also known as FLK-1/KDR). Since CD34 is not solely expressed on hematopoietic stem cells (expression is detected at a lower level on mature endothelial cells), further selection of EPCs using the more immature hematopoietic stem cell marker CD133 to distinguish cells capable of differentiating into endothelial cells in vitro was proposed. CD133 (also known as prominin and AC133) is a highly conserved antigen with unknown biologic activity, which is expressed on hematopoietic stem cells but is absent on mature endothelial cells and monocytic cells.[29] CD133$^+$ cells engrafted in rats on the 10th day post infarction have been shown to improve the ventricular ejection fraction as assessed 1 month after transplantation.[30]

Mesenchymal stem cells

Mesenchymal stem cells (MSCs) are a rare population of CD34$^-$ and CD133$^-$ cells that represent self-renewing clonal precursors of non-hematopoietic tissue. This class of progenitors resides in bone marrow and around blood vessels (as pericytes), in fat, skin, muscle, and other locations. MSCs exhibit multipotent differentiation potential and can give rise to mesodermal-derived tissue, including astrocytes, neurons, osteocytes, chondrocytes, adipocytes, and skeletal muscle.[31] MSCs lack unique surface antigens, so multiple expression markers (including CD29, CD71, CD90, CD106, and CD117) are relied upon to fully characterize this cell type. Detailed characterizations of MSCs can be found elsewhere.[32] The potential application of MSCs for cardiac repair became of interest when these cells were discovered to become cardiomyocytes in vitro, although the necessity of inducing regimens such as 5-acacytidine limits the clinical applicability of such strategies. One advantage of MSCs is that they are considered to be immune-privileged and have been successfully transplanted into hearts without the need for immunosuppression.[33] It is also apparent that MSCs home to areas of injury. In a study by Bittira et al,[34] rat MSCs labeled with *lacZ*, administered by tail vein injection, localized primarily to bone marrow. When the animals were subjected to myocardial infarction, however, *lacZ*$^+$ cells were found within the healing infarction, indicating that these cells were capable of seeking sites of injury.[34]

Purified human MSCs have been shown to differentiate to a cardiomyocyte phenotype in both normal[35] and infarcted[36] myocardium. The long-term survival of MSCs in the setting of a myocardial infarction has recently been studied. Interestingly, allogeneic MSCs transplanted into rat hearts 7 days post myocardial infarction survived in infarcted myocardium for as long as 6 months and expressed markers that suggested muscle (α-actinin, tropomyosin, MF-20, and phospholamban) and endothelial (vWF) phenotypes.[37] Although ventricular function was improved at 1 month, labeled MSCs failed to show muscle-specific marker proteins, indicating that mechanisms aside from differentiation contributed to the early functional effects of transplanted MSCs. Moreover, at 6 months, there was no longer any improvement in ventricular function – perhaps because only immature myofibrillar organization was detected, suggesting that MSCs lack the potential to acquire a mature cardiomyocyte phenotype.

Skeletal myoblasts

Cell-based cardiac repair began with the transplantation of autologous skeletal muscle satellite cells, commonly referred to as myoblast progenitor cells, which normally mediate the regeneration of skeletal muscle.[38–40] Although some investigators originally hoped that engrafted myoblasts would transdifferentiate into cardiomyocytes, several lines of evidence now indicate that these cells remain committed to a skeletal muscle fate (with the exception of rare fusion events at the graft–host interface). These cells, however, do not express the adhesion or gap junction proteins required to couple electromechanically with one another or with host myocardium.[41]

Resident cardiac stem cells

Although the major pathophysiologic response to myocardial damage was thought to be hypertrophy of still-viable cardiomyocytes, emerging data suggest that newly discovered populations of resident cardiac cells possess the ability to undergo mitosis and cytokinesis under certain conditions.[42] In a seminal study, Hierlihy et al,[43] showed that a specific cell type referred to as the "side population" could be isolated from the adult rat heart and cultured in vitro.[43] These cells showed stem cell-like behavior, with a restricted ability to differentiate into the cardiomyocyte lineage. Other studies have shown Lin^- $c\text{-}Kit^+$ cell clusters in the interstitium of the adult rat heart, many of which express markers for cell proliferation and transcription (GATA-4 and Nkx 2.5) associated with early cardiac development.[44] A similar potential is shown for $Sca\text{-}1^+$ cells isolated from adult murine hearts, with an expression profile equivalent to $c\text{-}Kit^+$ after stimulation with oxytocin[45] or 5-azacytidine[46] in vitro. When injected intravenously into reperfused hearts, $Sca\text{-}1^+$ cells were shown to target the border zone of the infarct and differentiate into cardiomyocytes.[46] In the adult human heart, clusters of stem cell-like cells expressing stem cell markers (such as Sca-1, c-Kit, and MSR-1) and harboring telomerase activity (a marker of replicating cells) have been identified. In the hypertrophied myocardium of aortic stenosis patients, the number of cardiac stem cells is increased almost 13-fold.[47] In a more recent study, a novel cardiac cell type was identified in postnatal rat, mouse, and human myocardium using the LIM-homeodomain transcription factor islet-1 (isl1).[48] This marker identifies a cell population of the embryonic heart, comprising most cells in the right ventricle, both atria, the outflow tract, and also specific regions of the left ventricle.[49] Currently, all resident cardiac progenitor cell types are thought to be clearly distinct from each other, such that $Sca\text{-}1^+$ cells lack c-Kit expression, $c\text{-}Kit^+$ cells lack Sca-1 expression, and $isl1^+$ cells lack Sca-1 and c-Kit expression. Cardiac progenitor cells have been isolated from small samples of human myocardium and can be expanded in vitro without losing cardiac cell lineage differentiation.[50]

Embryonic stem cells

Despite current ethical and political concerns, embryonic stem cells (ESCs) are considered prime candidates for cell-based therapies, since they possess unlimited capacity for self-renewal. Moreover, ESCs possess a vigorous cardiac potential, as ESC-derived cardiomyocytes express the molecular elements required for successful electromechanical coupling with host myocardium. A series of well-defined endogenous growth and differentiation factors and an increasing number of small molecules, including retinoic acid,[51] ascorbic acid,[52] and dynorphin B,[53] have been reported to promote cardiogenesis in mouse ESCs, which are highly dependent on concentration and timing of application.[51] Although, to date, a precise recipe for optimal ESC cardiac differentiation is lacking, there is much current interest in enriching mouse ESC-derived cardiomyocytes from spontaneously differentiating embryoid bodies using genetic selection techniques, since cardiomyocytes represent only a few percent of this total cell population.[54] Several investigators have successfully implanted ESC progeny into various models of myocardial injury, demonstrating sustained improvements in contractile function on echocardiography. It is still not confirmed, however, whether immune recognition plays a role in the acceptance of undifferentiated ESCs. Further, in recipient hearts, potential signaling mechanisms for selectively directing the implanted undifferentiated ESCs through cardiogenesis are not well characterized.

Characterization of cardiomyocytes

True regeneration of myocytes derived from cell-based cardiac repair requires phenotypic characterization by specific cardiac markers such as sarcomeric actins and myosins, myosin light chain 2v (MLC-2v), cardiac troponin I, GATA-4, and atrial natriuretic peptide.[55] Expression of N-cadherin and connexin 43 (major proteins of adherence junctions) is suggestive of electrophysiologic coupling with surrounding cells. In addition, regenerating myocytes are typically negative for vimentin, whereas fibroblasts are identified by the expression of procollagen and vimentin.[56]

Potential microscopic artifacts in the recognition of stem cell-derived myocytes

Some common artifacts of circulating progenitors include the accumulation of resident leukocytes and the high intrinsic autofluorescence of infarcted myocardial tissue. Autofluorescence is a recognized problem with normal striated muscle and can be mistaken for transgene expression of enhanced green fluorescent protein (EGFP) or a fluorescent immunostain.[55] Following injury, autofluorescence increases as a result of accumulated lipofuscin, blood-derived pigments, and other intrinsic fluors, including flavins and reduced nicotinamide adenine dinucleotide (NADH). In the case of EGFP, confusion with autofluorescence can be minimized by immunolabeling with a specific anti-EGFP antibody rather than relying on intrinsic fluorescence alone. The advantage of an immunohistochemical approach is the apparent amplification of the signal, reducing the signal-to-background ratio by about 300-fold.[56] It is essential to stain samples in the presence of a well-established positive and negative control, along with determination of the background fluorescence generated by the secondary antibody. The intense background autofluorescence in formaldehyde-fixed myocardial sections may be further controlled by exposure to 0.1% Sudan Black B after fluorescence staining.[57] Finally, the engulfment of necrotic cells by leukocytes may also hinder recognition of stem cell-derived myocytes, since these cells may show remnants of myocyte nuclei and/or cardiac myofibrils.[55] Inflammatory cell markers such as CD45 and CD68 or further characterization by transmission electron microscopy may help rule out the presence of leukocytes.

Myocyte fusion

Myocardial regeneration could result from fusion of the transplanted stem cell with existing cardiac cells, resulting in the formation of hybrid cells. The formation of a hybrid cell may contribute to the development or maintenance of these key cell types. Cell fusion should generate binucleated myocytes with one tetraploid and one diploid nucleus or myocytes with three diploid nuclei. Evidence for fusion between cardiac and stem cells has been obtained with, selective fluorophore low-molecular-weight tracers such as calcein-AM,[58] nanocrystal labeling,[59] combined EGFP and transgender cardiac transplantation,[56] and Cre–*lox* donor/recipient pairs.[46,60,61] The use of the latter technique, however, may generate false-positive results, since the phenomenon of metabolic cooperation[62] between biochemically marked cells may allow the diffusion of Cre

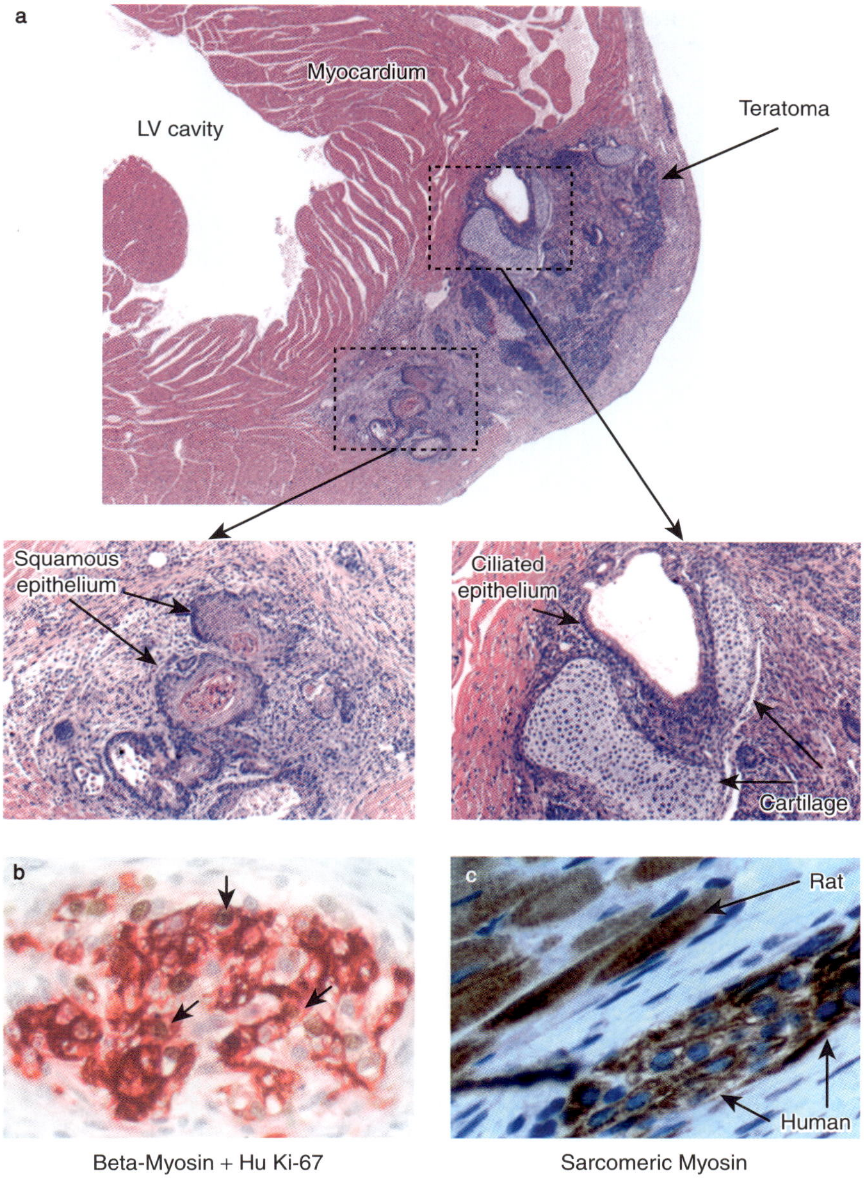

Figure 5.4 *Embryonic stem cell (ESC) grafts. (a) Grafting of undifferentiated mouse ESCs. Undifferentiated mouse ESCs consistently formed teratomas when implanted into the hearts of immunotolerant hosts. The teratoma replaced much of the left ventricular wall. The boxed insets show ectoderm-derived keratinizing squamous epithelium (left), mesoderm-derived cartilage (right), and endoderm-derived ciliated columnar epithelium (right). The tissue was stained with hematoxylin–eosin. LV, left ventricle. (b,c) Grafting of human ESC-derived cardiomyocytes. Human ESCs were differentiated as embryoid bodies, and cultures enriched for cardiomyocytes were transplanted into the hearts of nude rats. (b) One week later, the human cardiomyocytes could be identified by β-myosin heavy chain (β-MHC) expression (red) and showed substantial proliferative activity, as evidenced by staining with a human-specific Ki-67 antibody (brown, arrows). (c) By 4 weeks, the human cardiomyocytes (identified in serial sections with human-specific genomic probes) showed early sarcomere formation (sarcomeric myosin staining, brown). Reproduced with permission from Laflamme MA, Murry CE. Nat Biotechnol 2005;23:845–56.[55] (c) 2005 Nature Publishing Group (http://www.nature.com).*

recombinase to a recipient cell through intercellular junctions in the absence of cell fusion.[56] Myocyte volume size is another potential determinant of cell fusion, with expected new myocytes of equal or greater volume.[56] Although the incidence of cell fusion in the postinfarcted myocardium is not well defined, critical evaluation of current reports indicates that cell fusion is a non-dominant (or perhaps a non-existent) mechanism and may be considered essentially an in vitro phenomenon with few implications in vivo.[63]

Potential Complications of Cell-Based Therapy

As with most other controversial therapies, valid concerns have been raised about potential adverse effects, such as tumorigenicity or unregulated differentiation after stem cell transplantation in vivo. Along these lines, a few reports have documented teratoma formation after implantation of undifferentiated embryonic stem cells in knee joints[64] and hearts of immunotolerant hosts (Figure 5.4).[55] Notably, intramyocardial teratomas are rare, with only six reported cases in humans[65] and one additional case in the Armed Forces Institute of Pathology files; most such lesions occur in newborns, and all occur during the first 6 years of life. The majority of patients present with congestive heart failure; sudden death precipitated by acute arrhythmias caused by the tumor's interventricular location may be the first symptom.[65] Other reported complications of experimental cell-based therapy involve ventricular calcification after local transplantation of unselected bone marrow cells in rats with acute myocardial infarction.[66] The clinical consequences of severe ventricular calcification in the post-infarction patient are unknown. Other potential complications of cell transplantation into the heart include arrhythmias, coronary plaque angiogenesis with plaque rupture, hemorrhagic pericarditis, and infarct extension.

Summary Perspectives

Acute or healed myocardial infarction remains the primary cause of high morbidity and mortality in patients presenting with acute coronary syndromes or congestive heart failure. This has led to a search for new therapies beyond the use of pharmacologic agents alone. Cell-based transplantation is one potential approach to treating acute myocardial infarction by repopulating lost myocytes. One must be aware, however, that myocardial reperfusion can leave viable islands of myocytes within the scarred tissue in addition to inherently giving rise to an angiogenic/vasculogenic response, which presents a challenge to the successful identification of cell engraftment. In order to evaluate the effectiveness of cell therapy, it is imperative to carefully monitor cell plasticity and/or the ability of transplanted cells to integrate into a functional myocardium and to recognize potential artifacts that may cause misleading results. Critical issues concerning the utility of differentiated or multipotent cell types are as yet unresolved, and no universal markers identifying optimal stem cell types are available. Establishment of cell-derived viable myocytes without functional improvement is of no clinical significance, and the optimal goal is to provide long-term therapeutic benefit with minimal risk. This rapidly advancing field is still in its infancy, and serious progress towards providing clinically effective cell-based therapy will likely require a more comprehensive understanding of regenerative biology.

References

1. Hellermann JP, Goraya TY, Jacobsen SJ, et al. Incidence of heart failure after myocardial infarction: Is it changing over time? Am J Epidemiol 2003;157:1101–7.
2. Miura T, Shizukuda Y, Ogawa S, Ishimoto R, Iimura O. Effects of early and later reperfusion on healing speed of experimental myocardial infarct. Can J Cardiol 1991;7:146–54.
3. Heymans S, Luttun A, Nuyens D, et al. Inhibition of plasminogen activators or matrix metalloproteinases prevents cardiac rupture but impairs therapeutic angiogenesis and causes cardiac failure. Nat Med 1999;5:1135–42.
4. Virag JI, Murry CE. Myofibroblast and endothelial cell proliferation during murine myocardial infarct repair. Am J Pathol 2003;163:2433–40.
5. Luttun A, Carmeliet P. De novo vasculogenesis in the heart. Cardiovasc Res 2003;58:378–89.

6. Carmeliet P, Ng YS, Nuyens D, et al. Impaired myocardial angiogenesis and ischemic cardiomyopathy in mice lacking the vascular endothelial growth factor isoforms VEGF164 and VEGF188. Nat Med 1999;5:495–502.
7. Young PP, Hofling AA, Sands MS. VEGF increases engraftment of bone marrow-derived endothelial progenitor cells (EPCs) into vasculature of newborn murine recipients. Proc Natl Acad Sci USA 2002;99:11951–6.
8. Stoker ME, Gerdes AM, May JF. Regional differences in capillary density and myocyte size in the normal human heart. Anat Rec 1982;202:187–91.
9. Richard V, Murry CE, Reimer KA. Healing of myocardial infarcts in dogs. Effects of late reperfusion. Circulation 1995;92:1891–901.
10. Fishbein MC, Maclean D, Maroko PR. The histopathologic evolution of myocardial infarction. Chest 1978;73:843–9.
11. Jugdutt BI. Ventricular remodeling after infarction and the extracellular collagen matrix: When is enough enough? Circulation 2003;108:1395–403.
12. Alberts B, Johnson A, Lewis J, Raff M, Roberts K, Walter P. Molecular Biology of the Cell, 4th edn. New York: Garland, 2001.
13. Philips C, Wenstrup RJ. Biosynthetic and genetic disorders of collagen. In: Cohen IK, Diegelmann RF, Lindblad WJ (eds). Wound Healing: Biochemical and Clinical Aspects. Philadelphia: Saunders, 1992:152–71.
14. Mathur A, Martin JF. Stem cells and repair of the heart. Lancet 2004;364:183–92.
15. von Harsdorf R, Poole-Wilson PA, Dietz R. Regenerative capacity of the myocardium: implications for treatment of heart failure. Lancet 2004;363:1306–13.
16. Muller-Ehmsen P, Beltrami AP, Cesselli D, Pfeiffer P, Kazakov A, Bohm M. Myocardial regeneration by endogenous adult progenitor cells. J Mol Cell Cardiol 2005;39:377–87.
17. Ishii M, Koike C, Igarashi A, et al. Molecular markers distinguish bone marrow mesenchymal stem cells from fibroblasts. Biochem Biophys Res Commun 2005;332:297–303.
18. Yang AX, Mejido J, Luo Y, et al. Development of a focused microarray to assess human embryonic stem cell differentiation. Stem Cells Dev 2005;14:270–84.
19. Shen X, Collier JM, Hlaing M, et al. Genome-wide examination of myoblast cell cycle withdrawal during differentiation. Dev Dyn 2003;226:128–38.
20. Feldmann RE, Jr., Bieback K, Maurer MH, et al. Stem cell proteomes: a profile of human mesenchymal stem cells derived from umbilical cord blood. Electrophoresis 2005;26(14):2749–58.
21. Rafii S, Lyden D. Therapeutic stem and progenitor cell transplantation for organ vascularization and regeneration. Nat Med 2003;9:702–12.
22. Hristov M, Erl W, Weber PC. Endothelial progenitor cells: mobilization, differentiation, and homing. Arterioscler Thromb Vasc Biol 2003;23:1185–9.
23. Yeh ET, Zhang S, Wu HD, Korbling M, Willerson JT, Estrov Z. Transdifferentiation of human peripheral blood $CD34^+$-enriched cell population into cardiomyocytes, endothelial cells, and smooth muscle cells in vivo. Circulation 2003;108:2070–3.
24. Asahara T, Murohara T, Sullivan A, et al. Isolation of putative progenitor endothelial cells for angiogenesis. Science 1997;275:964–7.
25. Masuda H, Asahara T. Post-natal endothelial progenitor cells for neovascularization in tissue regeneration. Cardiovasc Res 2003;58:390–8.
26. Hill JM, Zalos G, Halcox JP, et al. Circulating endothelial progenitor cells, vascular function, and cardiovascular risk. N Engl J Med 2003;348:593–600.
27. Massa M, Rosti V, Ferrario M, et al. Increased circulating hematopoietic and endothelial progenitor cells in the early phase of acute myocardial infarction. Blood 2005;105:199–206.
28. Dimmeler S, Zeiher AM. Vascular repair by circulating endothelial progenitor cells: the missing link in atherosclerosis? J Mol Med 2004;82:671–7.
29. Handgretinger R, Gordon PR, Leimig T, et al. Biology and plasticity of $CD133^+$ hematopoietic stem cells. Ann NY Acad Sci 2003;996:141–51.
30. Agbulut O, Vandervelde S, Al Attar N, et al. Comparison of human skeletal myoblasts and bone marrow-derived $CD133^+$ progenitors for the repair of infarcted myocardium. J Am Coll Cardiol 2004;44:458–63.
31. Caplan AI, Bruder SP. Mesenchymal stem cells: building blocks for molecular medicine in the 21st century. Trends Mol Med 2001;7:259–64.
32. Deans RJ, Moseley AB. Mesenchymal stem cells: biology and potential clinical uses. Exp Hematol 2000;28:875–84.
33. Pittenger MF, Martin BJ. Mesenchymal stem cells and their potential as cardiac therapeutics. Circ Res 2004;95:9–20.
34. Bittira B, Shum-Tim D, Al-Khaldi A, Chiu RC. Mobilization and homing of bone marrow stromal cells in myocardial infarction. Eur J Cardiothorac Surg 2003;24:393–8.
35. Toma C, Pittenger MF, Cahill KS, Byrne BJ, Kessler PD. Human mesenchymal stem cells differentiate to a cardiomyocyte phenotype in the adult murine heart. Circulation 2002;105:93–8.
36. Shake JG, Gruber PJ, Baumgartner WA, et al. Mesenchymal stem cell implantation in a swine myocardial infarct model: engraftment and functional effects. Ann Thorac Surg 2002;73:1919–25; discussion 1926.
37. Dai W, Hale SL, Martin BJ, et al. Allogeneic mesenchymal stem cell transplantation in postinfarcted

rat myocardium: short- and long-term effects. Circulation 2005;112:214–23.
38. Marelli D, Desrosiers C, el-Alfy M, Kao RL, Chiu RC. Cell transplantation for myocardial repair: an experimental approach. Cell Transplant 1992;1:383–90.
39. Chiu RC, Zibaitis A, Kao RL. Cellular cardiomyoplasty: myocardial regeneration with satellite cell implantation. Ann Thorac Surg 1995;60:12–18.
40. Koh GY, Klug MG, Soonpaa MH, Field LJ. Differentiation and long-term survival of C2C12 myoblast grafts in heart. J Clin Invest 1993;92: 1548–54.
41. Reinecke H, Poppa V, Murry CE. Skeletal muscle stem cells do not transdifferentiate into cardiomyocytes after cardiac grafting. J Mol Cell Cardiol 2002;34:241–9.
42. Anversa P, Nadal-Ginard B. Myocyte renewal and ventricular remodelling. Nature 2002;415:240–3.
43. Hierlihy AM, Seale P, Lobe CG, Rudnicki MA, Megeney LA. The post-natal heart contains a myocardial stem cell population. FEBS Lett 2002;530: 239–43.
44. Beltrami AP, Barlucchi L, Torella D, et al. Adult cardiac stem cells are multipotent and support myocardial regeneration. Cell 2003;114:763–76.
45. Matsuura K, Nagai T, Nishigaki N, et al. Adult cardiac Sca-1-positive cells differentiate into beating cardiomyocytes. J Biol Chem 2004;279:11384–91.
46. Oh H, Bradfute SB, Gallardo TD, et al. Cardiac progenitor cells from adult myocardium: homing, differentiation, and fusion after infarction. Proc Natl Acad Sci USA 2003;100:12313–18.
47. Urbanek K, Quaini F, Tasca G, et al. Intense myocyte formation from cardiac stem cells in human cardiac hypertrophy. Proc Natl Acad Sci USA 2003;100:10440–5.
48. Laugwitz KL, Moretti A, Lam J, et al. Postnatal isl1$^+$ cardioblasts enter fully differentiated cardiomyocyte lineages. Nature 2005;433:647–53.
49. Cai CL, Liang X, Shi Y, et al. Isl1 identifies a cardiac progenitor population that proliferates prior to differentiation and contributes a majority of cells to the heart. Dev Cell 2003;5:877–89.
50. Messina E, De Angelis L, Frati G, et al. Isolation and expansion of adult cardiac stem cells from human and murine heart. Circ Res 2004;95: 911–21.
51. Wobus AM, Kaomei G, Shan J, et al. Retinoic acid accelerates embryonic stem cell-derived cardiac differentiation and enhances development of ventricular cardiomyocytes. J Mol Cell Cardiol 1997;29:1525–39.
52. Takahashi T, Lord B, Schulze PC, et al. Ascorbic acid enhances differentiation of embryonic stem cells into cardiac myocytes. Circulation 2003;107: 1912–16.
53. Ventura C, Zinellu E, Maninchedda E, Maioli M. Dynorphin B is an agonist of nuclear opioid receptors coupling nuclear protein kinase C activation to the transcription of cardiogenic genes in GTR1 embryonic stem cells. Circ Res 2003;92:623–9.
54. Klug MG, Soonpaa MH, Koh GY, Field LJ. Genetically selected cardiomyocytes from differentiating embronic stem cells form stable intracardiac grafts. J Clin Invest 1996;98:216–24.
55. Laflamme MA, Murry CE. Regenerating the heart. Nat Biotechnol 2005;23:845–56.
56. Kajstura J, Rota M, Whang B, et al. Bone marrow cells differentiate in cardiac cell lineages after infarction independently of cell fusion. Circ Res 2005;96:127–37.
57. Baschong W, Suetterlin R, Laeng RH. Control of autofluorescence of archival formaldehyde-fixed, paraffin-embedded tissue in confocal laser scanning microscopy (CLSM). J Histochem Cytochem 2001;49:1565–72.
58. Driesen RB, Dispersyn GD, Verheyen FK, et al. Partial cell fusion: a newly recognized type of communication between dedifferentiating cardiomyocytes and fibroblasts. Cardiovasc Res 2005;68:37–46.
59. Murasawa S, Kawamoto A, Horii M, Nakamori S, Asahara T. Niche-dependent translineage commitment of endothelial progenitor cells, not cell fusion in general, into myocardial lineage cells. Arterioscler Thromb Vasc Biol 2005;25:1388–94.
60. Alvarez-Dolado M, Pardal R, Garcia-Verdugo JM, et al. Fusion of bone-marrow-derived cells with Purkinje neurons, cardiomyocytes and hepatocytes. Nature 2003;425:968–73.
61. Reinecke H, Minami E, Poppa V, Murry CE. Evidence for fusion between cardiac and skeletal muscle cells. Circ Res 2004;94:e56–60.
62. Subak-Sharpe H, Burk RR, Pitts JD. Metabolic co-operation between biochemically marked mammalian cells in tissue culture. Rev Med Virol 2002;12:69–78; discussion 79–80.
63. Harris RG, Herzog EL, Bruscia EM, Grove JE, Van Arnam JS, Krause DS. Lack of a fusion requirement for development of bone marrow-derived epithelia. Science 2004;305:90–3.
64. Wakitani S, Takaoka K, Hattori T, et al. Embryonic stem cells injected into the mouse knee joint form teratomas and subsequently destroy the joint. Rheumatology 2003;42:162–5.
65. Swalwell CI. Benign intracardiac teratoma. A case of sudden death. Arch Pathol Lab Med 1993;117: 739–42.
66. Yoon YS, Park JS, Tkebuchava T, Luedeman C, Losordo DW. Unexpected severe calcification after transplantation of bone marrow cells in acute myocardial infarction. Circulation 2004;109:3154–7.

PART 2

Understanding Translational Cardiac Stem Cell Research

chapter 6

Large Animal Models of Myocardial Ischemia for Cardiac Cell Therapy

Edie M Oliveira and Franca Stedile Angeli

Introduction

Despite advances in pharmacologic therapies, as well as catheter-based and surgical revascularization techniques, coronary artery disease (CAD) is the leading cause of mortality in the industrialized world.[1] Therefore, emerging alternative treatments such as stem cell therapy may have an important therapeutic role to play in this patient population.

Stem cell therapy for cardiac diseases has been used in clinical studies, but many key questions regarding this novel therapy remain unanswered. Further preclinical studies are needed in order to assess its safety and efficacy.

To date, the regenerative potential of a number of cells has been investigated in various animal models. Table 6.1 lists some of those studies. Most of them have shown an improvement in cardiac function, coronary blood flow, or the healing process after an ischemic event.[2–7] Some of the preclinical studies were followed by clinical trials to confirm the efficacy and safety of the same approach in humans.

This chapter presents a brief overview of large animal models of myocardial ischemia for cardiac cell therapy.

Animal Model Selection

Few studies have compared the various in vivo large animal models of myocardial ischemia.[8,9] Because CAD is a multifactorial and heterogeneous disease, it is hard to reproduce accurately, even in large animals. However, despite the limitations of current large animal models, they are the most reliable way to predict outcomes before clinical protocols are initiated.

The first key aspect in large animal model research is to understand the differences between the available species and their potential to elicit the desired results. Although canines are frequently used, their basic anatomy and physiology differ from those of human beings, possibly limiting the interpretation of results. On the other hand, swine closely resemble humans with respect to cardiovascular anatomy, ventricular performance, electrical properties, and coronary artery distribution.

Cardiovascular anatomy

For many decades, canines have been the most commonly used species in studies of myocardial ischemia. They have a two-vessel coronary artery system, usually with a nondominant right coronary artery that supplies the right ventricle. The right coronary artery rarely supplies the heart's posterior surface and usually has only one major septal branch that arises from the left anterior descending (LAD) coronary artery. Moreover, canines have a larger left ventricle than humans and an unpredictable, though often substantial, collateral circulation network that can provide up to 40% of normal flow to the perfusion bed

Table 6.1 Stem cell therapy for cardiovascular disease: preclinical studies

Target	*Donor*	*Recipient*	*Cell type and source*	*Method of delivery*	*Therapeutic effects*	*Ref*
Myocardial ischemia	Swine	Autologous	$CD31^+$, peripheral blood	Transendocardial with NOGA system	↑Rentrop Score, ↑EF, ↑ capillary density	2
Myocardial ischemia	Swine	Autologous	MNCs, bone marrow	Transendocardial	↑capillary density, ↑collateral flow, ↑myocardial contractility	3
Myocardial ischemia	Canine	Allogeneic	MSCs	Intramyocardial	↑capillary density, ↑myocardial contractility	4
Myocardial ischemia	Rat	Autologous	MNCs, bone marrow	Intramyocardial	↑capillary density	—
Myocardial infarction	Human	Nude rat	$CD34^+$, peripheral blood	Intravenous	Transdifferentiation into cardiomyocytes, smooth muscle cells, and endothelial cells	5
Myocardial infarction	Human	Nude rat	$CD34^+$, bone marrow	Tail vein injection	↑EF, ↑capillary density, ↓fibrosis, ↓apoptosis, ↓infarct size	6
Myocardial infarction	GFP-mouse	Syngeneic mouse	$Lin^-c\text{-}Kit^+$, bone marrow	Intramyocardial	↑LVDP, ↑capillary density, ↓infarct	7

EF, ejection fraction; GFP, green fluorescent protein; LVDP, left ventricular diastolic pressure; MNCs, mononuclear cells; MSCs, mesenchymal cells.

of an acutely occluded epicardial coronary artery.[10]

Compared with swine, canines have somewhat similar coronary flow at rest but significantly higher coronary flow at a maximal heart rate. This may reflect the higher heart-size/bodyweight ratio of canines or the greater vascular capacity of the canine heart. Pathologic assessment has shown that left ventricular capillary density is also significantly greater in canines than in swine.[11]

Swine have three major coronary arteries, organized in a typically right-dominant coronary system, with minimal preexisting collateral vessels.[10,12] The swine commonly used in the laboratory weigh an average of 25–30 kg and have a heart-size/bodyweight ratio identical to that of a human ($p<0.005$). However, adult pigs that weigh more than 100 kg have a very low heart-size/bodyweight ratio, because their hearts do not increase proportionally to their corporeal mass.

Electrical properties

Although cardiac electrophysiology studies have been performed in animals since the beginning of the 20th century, these studies have yielded discrepant data. In examining the studies involving canines, one might find it hard to compare the results, because various researchers have used different terminology for electrocardiography (ECG) leads, different locations for electrode placement, and even different breeds of dogs.[13] Nevertheless, one would expect that the P-wave amplitude would always be positive in standard leads I and II and negative in leads aVF and V6. However, the Q- and R-wave amplitudes of the QRS complex are related to the dog's breed and age and do not follow the human patterns.

The ECG morphology in swine also differs from that in humans and canines, owing to deeper penetration of the ventricular free walls by the Purkinje fibers, which yields a different left ventricular activation sequence. In addition, as swine age, the QRS complex undergoes morphologic changes that indicate work overload. Rhythm disturbances, including Wenckebach's phenomenon, transient atrioventricular (AV) block, and sinus arrhythmia, are also common. More importantly, to a greater extent than in any other nonprimate animal, the normal intracardiac electrophysiologic parameters in swine resemble those in humans.

Swine are susceptible to ventricular fibrillation, whether spontaneous or induced. The high incidence of this arrhythmia makes cardiac surgery somewhat difficult. Unlike in dogs, ligation of a major coronary artery such as the LAD in pigs will frequently lead to ventricular fibrillation, which entails a mortality rate of more than 70%.[11]

Differences in cardiac physiology

The increased use of swine models in recent years can be attributed to the fact that the cardiac conduction system and the distribution of the coronary artery blood supply of swine are very similar to those in humans. Moreover, swine myocardial metabolism follows human pathways, relying on nonesterified fatty acids as the preferred substrate for energy production under normal conditions.[14] A second advantage of swine is that they adapt to exercise much as a human does; in contrast, the dog's superior exercise capacity is unique.[15]

Animal care: the ideal is not always easy

Dogs are naturally friendly and cooperative. They are sufficiently large to permit instrumentation for detailed measurement of hemodynamic parameters, even in a conscious animal, and they are much less prone than swine to develop cardiac arrhythmias and sudden death.

The major constraint on wider acceptance of swine as research animals is related to difficulties in care and handling. Also, the early mortality is usually much higher in porcine ischemic models than in canine models. Multiple interventions and even noninvasive monitoring are much harder to achieve in swine, as the need for repeat sedation increases morbidity.

Models of Myocardial Ischemia

Acute ischemia

Rapid occlusion of a coronary artery in a human or pig, whose collateral vessels are sparse, almost always results in complete infarction of the vascular bed at risk. This is not true of a canine model, in which collaterals are already abundant and develop rapidly during ischemia. Therefore, occlusion of the main side branches is usually necessary to create a considerable area of ischemia in dogs.

Coronary ligation

Ligation is a simple means of producing transient (3-hour) or permanent occlusion of the target artery. In the canine model, the proximal LAD can be ligated. In addition, a diagonal branch should be ligated to decrease collateral flow to the infarcted area and produce a transmural infarction.[16] In a porcine model, occlusion of the circumflex artery or another minor branch is preferred, as the mortality is unacceptable after LAD occlusion.[11]

Coronary balloon occlusion

As in the above-described model of intermittent ligation, arterial occlusion can be produced by placing an inflated balloon on the target vessel.

The advantage of this method is avoidance of open-chest surgery.

Microsphere embolization

A porcine model of coronary microembolization was first described by Mohri and Schaper[17] in 1993, based on the unique model introduced by Chilian et al[18] for studying the pathophysiology of vascular growth. In that model, ischemia begins at the moment of microsphere injection. The microspheres can be injected via a coronary artery catheter either with or without the use of a thoracotomy. This method produces areas of patchy necrosis in the left ventricle. Regional ischemia is usually less severe than complete blockage at a more proximal point.

Zimmermann et al[19] used 25-µm nonradioactive polystyrene microspheres to produce ischemia. The quantity of microspheres injected is usually adjusted to abolish the coronary blood flow reserve, and the diameter of the beads corresponds to the diameter of the target vessel, ranging from arteries to capillaries. Repetitive microembolization can also be used to produce chronic ischemia.

Inorganic mercury thrombosis

After the animal has been anesthetized, an acute myocardial infarction can be created by injecting a small amount of inorganic mercury (usually 0.1 ml), which is not ionized and will not cause an in vivo chemical reaction, into the target coronary artery. Mercury can be used to produce multiple infarcts in different layers of the left ventricle.[20] Approximately 30 minutes after coronary embolization, targeted segments of the left ventricle will contract and the ejection fraction will decrease.

Thrombus

Another way to create an acute infarction is by injecting an artificial thrombus[21] consisting of a combined arterial blob, fibrinogen, and thrombin. This model requires that the artery first undergo laser intimal ablation to create a stenotic lesion. The thrombus is then placed in the stenotic portion of the coronary artery to occlude it altogether.

Cryothermia

After exposure of the heart through a medium sternotomy, cryothermia can be used to produce an acute myocardial infarction. With a 5-mm diameter cylindrical cryoprobe, the ventricular free wall is cooled to –160°C with internally circulating liquid nitrogen. This usually involves five freezing cycles lasting 1 minute each, separated by 1-minute thawing intervals.[22,23]

Chronic myocardial ischemia

Most chronic ischemic models have used one of the following methods for producing stenosis or occlusion of an epicardial coronary artery.

Ameroid constriction

The ameroid constrictor is probably the most widely used device for producing chronic ischemia (Figure 6.1).[9] Originally described by Litvak et al[24] in 1957, these constrictors consist of a hygroscopic material (casein) within a steel sleeve. When placed around the artery, the constrictor absorbs water and swells, compressing the artery and producing a total coronary occlusion over 14–30 days or more.[25] When the constrictor is coated with petrolatum, water absorption is slowed, and the time to occlusion can be prolonged.[26]

The common perception that ameroid constrictors cause gradual coronary occlusion leading to myocardial ischemia and eventual collateral development may be an oversimplification. Whereas ameroid-induced coronary occlusion is indeed progressive, it is not necessarily gradual. These devices also cause mechanical trauma, which may lead to endothelial damage, platelet aggregation, and/or thrombus formation, and may cause a foreign body reaction and local scar formation.[27]

The degree to which ameroid devices cause ischemia depends on the general coronary artery topography, the location of the constrictor on the artery (i.e., proximal versus distal), device placement relative to side branches, the extent of preexisting collaterals, the animal's level of activity, and genetic/species differences.

As we have already emphasized, each model has its own strengths and weaknesses in terms

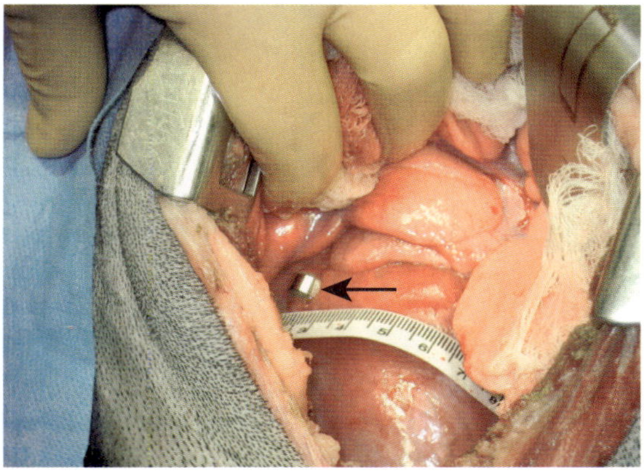

Figure 6.1 Placement of an ameroid constrictor in a canine model of chronic ischemia.

of its utility for preclinical trials. With ameroid constrictors, an important advantage is simplicity: once placed on a coronary artery, the device results in progressive arterial occlusion and creates a satisfactory model of chronic ischemia.

Limitations of this method include the fact that ameroid-induced coronary occlusion may be influenced by vascular tone, platelet aggregability, thrombogenicity, inflammation, and fibrosis. Also, ameroid devices cause a variable degree of infarction (generally subendocardial)[28] and lead to sudden death in a significant number of animals. Production of scarring, which is uneven in extent, has an important effect on the overall variability of the ameroid model.

Intermittent coronary occlusion

This model, often referred to as the "Franklin" model, is based on the demonstration that brief, repetitive total coronary occlusion is a potent stimulus for coronary collateral development as well as chronic cardiac ischemia.[29] Through brief, periodic inflations of a chronically implanted hydraulic balloon occluder, a coronary artery is subjected to repetitive proximal occlusion. The principal feature of this model is that no irreversible injury occurs. The major disadvantages are technical complexity and labor intensiveness.

Bone Marrow Harvest in Porcine Models

Bone marrow transplantation is one of the most powerful strategies for treating leukemia, aplastic anemia, congenital immunodeficiency, and autoimmune diseases.[27–29] Furthermore, gene therapy and organ transplantation using bone marrow cells have recently been carried out.[30–34] In humans, bone marrow cells are usually collected by means of multiple aspirations from the iliac crest, according to the method established by Thomas et al.[35] However, the literature contains few descriptions of bone marrow cell harvest in porcine models.

To develop a technique for this purpose, we conducted a cell therapy study in a porcine model of chronic ischemic cardiac disease. The study was performed in the cardiac catheterization laboratory. After being sedated, the animal was positioned in the prone position. The area over both posterior iliac crests was prepared with iodine and draped in a sterile fashion. Heparin sodium (1000 USP units/ml) – in 20 ml Monoject syringes (×6), each holding 2 ml of heparin – was given to prevent clotting. A sterile aspiration needle (provided in the Kendall Monoject Bone Marrow Biopsy/Aspiration Kit; Kendall, Mansfield, MA) was inserted into the marrow cavity in the target area (Figure 6.2). Marrow was then aspirated from the posterior iliac crests in no more than 20-ml aliquots with a disposable syringe (Figure 6.3). A total of 100 ± 20 ml of bone marrow was collected into seven 20-ml syringes. After the procedure, the area over the puncture site was cleaned and dressed with an adhesive bandage.

Delivery of Cell Therapy

Despite much discussion about the optimal protocol for cell delivery in animal protocols, researchers generally use the most convenient method, depending on physician expertise, accessibility of the target region, available delivery systems, cost, and personal preference. All experimental procedures and protocols must conform to institutional guidelines for the care

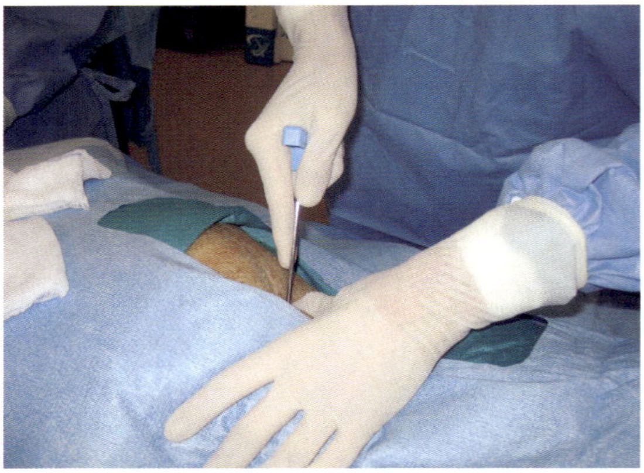

Figure 6.2 Iliac puncture in a swine model of chronic ischemia.

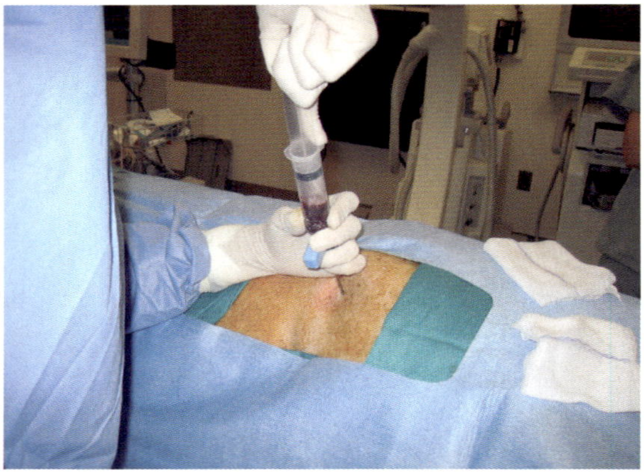

Figure 6.3 Bone marrow aspiration in a swine model of chronic ischemia.

and use of animals in research. At this time, the best approach is the most convenient one or the one most likely to fulfill researchers' expectations. With animal models, the cost is often relatively high because they require special equipment, supplies, infrastructure, and staff. At the Texas Heart Institute, we have had extensive experience with direct surgical delivery and transendocardial delivery. Delivery strategies will be discussed in detail in later chapters of this book. Therefore, we will focus on the particularities of direct surgical and transendocardial delivery in the above-described animal models.

Open surgical transmyocardial injection

Open transmyocardial injection is the most frequently used approach because of its practicality, familiarity, and certainty of delivery. This method not only provides adequate accessibility and localization but is also cost-efficient. A large number of our preclinical experiments used this approach, in both dogs and pigs. Once the animals were anesthetized and placed on a mechanical respirator, the heart was exposed through a left lateral thoracotomy (Figure 6.4). Using ameroid constriction (Figure 6.1), we ligated the LAD in dogs and the left circumflex coronary artery in pigs. To assure the presence of an ischemic area, we ligated collateral vessels in dogs and implanted an extra ameroid constrictor in pigs if the first marginal branch was bigger. Subsequent surgical closure was performed in the usual fashion, and the animals were closely observed in the postanesthesia recovery period. After surgery, the animals were treated with antibiotics and analgesics and were followed up for 4 weeks or more, depending on the protocol.

In another study, pigs underwent surgical transepicardial injection with gene-encoding adenovirus vascular endothelial growth factor 121 (Ad.VEGF121), using 1×10^{10} viral particles at six sites. After 24 hours, the animals were sacrificed, and their Ad.VEGF121 levels were found to be comparable with those in the transendocardially injected animals ($p=0.62$) (Figure 6.4).[36] Therefore, the open-chest approach is at least equivalent to the transmyocardial technique in terms of accessibility and is comparable in terms of outcomes.

Percutaneous approach

The percutaneous approach includes the intracoronary, retrograde (via the venous sinus), and transendocardial routes. Percutaneous delivery is less invasive and less complex than the surgical approach, involving less postoperative care and fewer complications. However, it may be less effective for accessing the targeted area. Also, it necessitates more specialized equipment so is much more expensive.

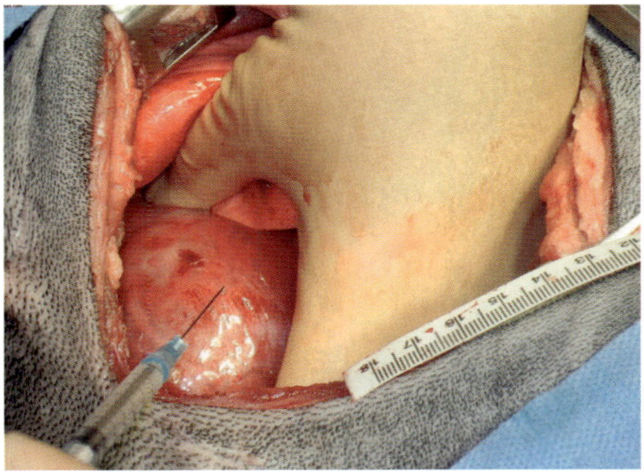

Figure 6.4 *Stem cell injection in the anterior left ventricular wall via a thoracotomy in a canine model.*

Transendocardial injection: mapping and injection

Targeting the endocardial wall is relatively easy and may be one of the most widely used methods of delivering genetic or angiogenic therapy. Multiple methods use the transendocardial approach to deliver a therapeutic substrate within the cardiac muscle. However, only one method – electromechanical mapping (EMM) with Biosense NOGA (Biosense-Webster, Waterloo, Belgium) – has a capacity for localizing the target area within the left ventricle, permitting precise therapeutic delivery. This method has been described in detail elsewhere.[37,38] It provides a three-dimensional (3D) image of the left ventricle by using a low magnetic field generated by three external magnetic field emitters placed beneath the operating table. Additional sensors are integrated into electrophysiologic deflectable-tip catheters (NogaStar; Biosense-Webster), one of which serves as the reference catheter and the other as the mapping catheter. The data acquired by the sensor are sent to a processing unit, enabling accurate real-time tracking of the catheter tip within the left ventricular cavity with minimal use of fluoroscopy.

To obtain a map in an animal model, we affix a reference catheter to the animal's back, then introduce a mapping catheter into the left ventricle under fluoroscopic guidance. While the mapping catheter is moved over multiple left ventricular endocardial sites, the system uses a triangular algorithm to reconstruct the left ventricular anatomy; the result is presented in real time on a Silicon Graphics workstation (Silicon Graphics, Inc., Mountain View, CA). Unipolar and bipolar endocardial potentials are recorded from the tip electrodes, and 3D electrical maps are reconstructed by displaying the voltage potentials on a graded color scale. From the mechanical data, regional contractility is obtained by using local endocardial shortening, calculated as the distance of an index point from its neighbors at end-diastole and end-systole (normalized to end-diastole).[39] The EMM workstation displays a unipolar voltage and a local shortening bullseye side by side. This integration of electrical and mechanical data yields a distinctive technique for analyzing left ventricular function (Figure 6.5).[40] On the basis of the resulting variables, we make the final diagnosis of normal, ischemic, borderline ischemic, or scar tissue. This method is explained further in another chapter of this book.

Mapping parameters

Preclinical studies, using a nonfluoroscopic 3D left ventricular mapping system, have revealed a reduction in the endomyocardial voltage potentials in nonviable and ischemic, noninfarcted myocardium. Since performing the first experiments, we have known that a good correlation exists between noninvasive indices of viability as assessed by single- and dual-isotope perfusion imaging, positron emission tomography (PET), and 3D left ventricular mapping.[41,42] Those observations set the parameters for later studies of electromechanically guided transendocardial injections of angiogenic growth factors, based on the presumption that reduced electrical activity indicated viable territories with reduced perfusion. Many studies have documented significant differences in the mean endocardial voltage amplitude between viable and infarcted myocardium.[43] Although some of these studies have suggested that bipolar measurements are superior,[44] unipolar voltage continues to be widely used. In our canine and swine models, the results have been similar to those of other

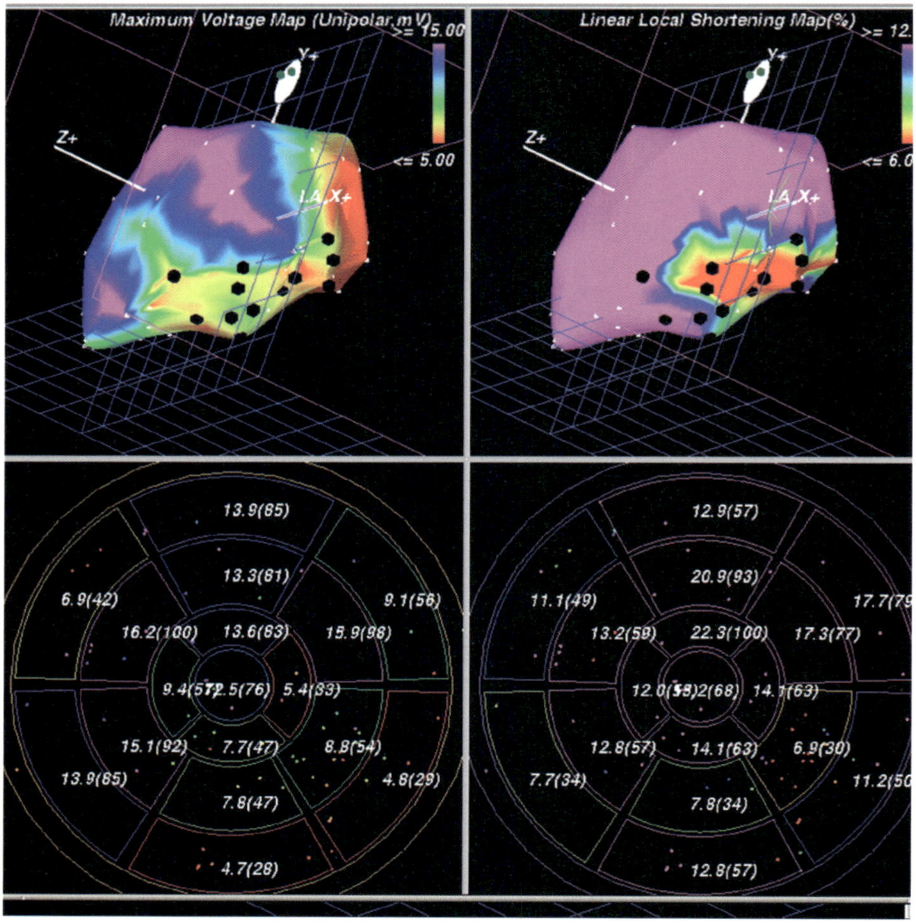

Figure 6.5 *Electromechanical map of a swine subjected to ameroid constrictor placement. The left panels depict the three-dimensional reconstruction of the unipolar voltage map (viability) and its correspondent polar map. The right panels depict the three-dimensional reconstruction of the linear local shortening map (LLS) (mechanical function) and its correspondent polar map. Abnormal values are represented in red and normal values in purple. The voltage map reveals a small area of inferior wall necrosis surrounded by a larger area of ischemia represented by the low LLS values in the right panels. The black dots represent the points that were injected.*

researchers, and confirm the rule that reduced local endocardial shortening or electrical voltage indicates alterations in perfusion or contractility.

Kornowski et al[37] described a left ventricular endocardial mapping study (involving unipolar voltage, bipolar voltage, and local endocardial shortening) in a canine model of acute occlusion. Electromechanical function was assessed in infarcted versus healthy myocardial regions at baseline and at 24 hours and 3 weeks after left LAD occlusion in both ischemic and nonischemic animals.[37] A significant reduction in voltage potentials was noticed in the myocardial infarction zone versus remote zones. Compared with control subjects, canine models had significantly impaired linear local shortening in infarcted zones. In our experience with chronic swine and canine models, we also have concluded that it is possible to differentiate ischemic from nonischemic tissue. In preclinical studies, catheter-based EMM provides real-time assessment of myocardial function in the animal laboratory, where other methods are seldom available for this purpose.

Conclusions

Each of the above-described animal models of myocardial ischemia has its own strengths and limitations. In cell therapy, reproducible results are directly related to the use of standardized preclinical animal models. At this point, given their anatomic similarity to humans, swine should be the preferred species utilized in stem cell research.

References

1. American Heart Association. Conference Proceedings. Atherosclerotic Vascular Disease Conference Writing Group I: Epidemiology. Circulation 2004; 109:2605–12.
2. Kawamoto A, Tkebuchava T, Yamagichi J, et al. Intramyocardial transplantation of autologous endothelial progenitor cells for therapeutic neovascularization of myocardial ischemia. Circulation 2003;107:461–8.
3. Fuchs S, Baffour R, Zhou YF, et al. Transendocardial delivery of autologous bone marrow enhances collateral perfusion and regional function in pigs with chronic myocardial ischemia. J Am Coll Cardiol 2001;37:1726–32.
4. Silva GV, Litowsky S, Assad JA, et al. Mesenchymal stem cells differentiate into an endothelial phenotype, enhance vascular density and improve heart function in a chronic myocardial ischemia model. Circulation 2005;111:150–6.
5. Yeh ETH, Zhang S, Wu HD, et al. Transdifferentiation of human peripheral blood CD34$^+$-enriched cell population into cardiomyocytes, endothelial cells, and smooth muscle cells in vivo. Circulation 2003;108:2070–3.
6. Kocher AA, Schuster MD, Szabolcs MJ, et al. Neovascularization of ischemic myocardium by human bone-marrow derived angioblasts prevents cardiomyocyte apoptosis, reduces remodeling and improves cardiac function. Nat Med 2001;7:430–6.
7. Orlic D, Kajstura J, Chimenti S, et al. Bone marrow cells regenerate infarcted myocardium. Nature 2001;410:701–5.
8. Verdouw PD, van den Doel MA, de Zeeuw S, Duncker DJ. Animal models in the study of myocardial ischaemia and ischaemic syndromes. Cardiovasc Res 1998;39:121–35.
9. Hughes GC, Post MJ, Simons M, Annex BH. Translational physiology: porcine models of human coronary artery disease: implications for clinical trials of therapeutic angiogenesis. J Appl Physiol 2003;94:1689–701.
10. Hearse DJ. The elusive coypu: the importance of collateral flow and the search for an alternative to the dog. Cardiovasc Res 2000;45:215–19.
11. White FC, Roth DM, Bloor CM. The pig as a model for myocardial ischemia and exercise. Lab Anim Science 1986;36:351–6.
12. Schaper W, Jageneau A, Xhonneux R. The development of collateral circulation in the pig and dog heart. Cardiologia 1967;51:321–55.
13. Ulloa HM, Houston BJ, Altrogge DM. Arrhythmia prevalence during ambulatory electrocardiographic monitoring of beagles. Am J Vet Res 1995; 56:275–81.
14. Hughes HC. Swine in cardiovascular research. Lab Anim Sci 1986;36:348–50.
15. Hastings AB, White FC, Sanders TM, Bloor CM. Comparative physiological responses to exercise stress. J Appl Physiol 1982;52:1077–83.
16. Li J, Brown LF, Hibberd MG, et al. VEGF, flk-1, and flt-1 expression in a rat myocardial model of angiogenesis. Am J Physiol 1996;270:H1803–11.
17. Mohri M, Schaper W. Angiogenesis in porcine hearts with coronary microembolization. In: Schaper J (ed). Collateral Circulation. Boston: Kluwer,1993:103–21.
18. Chilian WM, Mass HJ, Williams SE, Layne SM, Smith ES, Scheel KW. Microvascular occlusions promote coronary collateral growth. Am J Physiol 1990;258:H1103–11.
19. Zimmermann R, Arras M, Ullmann C, et al. Time course of mitosis and collateral growth following coronary microembolization in the porcine heart. Cell Tissue Res 1997;287:583–90.
20. Uchida Y, Yanigisawa-Miwa A, Nakamura F, et al. Angiogenic therapy of acute myocardial infarction by intrapericardial injection of basic fibroblast growth factor and heparin sulfate: an experimental study. Am Heart J 1995;130:1182–8.
21. Yanagisawa-Miwa A, Uchida Y, Tomaru T, et al. Salvage of infarcted myocardium by angiogenic action of basic fibroblast growth factor. Science 1992;257:1401–3.
22. Huwer H, Winning J, Vollmar B, et al. Microvascularization and ventricular function after local alginate-encapsulated angiogenic growth factor treatment in a rat cryothermia-induced myocardial infarction model. Microvasc Res 2001; 62:211–14.
23. Huwer H, Risslar J, Vollmar B, et al. Angiogenesis and microvascularization after cryothermia-induced myocardial infarction: a quantitative fluorescence microscopic study in rats. Basic Res Cardiol 1999;94:85–93.

24. Litvak J, Siderides LE, Vineberg A. The experimental production of coronary artery insufficiency and occlusion. Am Heart J 1957;53:505–18.
25. Elzinga WE. Ameroid constrictor: uniform closure rates and calibration procedure. J Appl Physiol 1969;27:419–21.
26. Vineberg A, Mahanti B, Litvak J. Experimental gradual coronary artery constriction by ameroid constrictors. Surgery 1960;47:765–71.
27. Unger EF. Experimental evaluation of coronary collateral development. Cardiovasc Res 2001;49: 497–506.
28. Schaper W. Development and role of coronary collaterals. Trends Cardiovasc Med 1991;1:256–61.
29. Thomas ED. Does bone marrow transplantation confer a normal life span? N Engl J Med 1999;341: 50–1.
30. Marmont AM. Immune ablation followed by allogeneic or autologous bone marrow transplantation: a new treatment for severe autoimmune diseases? Stem Cells 1994;12:125–35.
31. Ikehara S. Bone marrow transplantation for autoimmune diseases. Acta Haematol 1998;99: 116–32.
32. Matsuda KM, Kume A, Ueda Y, et al. Development of a modified selective amplifier gene for hematopoietic stem cell gene therapy. Gene Ther 1999; 6:1038–44.
33. Sachs DH. Mixed chimerism as an approach to transplantation tolerance. Clin Immunol 2000;95: S63–8.
34. Chatzipetrou MA, Mathew JM, Kenyon NS, et al. Analysis of post-transplant immune status in recipients of liver/bone marrow allografts. Hum Immunol 1999;60:1281–8.
35. Thomas JM, Verbanac KM, Smith JP, et al. The facilitating effect of one-DR antigen sharing in renal allograft tolerance induced by donor bone marrow in rhesus monkeys. Transplantation 1995;59:245–55.
36. Kornowski R, Leon MB, Fuchs S, et al. Electromagnetic guidance for catheter-based transendocardial injection: a platform for intramyocardial angiogenesis therapy results in normal and ischemic porcine models. J Am Coll Cardiol 2000; 35:1031–9.
37. Kornowski R, Hong MK, Gepstein L, et al. Preliminary animal and clinical experiences using an electromechanical endocardial mapping procedure to distinguish infarcted from healthy myocardium. Circulation 1998;98:1116–24.
38. Gepstein L, Golden A, Lessick J, et al. Electromechanical characterization of chronic myocardial infarction in the canine coronary occlusion model. Circulation 1998;98:2055–64.
39. Fuchs S, Kornowski R. Correlation between endocardial voltage mapping and myocardial perfusion: implications for the assessment of myocardial ischemia. Coron Artery Dis 2005;16: 163–7.
40. Sarmento-Leite R, Silva GV, Vaughn WK, Gottschall CAM, Perin EC. Predicting LV ejection fraction from electromechanical mapping: correlation with angiographic parameters. Am J Cardiol 2000;86(Suppl 8A):108i (Abst TCT-283).
41. Perin EC, Silva GV, Sarmento-Leite R, et al. Assessing myocardial viability and infarct transmurality with left ventricular electromechanical mapping in patients with stable coronary artery disease: validation by delayed-enhancement magnetic resonance imaging. Circulation 2002;106: 957–61.
42. Fuchs S, Hendel RC, Baim DS, et al. Comparison of endocardial electromechanical mapping with radionuclide perfusion imaging to assess myocardial viability and severity of myocardial ischemia in angina pectoris. Am J Cardiol 2001; 87:874–80.
43. Fallavollita JA, Valeti U, Oza S, Canty JM Jr. Spatial heterogeneity of endocardial voltage amplitude in viable, chronically dysfunctional myocardium. Basic Res Cardiol 2004;99:212–22.
44. Champagne S, Su JB, Unterseeh T, Elamine S, et al. Electromechanical mapping of myocardial ischemia in coronary occlusion in the pig. Arch Mal Coeur Vaiss 2003;96:332–8.

chapter 7

The Basics of Pathologic Assessment in Experimental Models of Stem Cell Therapy

Deborah Vela, L Maximilian Buja, and Silvio Litovsky

Introduction

Pathologic assessment plays a crucial role in cardiac stem cell therapy research both in vitro and in vivo. It allows researchers to quantify and evaluate the safety and effectiveness of stem cell transplantation in cardiac tissues. In this chapter, which is intended mainly for the clinician and clinical scientist, we will review the more commonly used tools of pathology as they apply to stem cell therapy research, including myocardial injury models, experimental stem cell types, and techniques for pathologic assessment of tissues that have undergone stem cell transplantation.

Animal Models

Much current knowledge of stem cells and their therapeutic potential has been acquired through in vitro studies. In vivo models were developed to gain insight into *how*, and even *if*, transplanted stem cells would indeed engraft and transdifferentiate into a specific cell type in a specific organ and in a certain environment.

Whole-animal experimentation in the field of cardiac stem cell therapy has involved small (mouse and rat) and large (dog, pig, and sheep) animal models. Smaller models – particularly the mouse – offer the advantage of a great variety of backgrounds and transgenic species (e.g., severe combined immunodeficiency, nude, and green fluorescent protein mice). The large animals allow injury models and delivery routes that more closely simulate actual clinical settings (e.g., chronic ischemic injury and intracoronary and transendocardial delivery). It is important to note, however, that the coronary arteries of dogs, unlike those of humans or pigs, are not terminal arteries; instead, they provide a rich collateral circulation. This should be kept in mind when selecting and assessing myocardial ischemia models.

Myocardial Injury Models

Although a few of the earlier cell engraftment experiments were carried out in normal hearts, models designed to replicate myocardial injury – particularly ischemic injury – are now widely used. These studies have given rise to the concept that the microenvironment can induce the transdifferentiation of engrafted cells.

Cryoinjury

Cryoinjury, also known as freeze–thaw injury, is used mostly in small animal models.[1,2] A

Table 7.1 Phenotypic characteristics of stem cell types used for stem cell therapy

Cell type	*Positive for*	*Negative for*
Embryonic	Oct-4, SSEA-1, SSEA-3, SSEA-4, TRA-1-60, TRA-1-80, Nanog, alkaline phosphatase, telomerase[78–80]	—
Adult		
Skeletal myoblasts	Sarcomeric myosin, desmin, myogenin, myoD, MRF4, c-Met[1,24]	—
Bone marrow stem cells:		
Hematopoietic stem cells	c-Kit, Sca-1, CD45[25,26,81]	Lin
Endothelial progenitor cells	VEGFR-2, CD34, CD133 (AC133)[82,83]	—
Mesenchymal stem cells	SH2, SH3, SH4, Stro-1, CD44, CD90 (Thy1)[32,84,86]	Lin, CD34, CD45
Cardiac stem cells	c-Kit, GATA-4, MEF2C, Csx/Nkx 2.5[42]	Lin, CD34, CD45

metallic rod is first cooled (usually with liquid nitrogen) and then placed directly on the anterior surface of the heart (i.e., the left ventricle, LV) for several seconds. The resulting lesion is typically a disk-shaped region of coagulation necrosis that extends into the myocardium but is not transmural.

Acute ischemia

This form of injury is intended to closely replicate an acute myocardial infarction. Coronary artery occlusion (e.g., ligation) is performed on one of the main coronary vessels [usually the left anterior descending (LAD), although the left circumflex is sometimes used in pigs]. When using canine models, ligation of collaterals is sometimes performed as well.

Chronic ischemia

This model applies mainly to large animals and usually involves the placement of an ameroid constrictor around one coronary artery. An ameroid constrictor consists of an inner ring of casein, a milk protein, surrounded by a stainless steel sheath. Casein is a hygroscopic substance that gradually swells as it slowly absorbs body fluid. The stainless steel sheath forces the casein to swell inward, eventually closing the ring and obliterating the vessel it is placed upon. Ameroid constrictors gradually close over 4–5 weeks. The time to occlusion of the vessel depends on the size of the vessel and constrictor and the rigidity of the outer ring. Closure is most rapid during the first 3–14 days after implantation; the rate of closure declines thereafter.

Stem Cell Types Used in Cardiovascular Research

The search for the ideal stem cell type to use in restoring damaged cardiac tissue has involved a variety of stem and progenitor cells. A detailed description of each is beyond the scope of this chapter. Nevertheless, a few highlights about each type are briefly mentioned below, and their main phenotypic markers are listed in Table 7.1.

Embryonic and fetal stem cells

Embryonic stem cells (ESCs) are derived from the inner cell mass of the blastocyst. Of all stem cell types, they have the greatest potential to become cardiomyocytes.[3] Host paracrine signaling supports cardiac-specific differentiation in the cardiac environment. Ethical and political considerations, however, make it unlikely that ESCs will be used in the near future in humans. A number of studies have shown the potential of ESCs for cardiac regeneration in experimental animals.[4–8] Fetal and neonatal cardiomyocytes have been successfully used since the mid 1990s.[9–12]

Adult stem cells

Skeletal myoblasts

Skeletal myoblasts (also known as satellite cells)[1,13–17] and bone marrow-derived cells are the only stem cell types presently available for clinical use in the USA. Several small clinical studies of myoblast transplantation in patients with heart disease have been published.[18–21] Myoblasts are the only progenitor cells in the human body that normally develop a contractile apparatus, which makes them an attractive candidate to restore contractile function in the heart. They are also relatively resistant to ischemia. Myofibers are essentially fast-twitch skeletal muscle, but after transplantation and as wound healing progresses, some of them develop a slow-twitch phenotype similar to that of cardiac muscle. Isolation and expansion of myoblasts is relatively easy, and after 2–3 weeks of cell culture, they can be transplanted in large numbers.[22] It should be remembered that markers evolve over time after skeletal myoblast transplantation.[23] However, despite these beneficial features, skeletal myoblasts do not achieve electromechanical coupling with cardiac myocytes in vivo.[24]

Bone marrow stem cells

The potential ability of *hematopoietic stem cells* (HSCs) to transdifferentiate into a wide variety of phenotypes, including cardiomyocytes, is a matter of intense debate. While some groups[25] have reported prominent regeneration of infarcted myocardium, others have been unable to reproduce these findings,[26–28] despite using largely similar cell populations and protocols.

Endothelial progenitor cells (EPCs) have been shown to increase perfusion of ischemic organs.[29,30] The potential of EPCs to transdifferentiate into cardiac myocytes in vivo has not been reported. However, one isolated report noted the transdifferentiation of human EPCs into functionally active cardiomyocytes in vitro when cocultivated with rat cardiomyocytes.[31] Cell fusion was not seen between the cell types.

Mesenchymal stem cells (MSCs), also called *marrow stromal cells*, are actually adult mesenchymal progenitor cells that can potentially give rise to a variety of mesenchymal cell types (e.g., fibroblasts, muscle, bone, and adipose tissue).[32] They are being actively investigated at present as a source of stem cells in the cardiology field.[33–40] The results reported so far have been generally supportive of the potential of these stem cells. Increased vascularity appears to be a prominent finding in most studies and is probably a significant reason for the reported beneficial effect. Differentiation into cardiomyocytes has also been reported, but the relative importance of this factor to the overall physiologic effect remains unclear. The isolation and preparation of these cells appears to be straightforward.[37,38]

Cardiac stem cells

There is evidence that certain primitive cardiac myocytes are capable of dividing in the normal and pathologic human heart.[41] Like MSCs, these cells are $CD34^-$ and $CD45^-$. Beltrami et al[42] have shown that these cells support regeneration after myocardial infarction in the rat. Why these cells fail to regenerate the human myocardium after injuries such as a myocardial infarction is unknown. Research is focused on ways to boost the magnitude of the regenerative response of these endogenous cardiac stem cells.

Preparation and Labeling

The cell type selected for stem cell therapy must be appropriately harvested, isolated, and expanded before it can be labeled. Cell preparation procedures may involve the use of transdifferentiation enhancers, such as 5-azacytidine[2,43,44] or oxytocin (considered by some to be a stronger inducer of cardiac differentiation than 5-azacytidine).[45] Labeling procedures are of utmost importance to the experimental design because they allow the fate of implanted stem cells to be tracked and monitored in order to confirm or rule out cell engraftment and transdifferentiation. There are several particularly useful labeling procedures.

BrdU incorporation

The thymidine analogue 5-bromo-2′-deoxyuridine (BrdU) is used to identify cells undergoing DNA synthesis. Because newly synthesized DNA thymidine is partly replaced by BrdU, BrdU can serve as a proliferation marker. BrdU is added in high concentrations to the cell culture.[1,46]

Fluorescence labeling and dye marking

Vital fluorescent dyes are used to mark cells temporarily. These markers can be divided into nuclear and cytoplasmic dyes.

Nuclear dyes

A number of DNA-binding dyes can be used to highlight the nucleus. These include Hoechst 33342, Hoechst 33258, 4′,6-diamidino-2-phenylindole (DAPI), mithramycin, propidium iodide, 7-aminoactinomycin D, SYTOX green, DRAQ5, and TO-PRO-3 iodide. They share many properties but vary in their excitation points.

The most popular of these nuclear dyes is DAPI, an ultraviolet (UV)-excited fluorescent dye that has been used as a cell marker since the 1980s.[47] Its high affinity for double-stranded DNA makes it an excellent nuclear labeling dye. It forms strong electrostatic interactions with adenine–thymine-rich regions of DNA. The fluorescence quantum yield of the free dye is very low, but the binding to DNA results in a highly fluorescent complex. DAPI is nontoxic and does not alter the ultrastructure of organelles. Its labeling efficiency is almost 100%, leaving virtually no DAPI fluorescence in the culture medium when performing in vitro experiments. Although DAPI is generally considered a reliable cell marker,[48,49] false-negative results may potentially arise from DAPI dilution in proliferating cells, and false-positive results may arise if large numbers of marked cells die and DAPI is taken up by other cells.[50]

Cytoplasmic dyes

Fluorescent labels can be used to mark a variety of cytoplasmic structures and components, such as the cell membrane, organelles, and ions. The cell membrane marker 1,1′-dioctadecyl-3,3,3′,3′-tetramethylindocarbocyanine perchlorate (DiI) is one of the most popular. Cell membranes labeled with DiI emit an orange–red fluorescence. This is due to the insertion of the two long (C_{18}) hydrocarbon chains of DiI into lipid bilayers. The popularity of this cross-linkable membrane dye is mostly due to its photostability and low toxicity, which allow long-term cell tracking both in vitro and in vivo.[51]

Genetic markers

Genetic markers of donor stem cells can be classified as endogenous (occurring naturally within the cell) or exogenous (introduced into the cell). Both types of genetic markers can signal the presence of a donor cell, but neither type can identify the type of cell into which the donor cell has differentiated. Thus, secondary criteria, such as morphology and colocalization with specific markers, are needed to establish cell identity.[52]

In some instances, donor cells that express a nuclear marker gene under the control of a cell type-specific promoter are used to improve detection of cell differentiation.[4,8,27,53] With this method, donor cells will not express the marker until they differentiate into the cell type of interest. Although this generates less disputable data, it does not reliably identify distinct phenotypes.[52] Hence, determining donor cell localization still requires colocalization with other cardiomyocyte or vascular markers (Figure 7.1).

Endogenous markers

A useful endogenous marker is the Y chromosome. In situ hybridization with Y-chromosome-specific probes can be used to identify male cells after engraftment in female recipients.[46,54] Visualization of the Y chromosome on regular histologic sections is straightforward. However, its usefulness as a marker is limited because it requires bridging between genders and species and because its histocompatibility antigen can elicit immune reactions.[25]

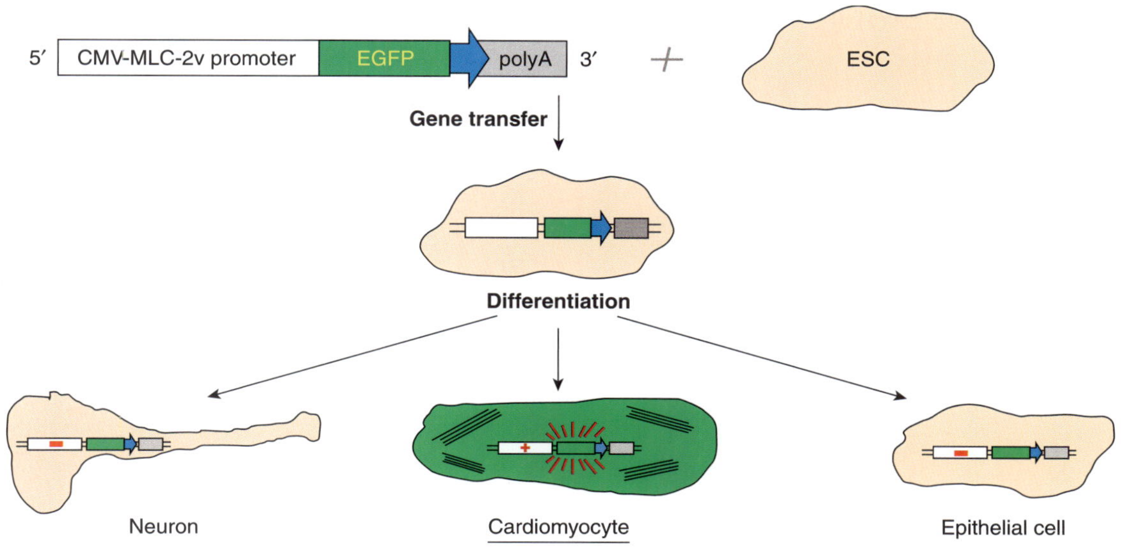

Figure 7.1 *Strategy for in vitro selection of cardiomyocytes from differentiated embryonic stem cells (ESCs) via expression of enhanced green fluorescent protein (EGFP) under control of the myosin light chain 2 ventricular (MLC-2v) promoter. A cytomegalovirus (CMV) enhancer element is introduced 5′ to the promoter to increase fluorescence. Reproduced from Nir SG, et al. Cardiovasc Res 2003; 58: 313–23*[8] *with permission from the European Society of Cardiology.*

Exogenous markers

Transgene-based exogenous genetic markers are versatile and widely used. So-called "active" exogenous genetic markers are obtained by transgenic reporter gene expression and consist mainly of two types: enzymatic (i.e., *lacZ*) and fluorescent [i.e., green fluorescent protein (GFP) and enhanced GFP (EGFP)]. So-called "passive" markers, such as a known DNA sequence that is inserted into the genome and can be detected by in situ hybridization or Southern blot analysis, are rarely used in the field.

β-Galactosidase (the enzyme encoded by the *lacZ* gene of *Escherichia coli*) is widely used because its expression is considered to have a neutral effect on cell physiology. β-Galactosidase is detected even in formalin-fixed, paraffin-embedded tissue sections by binding with its substrate X-gal, which is readily visible by its blue color. Insertion of *lacZ* is accomplished in many cell lines by gene trap insertion of *lacZ* into the endogenous locus Rosa26.[52]

GFP, which was originally isolated from its native host, the bioluminescent jellyfish *Aequorea victoria,* has become over the last decade one of the most widely used cell-tracking tools. This calcium-activated photoprotein fluoresces bright green when exposed to UV light. GFP has a number of properties that make it extremely useful as a biomarker and reporter gene. It is extremely stable, and its fluorescent properties are unaffected by relatively prolonged treatment with many proteases (e.g., trypsin, chymotrypsin, and pancreatin).[55,56] It is stable across a broad range of pH values (5.5–12). GFP has no physiologic effect on cell function and does not require a substrate to fluoresce. Its genetic expression allows it to be used as a noninvasive, real-time, transiently or stably expressed bioreporter both in vitro and in vivo. Despite these qualities, GFP has several limitations, including low expression level, photosensitivity, weak fluorescence, insolubility, and instability at high temperatures (an important limitation in vertebrate models). Many of these limitations have been overcome by the creation of mutant forms such as EGFP, which is more thermostable and more fluorescent.

Methods of Delivery

Routes of delivery are discussed in detail in other chapters of this book. For the purpose of our review, it is sufficient to point out that the method of delivery can have a major effect on cell viability. The delivery methods most commonly used in in vivo experimental models are intravenous/systemic, transmyocardial (via direct surgical injection), intracoronary, and transendocardial (via NOGA-mediated injection) (see Chapter 11).

Tools of Assessment

Planimetry and sonomicrometry

Planimetry, or the measurement of the area of a plane figure by measuring its boundary line, is used to quantify infarct size (see below).[57,58] Planimetry can be accomplished in several ways. Infarct boundaries can be traced on a sheet of paper, cut out, and measured by hand. They can also be traced and measured using analog planimeters, which provide moderately accurate results but require a fair amount of user skill. Most laboratories use a computer to digitally acquire and analyze tracings. Infarct tracings from dog or pig hearts can be digitized directly, but those from small animal hearts must be magnified. Because subjectivity can be an issue when recording tracings, a blinded investigator is recommended.

Sonomicrometry, or the ultrasonic measurement of an area or volume by piezoelectric crystals, is also used to quantify infarct size.[59,60] This approach has the advantage of allowing direct in vivo collection of both physiologic data (e.g., regional wall motion and segment shortening) and morphologic data (e.g., wall thickness and ventricular geometry and volume) from the heart in vivo. Crystal alignment (perpendicular to the LV circumference) is important for acquisition of accurate dimensional data.

Immunohistochemistry

This technique identifies cellular or tissue constituents (e.g., antigens) by means of antigen–antibody interactions. The site of antibody binding can be identified either by direct antibody labeling or, as is more often the case, by secondary antibody labeling that intensifies the interaction.

Light microscopy

Light microscopy involves examination of specimens under visible light. Limitations as to what can be seen are due less to magnification than they are to resolution, illumination, and contrast.

Transmission electron microscopy

Transmission electron microscopy (TEM) involves examination of specimens as an electron beam is passed through them. This reveals more information about the internal ultrastructure. The resolution of TEM is about 10 000 times greater than that of light microscopy. This allows resolution of structures as small as 3 nm. The greatest obstacle to examining biologic material by TEM is the nonphysiologic conditions to which specimens must be exposed. Specimens must be dried, fixed, and sliced into sections thin enough (50–100 nm) to allow electrons to pass through them; exposed to electron-opaque heavy metal salts (e.g., osmium) to allow visualization; and finally exposed to a high vacuum during examination.

Fluorescence and confocal microscopy

Both fluorescence and confocal microscopy are based on the physical principle that fluorescent molecules absorb light at one wavelength and emit it at another, longer wavelength. A fluorescence microscope is basically a conventional light microscope that uses a much more intense light to illuminate the sample. It is equipped with special "filter cubes," each of which allows light of a particular wavelength to reach the eyepiece.

In fluorescence microscopy, cells or tissues are stained with fluorescent dye molecules. Fixed cells are treated first with primary antibodies specific to proteins of interest and then with secondary antibodies conjugated with fluorescent dyes. The dyes differ in excitation and emission wavelength so that they can be excited independently and observed in separate fluorescent channels (Figure 7.2a,b). Colocalization is revealed by the overlapping of colors and is often demonstrated when images captured at different emission wavelengths are merged. In the most

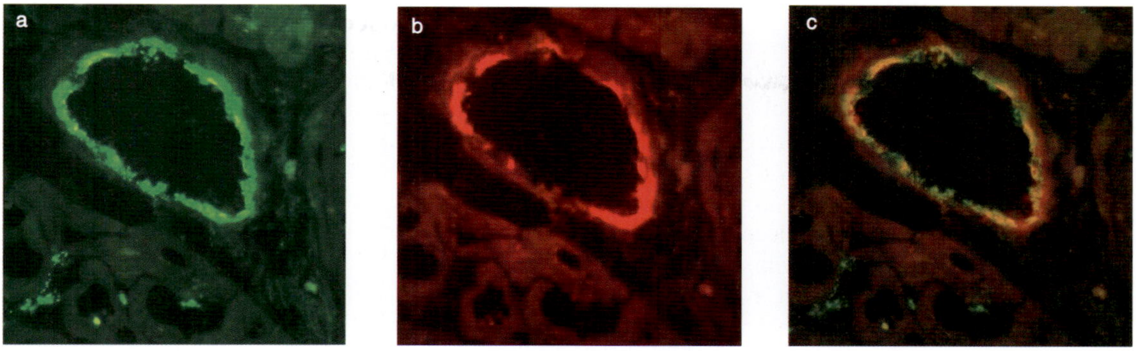

Figure 7.2 *(a) Fluorescein 5′-isothiocyanate (FITC) staining of factor VIII (green) in the endothelium of a canine myocardial vessel. (b) 1,1′-Dioctadecyl-3,3,3′,3′-tetramethylindocarbocyamine perchlorate (DiI) staining of mesenchymal stem cells (red). (c) Colocalization of FITC-stained endothelial cells and DiI-stained mesenchymal stem cells (yellow), indicating transformation of the stem cells into endothelial cells.*

common scenario, an antibody detected by a green emission colocalizes with an antibody detected by a red emission; when the emissions are merged, a yellow emission is seen (Figure 7.2c). Practically all investigators in the field of stem cell transplantation use this method to identify donor stem cell markers and antigens in mature cardiac myocytes and vascular structures.

The resolution of standard fluorescence microscopy can be compromised by fluorescence from outside the focal plane of interest, especially in tissues made up of multiple cell layers. In this regard, confocal microscopy (also referred to as confocal scanning laser microscopy) offers several advantages. Depth of field can be controlled, and discrete areas of tissue virtually free of out-of-focus fluorescence can be imaged. This reduces the chance of artifacts. Confocal microscopy also allows optical examination of serial sections from thick specimens.

Pathologic Assessment

Gross examination

Thorough pathologic examination of specimens from a heart that has received a stem cell transplant cannot be overemphasized. Although the major aim is to detect (or rule out) transdifferentiation of the stem cells into mature cardiac myocytes, capillaries, and larger vessels, meticulous gross examination can also provide invaluable information about the effect of the stem cell therapy.

Hearts of animals subjected to experimental interventions should be carefully weighed and compared with appropriate controls. In the context of acute ischemia models, higher experimental weights suggest remodeling, a serious complication of myocardial infarction. To obtain more information from the gross specimen, the heart must then be opened. This is usually done by cutting the heart transversely, from apex to base, into four or five slices ("breadloaf" technique). This allows for observation of the general geometry of the ventricle, classification of the infarct (e.g., transmural or subendocardial), detection of compensatory hypertrophy, measurement of LV wall thickness (thinning would suggest remodeling), and detection of aneurysms.

Freeze–thaw injury (cryoinjury) is a useful model in which to study myocardial repair.[1] Freeze–thaw injury and myocardial infarction both produce similar cellular patterns of coagulation necrosis, inflammation, phagocytosis, granulation tissue formation, and scarring. It should be noted, however, that infarcts and freeze–thaw lesions differ in important ways. Infarcts typically display irregular borders with viable peninsulas of subepicardial myocardium along penetrating vessels, whereas freeze–thaw lesions typically consist of areas of necrosis in the subepicardium confluent with viable myocardium in the subendocardium. Also, freeze–thaw lesions are not transmural and therefore are not usually associated with cardiac aneurysm formation.

Infarct size quantification

Quantification of infarct size is of paramount importance in the pathologic assessment of stem cell therapy, since a major goal of such therapy is to reduce the size of the myocardial infarct. In animal studies, infarct size is quantified by comparing tissue from treated and sham-treated animals. Tetrazolium staining has emerged as one of the most popular methods for early detection of myocardial infarction in a whole heart. This technique relies on the ability of dehydrogenase enzymes and cofactors in tissue to react with tetrazolium salts to form a pigment. Two forms of these salts are available: nitro blue tetrazolium, which does not cross cell membranes and therefore can only be used with sectioned tissue, and triphenyltetrazolium chloride (TTC), which does cross cell membranes and can be used both as a stain for sections and as a perfusate for the whole heart. Viable tissue should turn dark blue upon nitro blue tetrazolium staining and deep red upon TTC staining.

When a heart is subjected to regional ischemia, it becomes necessary to delineate the field of the occluded artery. This field is often referred to as the "risk zone" or "region at risk" of infarction. The risk zone is commonly marked by infusing a dye into the coronary tree while the coronary branch of interest is occluded. A number of dyes and particulate markers (e.g., radiolabeled microspheres that can be detected later radiographically, or fluorescent particles of zinc or cadmium sulfate) have been used. However, Evans blue dye is the most popular dye. An infarcted heart perfused with TTC and Evans blue dye and then sectioned would appear blue in the nonrisk zone, red in areas of the risk zone containing viable tissue, and white in areas of the risk zone containing necrotic tissue.[61]

When a heart has been subjected to global ischemia, the entire heart constitutes the risk zone. Stained sections are then either photographed or assessed by planimetry (see above).

It should be noted that TTC is toxic and causes tissues to contract. This may make accurate quantification of infarct size difficult, especially in smaller animal models. For example, in the rabbit, infarct size varies as a function of the size of the region at risk; however, no infarct occurs in risk areas of less than 0.3 cm^2. Thus, results of rabbit experiments in which the risk zone is smaller than 0.5 cm^2 are generally excluded.[62] On occasion, though, infarct size in small animal models has been measured by determining the number of lost cardiomyocytes.[63]

Gross quantification of infarct size is complemented by light-microscopic evaluation of collagen type I and III expression and healing. Trichrome staining is helpful for collagen evaluation because it differentiates areas of fibrosis from areas of residual necrosis. Satisfactory healing is important in the prevention of dyskinesia.

When evaluating infarct size and healing, it is also important to consider the type of injury (acute or chronic), duration of ischemia, timing and route of cell implantation, and length of survival.

Microscopic assessment

Cell characterization

Important cellular morphologic features (e.g., orientation in relation to host cells, size, and nuclear polymorphism[34,64]) can be discerned by standard hematoxylin–eosin (H&E) staining and light microscopy. These techniques can also be used to confirm the absence of nonmuscular and nonvascular cell types (e.g., chondrocytes, osteocytes, adipocytes, and fibroblasts), which is especially important when dealing with ESCs. Important ultrastructural details (e.g., the typical sarcomeric organization of myotubes, number of mitochondria, number of atrial granules, and presence of intercalated disks and gap junctions) that help typify a cell can be identified by TEM. However, TEM is infrequently used for this purpose because it is costly and because only very small tissue specimens can be studied.

For further characterization of engrafted cells, immunostaining is necessary. Immunohistochemistry plays a very important role in stem cell

Table 7.2 Mature cell markers

Skeletal muscle
α-Actinin, desmin, fast skeletal myosin heavy chain (MHC), myosin light chain (MLC), M-cadherin, titin, troponin T, troponin I, tropomyosin[1,24]

Cardiac muscle
α-Sarcomeric actin, α-actinin, α-MHC, β-MHC, atrial natriuretic peptide (ANP), cardiac titin, desmin, desmoplakin, lamin A/C, lamin B2, MLC-2a (atrial), MLC-2v (venticular), cardiac troponin T, cardiac troponin I, connexin 43, N-cadherin, phospholamban, tropomyosin[7,25,85]

Vascular
α-Smooth muscle actin (α-SMA), desmin, vimentin, Flk-1, CD31, intercellular adhesion molecule 2 (ICAM-2), VE-cadherin, vascular endothelial cell growth factor receptor 2 (VEGFR-2), von Willebrand factor (vWF), factor VIII, endothelial nitric oxide synthase (eNOS), E-selectin[31,82]

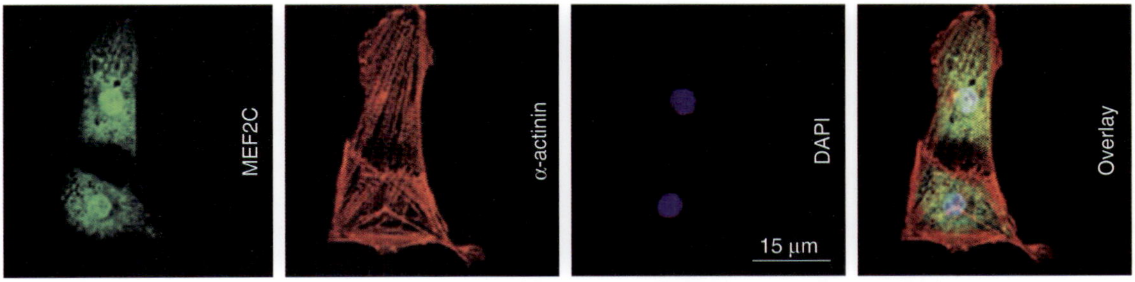

Figure 7.3 *Immunofluorescence demonstrating the expression of cardiac-specific markers in cardiomyocytes derived in vitro from a murine stem cell colony (GCR8). The transcription factor myosin enhancer factor 2C (MEF2C) appears green; the contractile protein a-actinin appears red. Stem cell nuclei stained with 4′,6-diamidino-2-phenylindole (DAPI) appear blue. The overlay image merges all three immunofluorescent stains. Reprinted from Hodgson DM et al. Am J Physiol Heart Circ Physiol 2004;287:H471–9[4] with permission from the American Physiological Society.*

therapy assessment. Each immunohistochemical marker mentioned above can be detected by labeling with a corresponding antibody. Structural proteins and unique phenotypic cellular components can be detected by the same means. Table 7.2 lists some common phenotypic markers of cell types found in the normal mature heart and skeletal muscle.

Other targets of immunostaining are proliferation and transcription factors. BrdU can be administered in vivo. Positive staining for BrdU confirms its uptake and demonstrates that active DNA synthesis (i.e., cell proliferation) has taken place. Ki-67 (also called MIB-1) is a nuclear antigen naturally expressed in proliferating cells but not quiescent ones. It is expressed in late G_1, S, G_2, and M phases but not in G_0. Transcription factors such as myocyte enhancer factor 2C (MEF2C), cardiac-specific GATA-4, and Csx/Nkx 2.5 can also be immunostained (Figure 7.3). The expression of all three of these factors is restricted to the initial phase of myocyte differentiation.

Fusion between donor stem cells and recipient mature differentiated cells is possible, but the effect of this phenomenon in vivo is still unclear.[65–69]

Angiogenesis and capillary density assessment

There is general consensus that most types of cell therapy increase myocardial vascularity.[70] Regardless of whether new blood vessels form de novo from precursor cells (vasculogenesis) or new capillaries sprout from preexisting vasculature (angiogenesis or neoangiogenesis), two important features of this new blood vessel growth (neovascularization) need to be determined: (a) the origin of its cellular components and (b) their density.

To determine origin, a tissue section from the area of interest (e.g., the infarct or peri-infarct area) can be immunostained to highlight *both* the label carried by the transplanted cells *and* a distinctive phenotypic marker (Table 7.2). Colocalization of these double stains will confirm an origin in transplanted stem cells. If the transplanted cells have previously been labeled with a fluorescent marker, then a fluorescent molecule (e.g., fluorescein 5′-isothiocyanate (FITC)) will be attached to the antibody that is highlighting the typical phenotype marker, and colocalization will yield a third color (e.g., green merged with red becomes yellow) (Figure 7.2).

Quantification of new vessels (referred to as capillary density assessment) can be done in many ways, although they all involve immunohistochemical staining of a chosen vascular component. Because most neovascularization occurs through angiogenesis, a preferred method of quantification involves the use of endothelial cell marker factor VIII. In this semiquantitative method, the results are usually expressed as number of vessels per high-power field (HPF). In reporting these results, the researcher should specify how the counting was done [e.g., magnification, inclusion criteria, and number of HPFs examined (usually 5)].

Depending on the experimental design, quantification of angiogenic factors [e.g., vascular endothelial cell growth factor (VEGF), fibroblast growth factor (FGF), and platelet-derived growth factor (PDGF)] by reverse transcriptase polymerase chain reaction (RT–PCR) may yield additional useful data.[67]

Combining tools and techniques

Using the tools and techniques described above, researchers have gained important insights into the processes of transdifferentiation, vasculogenesis, and neoangiogenesis that occur during stem cell therapy. Several examples are reviewed below.

Cultured ESCs are often transfected with GFP in order to track them after transplantation.[5] Some researchers have evaluated stem cells pathologically before transplanting them into recipient ischemic hearts in order to confirm that the stem cells have differentiated into electrically active cardiomyocytes (i.e., cells with action potentials similar to those of neonatal cardiomyocytes). This strategy was used by Kofidis and colleagues[71] in studies where insulin-like growth factor (IGF) was added to the ESC culture medium, and GFP^+ cells were shown to colocalize with the adult myocardial proteins connexin 43 and α-sarcomeric actin. It was also used by Min et al[5] in order to identify stem cells that had transdifferentiated into a mature cardiomyocyte phenotype.

The tools for immunohistochemical evaluation of cardiac stem cell therapy with ESCs or adult cells have also been used to evaluate cardiac therapy with fetal or neonatal cardiomyocyte xenografts. Li et al[12] studied the long-term survival of rat neonatal cardiomyocytes that had been transplanted into normal mouse hearts after first being treated with CTLA4-Ig to block the costimulatory pathway and with anti-CD40L monoclonal antibody to transiently block CD40. Immunohistochemical analysis confirmed the long-term survival of the xenografted cardiac myocytes and also identified a rare gap junction between the xenografts and native myocytes. This has raised interest in the possibility of xenografting animal fetal or neonatal cells into human hearts.

Immunofluorescence, PCR, and in situ hybridization have been used to evaluate pathologically the effectiveness of therapy with myoblast stem cells.[72,73] However, judicious selection of antibodies (Table 7.1) is mandatory for such examinations, since myoblast grafts gain some markers of cardiac differentiation but not others, and especially since fusion between skeletal and cardiac myocytes has been described.[72,73] The arrhythmogenic potential of skeletal myoblast grafts, possibly a result of the poor electrical connection with the surrounding myocardium, is a matter of concern.[74]

Use of transgenic mice in which a cardiac-specific protein drives expression of the β-galactosidase reporter[27,53] or a fluorescent marker[4] has been a major advance in the pathologic evaluation of stem cell therapy. Murry et al[27] used hematopoietic stem cells from a transgenic mouse line in which the cardiac-specific α-myosin heavy chain (α-MHC) drives expression of a β-galactosidase reporter, in order to monitor for differentiation into cardiomyocytes after injection into the peri-infarct area.[27] In that study, the lack of X-gal (blue) staining in the fixed heart strongly suggested that no stem cell differentiation had occurred. Agbulut et al[53] expanded on this technique to determine whether bone marrow cells from transgenic mice expressing *lacZ* under the control of either desmin or vimentin promoters differentiated respectively into muscle or mesenchymal cells. DiI-mediated red fluorescence colocalized focally with the green fluorescence of FITC-conjugated anti-vinculin antibodies, MHC, myosin binding protein C, and anti-caveolin 1a antibodies, rendering a yellow fluorescence. A mesenchymal cell phenotype was seen in the first week after transplantation; a muscular cell phenotype appeared 2 weeks after transplantation.

In addition, an ingenious protocol has been developed in which recipient hosts deficient in a donor-derived marker are used to detect donor-derived cells. Examples include the detection of dystrophin in *mdx*-recipient mice and δ-sarcoglycan in δ-sarcoglycan-null mice. Both conditions induce progressive cardiomyopathy and muscular dystrophy in humans and mice. The latter model was used by Lapidos et al,[75] who transplanted pluripotent bone marrow-derived cells from male mice into δ-sarcoglycan-null female mice. Despite successful engraftment, as demonstrated by fluorescent in situ hybridization (FISH) with a Y-chromosome-specific probe, no significant sarcoglycan positivity was seen in cardiomyocytes or skeletal myofibers, suggesting that expression of this key protein was lost during the engraftment process.

Lately, a large body of literature has focused on the use of mesenchymal bone marrow-derived stem cells. Wang et al[76] obtained mesenchymal progenitor cells from rats, labeled them with DAPI, and injected them into the myocardium of infarcted isogenic rats. Four weeks later, donor cells had the same histologic appearance as recipient myocytes and expressed sarcomeric MHC. Moreover, connexin 43 positivity demonstrated electrical connections with the surrounding myocardium. Davani et al[77] used a largely similar protocol. Thirty days after implantation, some engrafted (DAPI$^+$) cells expressed a smooth muscle or endothelial phenotype [α-smooth muscle actin (α-SMH) or CD31, respectively]. Increased vascular density was seen in treated animals as compared with controls.

Conclusions

Research has shown the potential of various types of stem cells to engraft in the injured heart. This chapter has provided a review of the use of pathology techniques to document the extent of myocardial damage and the evidence of stem cell engraftment and transdifferentiation. Application of these techniques is essential for any studies aimed at further characterizing the role of stem cells in myocardial regeneration.

References

1. Murry CE, Wiseman RW, Schwartz SM, Hauschka SD. Skeletal myoblast transplantation for repair of myocardial necrosis. J Clin Invest 1996;98:2512–23.
2. Tomita S, Li RK, Weisel RD, et al. Autologous transplantation of bone marrow cells improves damaged heart function. Circulation 1999;100:II247–56.
3. Mery A, Papadimou E, Zeineddine D, et al. Commitment of embryonic stem cells toward a cardiac lineage: molecular mechanisms and evidence for a promising therapeutic approach for heart failure. J Muscle Res Cell Motil 2003;24: 269–74.
4. Hodgson DM, Behfar A, Zingman LV, et al. Stable benefit of embryonic stem cell therapy in

myocardial infarction. Am J Physiol Heart Circ Physiol 2004;287:H471–9.
5. Min JY, Yang Y, Converso KL, et al. Transplantation of embryonic stem cells improves cardiac function in postinfarcted rats. J Appl Physiol 2002; 92:288–96.
6. Gepstein L. Derivation and potential applications of human embryonic stem cells. Circ Res 2002;91: 866–76.
7. Boheler KR, Czyz J, Tweedie D, Yang HT, Anisimov SV, Wobus AM. Differentiation of pluripotent embryonic stem cells into cardiomyocytes. Circ Res 2002;91:189–201.
8. Nir SG, David R, Zaruba M, Franz WM, Itskovitz-Eldor J. Human embryonic stem cells for cardiovascular repair. Cardiovasc Res 2003;58:313–23.
9. Soonpaa MH, Koh GY, Klug MG, Field LJ. Formation of nascent intercalated disks between grafted fetal cardiomyocytes and host myocardium. Science 1994;264:98–101.
10. Sakai T, Li RK, Weisel RD, et al. Fetal cell transplantation: a comparison of three cell types. J Thorac Cardiovasc Surg 1999;118:715–24.
11. Sakakibara Y, Tambara K, Lu F, et al. Combined procedure of surgical repair and cell transplantation for left ventricular aneurysm: an experimental study. Circulation 2002;106:I193–7.
12. Li TS, Ito H, Kajiwara K, Hamano K. Long-term survival of xenografted neonatal cardiomyocytes by adenovirus-mediated CTLA4-Ig expression and CD40 blockade. Circulation 2003;108:1760–5.
13. Chiu RC, Zibaitis A, Kao RL. Cellular cardiomyoplasty: myocardial regeneration with satellite cell implantation. Ann Thorac Surg 1995;60:12–18.
14. Yoon PD, Kao RL, Magovern GJ. Myocardial regeneration. Transplanting satellite cells into damaged myocardium. Tex Heart Inst J 1995;22:119–25.
15. Atkins BZ, Lewis CW, Kraus WE, Hutcheson KA, Glower DD, Taylor DA. Intracardiac transplantation of skeletal myoblasts yields two populations of striated cells in situ. Ann Thorac Surg 1999;67: 124–9.
16. Taylor DA, Atkins BZ, Hungspreugs P, et al. Regenerating functional myocardium: improved performance after skeletal myoblast transplantation. Nat Med 1998;4:929–33.
17. Reinecke H, MacDonald GH, Hauschka SD, Murry CE. Electromechanical coupling between skeletal and cardiac muscle. Implications for infarct repair. J Cell Biol 2000;149:731–40.
18. Ince H, Petzsch M, Rehders TC, Chatterjee T, Nienaber CA. Transcatheter transplantation of autologous skeletal myoblasts in postinfarction patients with severe left ventricular dysfunction. J Endovasc Ther 2004;11:695–704.
19. Menasche P, Hagege AA, Vilquin JT, et al. Autologous skeletal myoblast transplantation for severe postinfarction left ventricular dysfunction. J Am Coll Cardiol 2003;41:1078–83.
20. Pagani FD, DerSimonian H, Zawadzka A, et al. Autologous skeletal myoblasts transplanted to ischemia-damaged myocardium in humans. Histological analysis of cell survival and differentiation. J Am Coll Cardiol 2003;41:879–88.
21. Hagege AA, Carrion C, Menasche P, et al. Viability and differentiation of autologous skeletal myoblast grafts in ischaemic cardiomyopathy. Lancet 2003; 361:491–2.
22. van den Bos EJ, Davis BH, Taylor DA. Transplantation of skeletal myoblasts for cardiac repair. J Heart Lung Transplant 2004;23:1217–27.
23. Robinson SW, Cho PW, Levitsky HI, et al. Arterial delivery of genetically labelled skeletal myoblasts to the murine heart: long-term survival and phenotypic modification of implanted myoblasts. Cell Transplant 1996;5:77–91.
24. Reinecke H, Poppa V, Murry CE. Skeletal muscle stem cells do not transdifferentiate into cardiomyocytes after cardiac grafting. J Mol Cell Cardiol 2002;34:241–9.
25. Orlic D, Kajstura J, Chimenti S, et al. Bone marrow cells regenerate infarcted myocardium. Nature 2001;410:701–5.
26. Balsam LB, Wagers AJ, Christensen JL, Kofidis T, Weissman IL, Robbins RC. Haematopoietic stem cells adopt mature haematopoietic fates in ischaemic myocardium. Nature 2004;428:668–73.
27. Murry CE, Soonpaa MH, Reinecke H, et al. Haematopoietic stem cells do not transdifferentiate into cardiac myocytes in myocardial infarcts. Nature 2004;428:664–8.
28. Nygren JM, Jovinge S, Breitbach M, et al. Bone marrow-derived hematopoietic cells generate cardiomyocytes at a low frequency through cell fusion, but not transdifferentiation. Nat Med 2004;10:494–501.
29. Kawamoto A, Gwon HC, Iwaguro H, et al. Therapeutic potential of ex vivo expanded endothelial progenitor cells for myocardial ischemia. Circulation 2001;103:634–7.
30. Asahara T, Masuda H, Takahashi T, et al. Bone marrow origin of endothelial progenitor cells responsible for postnatal vasculogenesis in physiological and pathological neovascularization. Circ Res 1999;85:221–8.
31. Badorff C, Brandes RP, Popp R, et al. Transdifferentiation of blood-derived human adult endothelial progenitor cells into functionally active cardiomyocytes. Circulation 2003;107:1024–32.
32. Dennis JE, Caplan AI. Bone marrow mesenchymal stem cells. In: Sell S (ed). Stem Cells Handbook. Totowa, NJ: Humana Press, 2004:107–17.
33. Silva GV, Litovsky S, Assad JA, et al. Mesenchymal stem cells differentiate into an endothelial

phenotype, enhance vascular density, and improve heart function in a canine chronic ischemia model. Circulation 2005;111:150–6.
34. Hattan N, Kawaguchi H, Ando K, et al. Purified cardiomyocytes from bone marrow mesenchymal stem cells produce stable intracardiac grafts in mice. Cardiovasc Res 2005;65:334–44.
35. Shim WS, Jiang S, Wong P, et al. Ex vivo differentiation of human adult bone marrow stem cells into cardiomyocyte-like cells. Biochem Biophys Res Commun 2004;324:481–8.
36. Wang JA, Li CL, Fan YQ, He H, Sun Y. Allograftic bone marrow-derived mesenchymal stem cells transplanted into heart infarcted model of rabbit to renovate infarcted heart. J Zhejiang Univ Sci 2004;5:1279–85.
37. Alhadlaq A, Mao JJ. Mesenchymal stem cells: isolation and therapeutics. Stem Cells Dev 2004; 13:436–48.
38. Pittenger MF, Martin BJ. Mesenchymal stem cells and their potential as cardiac therapeutics. Circ Res 2004;95:9–20.
39. Airey JA, Almeida-Porada G, Colletti EJ, et al. Human mesenchymal stem cells form Purkinje fibers in fetal sheep heart. Circulation 2004;109: 1401–7.
40. Vulliet PR, Greeley M, Halloran SM, MacDonald KA, Kittleson MD. Intra-coronary arterial injection of mesenchymal stromal cells and microinfarction in dogs. Lancet 2004;363:783–4.
41. Beltrami AP, Urbanek K, Kajstura J, et al. Evidence that human cardiac myocytes divide after myocardial infarction. N Engl J Med 2001;344: 1750–7.
42. Beltrami AP, Barlucchi L, Torella D, et al. Adult cardiac stem cells are multipotent and support myocardial regeneration. Cell 2003;114:763–76.
43. Makino S, Fukuda K, Miyoshi S, et al. Cardiomyocytes can be generated from marrow stromal cells in vitro. J Clin Invest 1999;103:697–705.
44. Oh H, Bradfute SB, Gallardo TD, et al. Cardiac progenitor cells from adult myocardium: homing, differentiation, and fusion after infarction. Proc Natl Acad Sci USA 2003;100:12313–18.
45. Matsuura K, Nagai T, Nishigaki N, et al. Adult cardiac Sca-1-positive cells differentiate into beating cardiomyocytes. J Biol Chem 2004;279:11384–91.
46. Orlic D, Kajstura J, Chimenti S, Bodine DM, Leri A, Anversa P. Transplanted adult bone marrow cells repair myocardial infarcts in mice. Ann NY Acad Sci 2001;938:221–9; discussion 229–30.
47. Kapuscinski J. DAPI: a DNA-specific fluorescent probe. Biotech Histochem 1995;70:220–33.
48. Chedrawy EG, Wang JS, Nguyen DM, Shum-Tim D, Chiu RC. Incorporation and integration of implanted myogenic and stem cells into native myocardial fibers: anatomic basis for functional improvements. J Thorac Cardiovasc Surg 2002; 124:584–90.
49. Thompson RB, Parsa CJ, van den Bos EJ, et al. Video-assisted thoracoscopic transplantation of myoblasts into the heart. Ann Thorac Surg 2004; 78:303–7.
50. Borenstein N, Hekmati M, Bruneval P, Montarras D. Unambiguous identification of implanted cells after cellular cardiomyoplasty: a critical issue. Circulation 2004;109:e209–10; author reply e209–10.
51. Yoon YS, Park JS, Tkebuchava T, Luedeman C, Losordo DW. Unexpected severe calcification after transplantation of bone marrow cells in acute myocardial infarction. Circulation 2004;109: 3154–7.
52. Jackson KA, Majka SM, Wang H, et al. Regeneration of ischemic cardiac muscle and vascular endothelium by adult stem cells. J Clin Invest 2001;107: 1395–402.
53. Agbulut O, Menot ML, Li Z, et al. Temporal patterns of bone marrow cell differentiation following transplantation in doxorubicin-induced cardiomyopathy. Cardiovasc Res 2003;58:451–9.
54. Deten A, Volz HC, Clamors S, et al. Hematopoietic stem cells do not repair the infarcted mouse heart. Cardiovasc Res 2005;65:52–63.
55. Tsien RY. The green fluorescent protein. Annu Rev Biochem 1998;67:509–44.
56. Chiang CF, Okou DT, Griffin TB, Verret CR, Williams MN. Green fluorescent protein rendered susceptible to proteolysis: positions for protease-sensitive insertions. Arch Biochem Biophys 2001;394:229–35.
57. Palojoki E, Saraste A, Eriksson A, et al. Cardiomyocyte apoptosis and ventricular remodeling after myocardial infarction in rats. Am J Physiol Heart Circ Physiol 2001;280:H2726–31.
58. Kanno S, Lerner DL, Schuessler RB, et al. Echocardiographic evaluation of ventricular remodeling in a mouse model of myocardial infarction. J Am Soc Echocardiogr 2002;15:601–9.
59. Sebbag L, Verbinski SG, Reimer KA, Jennings RB. Protection of ischemic myocardium in dogs using intracoronary 2,3-butanedione monoxime (BDM). J Mol Cell Cardiol 2003;35:165–76.
60. Thompson RB, van den Bos EJ, Davis BH, et al. Intracardiac transplantation of a mixed population of bone marrow cells improves both regional systolic contractility and diastolic relaxation. J Heart Lung Transplant 2005;24:205–14.
61. Freeman I, Grunwald AM, Robin B, Rao PS, Bodenheimer MM. Effect of early reperfusion on use of triphenyltetrazolium chloride to differentiate viable from non-viable myocardium in area of risk. Cardiovasc Res 1990;24:109–14.
62. Ytrehus K, Liu Y, Tsuchida A, et al. Rat and rabbit heart infarction: effects of anesthesia, perfusate,

risk zone, and method of infarct sizing. Am J Physiol 1994;267:H2383–90.

63. Orlic D, Kajstura J, Chimenti S, et al. Mobilized bone marrow cells repair the infarcted heart, improving function and survival. Proc Natl Acad Sci USA 2001;98:10344–9.
64. Lanza R, Moore MA, Wakayama T, et al. Regeneration of the infarcted heart with stem cells derived by nuclear transplantation. Circ Res 2004;94:820–7.
65. Terada N, Hamazaki T, Oka M, et al. Bone marrow cells adopt the phenotype of other cells by spontaneous cell fusion. Nature 2002;416:542–5.
66. Alvarez-Dolado M, Pardal R, Garcia-Verdugo JM, et al. Fusion of bone-marrow-derived cells with Purkinje neurons, cardiomyocytes and hepatocytes. Nature 2003;425:968–73.
67. Liu Y, Guo J, Zhang P, et al. Bone marrow mononuclear cell transplantation into heart elevates the expression of angiogenic factors. Microvasc Res 2004;68:156–60.
68. Camargo FD, Chambers SM, Goodell MA. Stem cell plasticity: from transdifferentiation to macrophage fusion. Cell Prolif 2004;37:55–65.
69. Shi D, Reinecke H, Murry CE, Torok-Storb B. Myogenic fusion of human bone marrow stromal cells, but not hematopoietic cells. Blood 2004;104:290–4.
70. Kocher AA, Schuster MD, Szabolcs MJ, et al. Neovascularization of ischemic myocardium by human bone-marrow-derived angioblasts prevents cardiomyocyte apoptosis, reduces remodeling and improves cardiac function. Nat Med 2001;7: 430–6.
71. Kofidis T, de Bruin JL, Yamane T, et al. Insulin-like growth factor promotes engraftment, differentiation, and functional improvement after transfer of embryonic stem cells for myocardial restoration. Stem Cells 2004;22:1239–45.
72. Reinecke H, Minami E, Poppa V, Murry CE. Evidence for fusion between cardiac and skeletal muscle cells. Circ Res 2004;94:e56–60.
73. Agbulut O, Vandervelde S, Al Attar N, et al. Comparison of human skeletal myoblasts and bone marrow-derived CD133+ progenitors for the repair of infarcted myocardium. J Am Coll Cardiol 2004;44:458–63.
74. Siminiak T, Kalawski R, Fiszer D, et al. Autologous skeletal myoblast transplantation for the treatment of postinfarction myocardial injury: phase I clinical study with 12 months of follow-up. Am Heart J 2004;148:531–7.
75. Lapidos KA, Chen YE, Earley JU, et al. Transplanted hematopoietic stem cells demonstrate impaired sarcoglycan expression after engraftment into cardiac and skeletal muscle. J Clin Invest 2004;114:1577–85.
76. Wang JS, Shum-Tim D, Galipeau J, et al. Marrow stromal cells for cellular cardiomyoplasty: feasibility and potential clinical advantages. J Thorac Cardiovasc Surg 2000;120:999–1005.
77. Davani S, Marandin A, Mersin N, et al. Mesenchymal progenitor cells differentiate into an endothelial phenotype, enhance vascular density, and improve heart function in a rat cellular cardiomyoplasty model. Circulation 2003;108:II253–8.
78. Nichols J, Zevnik B, Anastassiadis K, et al. Formation of pluripotent stem cells in the mammalian embryo depends on the POU transcription factor Oct4. Cell 1998;95:379–91.
79. Thomson JA, Itskovitz-Eldor J, Shapiro SS, et al. Embryonic stem cell lines derived from human blastocysts. Science 1998;282:1145–7.
80. Mitsui K, Tokuzawa Y, Itoh H, et al. The homeoprotein Nanog is required for maintenance of pluripotency in mouse epiblast and ES cells. Cell 2003;113:631–42.
81. Goodell MA, Rosenzweig M, Kim H, et al. Dye efflux studies suggest that hematopoietic stem cells expressing low or undetectable levels of CD34 antigen exist in multiple species. Nat Med 1997;3:1337–45.
82. Hristov M, Erl W, Weber PC. Endothelial progenitor cells: mobilization, differentiation, and homing. Arterioscler Thromb Vasc Biol 2003;23: 1185–9.
83. Peichev M, Naiyer AJ, Pereira D, et al. Expression of VEGFR-2 and AC133 by circulating human CD34+ cells identifies a population of functional endothelial precursors. Blood 2000;95:952–8.
84. Pittenger MF, Mackay AM, Beck SC, et al. Multilineage potential of adult human mesenchymal stem cells. Science 1999;284:143–7.
85. Sachinidis A, Sauer H, Wartenberg M, Hescheler J. Transcription factors, growth factors, and signal cascades capable of priming cardiogenesis. In: Sell S (ed). Stem Cells Handbook. Totowa, NJ: Humana Press, 2004:239–49.
86. Jain M, Pfister O, Hajjar RJ, Liao R. Mesenchymal stem cells in the infarcted heart. Coron Artery Dis 2005;16:93–7.

PART 3

Clinical Utilization of Stem Cells in Cardiovascular Diseases

chapter 8

Cardiovascular Cell Therapy Overview: Realistic Targets in 2006

Doris A Taylor and Harald C Ott

Introduction

Cell transplantation is the first therapy designed to treat the underlying injury in heart failure[1]—cardiomyocyte and vessel cell death—and bring us closer to the ambitious goal of myocardial regeneration. The first 15 years of preclinical and early clinical research have left us with promising results, insights into using cells as a therapeutic tool, and an understanding of the complexity of cell-based repair and regeneration. Since 1998, when we first reported functional repair after injection of autologous skeletal myoblasts into the injured heart,[2] a variety of cell types have been proposed for transplantation in different stages of cardiovascular disease. The field has matured from an initial "out of the box" idea to one of the most active areas of cardiovascular research, yet many questions still remain. Now it is time to define realistic targets and to translate what we have learned.

Questions in the Field in 2006

As we move forward, several opportunities and hurdles remain. It is now obvious that cell-based cardiac and vascular repair is feasible, both early and later in the disease process. In fact, cell therapy may offer an unparalleled opportunity for improvement to millions of individuals living with cardiovascular disease. However, many questions about the technology remain. The mechanisms associated with cardiovascular repair remain unclear. Whether a best cell type, delivery method, or route of administration exists is unknown. Whether cell-based disease prevention is feasible is still unanswerable. And the potential for combined cell- and gene-based approaches remains largely unexplored.

Now is the time to delve deeply into these questions, even as we cautiously proceed clinically. Only by understanding the underlying mechanisms associated with repair will we be able to decrease unanticipated clinical effects, to choose the right cell for the right patient, and thus to potentially fulfill the promise of the most exciting opportunity yet to treat cardiovascular disease. As we do so, we must avoid uncontrolled, poorly planned studies, and until we understand the potential of cell therapy, we must limit "too good to be true" promises. Only by addressing unanswered questions, carefully limiting our promises, and rigorously performing preclinical and clinical studies can we provide the surest opportunity for safely moving the field forward.

The Goal: Regeneration vs Repair

Cardiac regeneration is our ultimate goal — literally regenerating contractile cardiac muscle, functional vasculature, and electrical conductance in a fibrous, dilated, and underperfused scar (Figure 8.1a). However, full regeneration is not currently possible and not likely to occur in the near future. Yet, in 2006, we face a growing population of patients, with limited options, who require that we formulate intermediate goals and develop

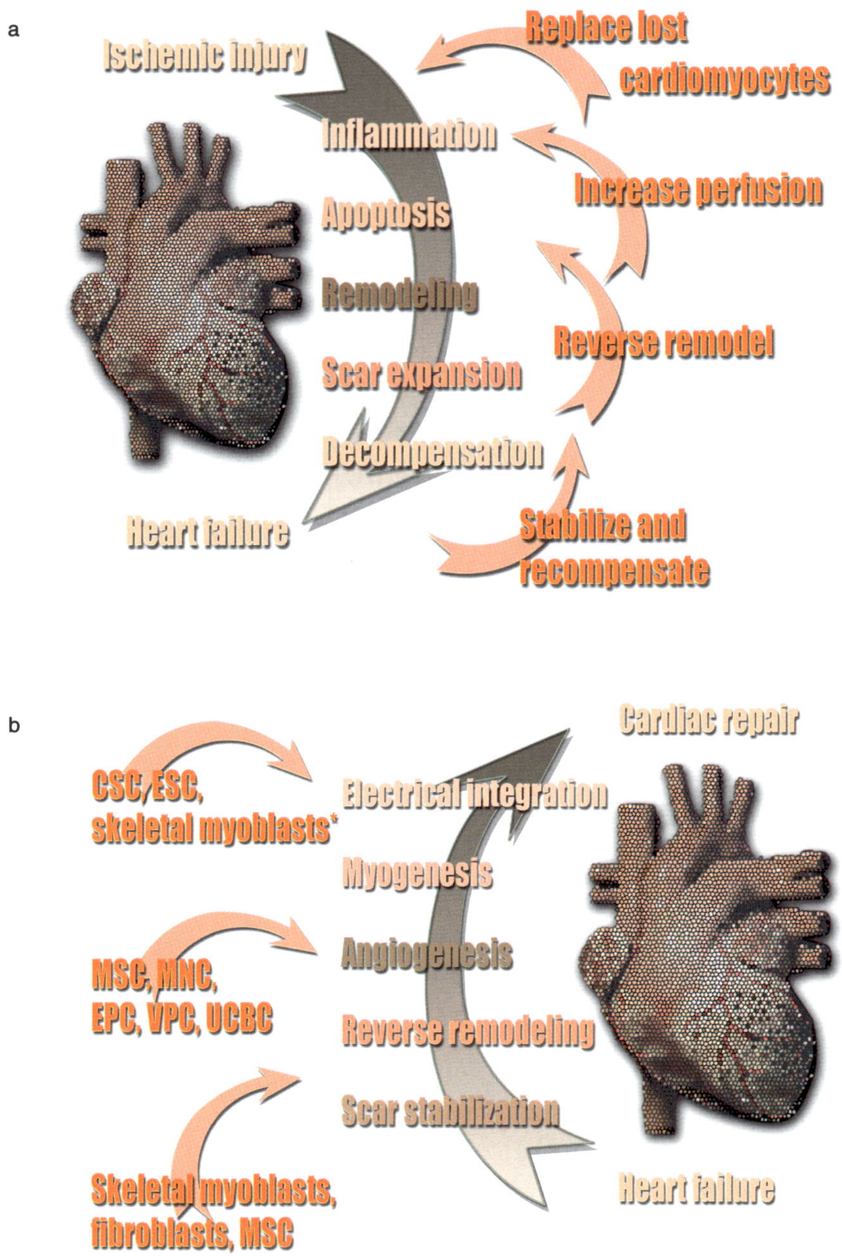

Figure 8.1 *(a) Targets for cell-based cardiac repair. We have to first, stabilize and recompensate the injured heart; second, reverse-remodel to improve left ventricular geometry; third, increase perfusion to allow, fourth, the replacement of lost cardiomyocytes. (b) Proposed mechanisms of currently tested cell therapies. Different mechanisms of function have been attributed to different tested cell types. Scar stabilization and reverse remodeling, angiogenesis, and ultimately myogenesis will all require certain cell properties. CSC, cardiac-derived stem cell; EPC, endothelial progenitor cell; ESC, embryonic stem cell; MNC, mononuclear cell; MSC, mesenchymal stem cell; UCBC, umbilical cord blood cell; VPC, vascular progenitor cell; *myogenesis.*

usable therapeutic tools. What *can* be truly claimed as a realistic goal of cell therapy is cardiac and vascular *repair—restoring mechanical function and perfusion to the dilated and decompensated heart* (Figure 8.1b), even in the absence of regeneration.

To date, the reported clinical studies (Table 8.1)[3] have focused on being "first in man" and thus primarily have served as feasibility attempts to promote this exciting field. Developing stepwise approaches to make critical decisions about trial design and patient treatment should be our current goal. This will necessarily involve developing criteria for several important choices that define each study: cell type, route of cell delivery, whether to use growth factors instead of (or in addition to) cells, whether cells can serve as vectors for genes, and which patient population should be included. The data now beginning to emerge should allow more informed decisions and should be considered as each new study is initiated.

Choosing a cell type: the implications

The most prevalent question in 2006 is the choice of cell type, which immediately forces us to acknowledge the heterogeneity of the patient populations facing cardiovascular disease. In addition, it requires that we acknowledge that cells have different inherent properties and likely different potential benefits and risks. Thus, the choice of cell type may ultimately depend greatly on the injury to be treated (Table 8.2) and on the routes of administration available.

Angiogenesis vs Myogenesis

In conditions where chronic ischemia prevails, or where reperfusion is the primary objective, the angiogenic potential of the cells may be of high priority. Under these conditions, bone marrow- or blood-derived mononuclear cells,[4] endothelial[5] or vascular[6] progenitor cells, marrow angioblasts,[7] or blood-derived multipotent adult progenitor cells[8] may be better choices than myogenic precursors. In patients where additional restoration of contractile function is the clinical goal—such as those with end-stage ischemic heart failure or those early post infarction, when blood flow has been restored but cardiocytes have died—delivering cells with contractile potential seems a more reasonable approach. Under these conditions, naturally myogenic cells (e.g., skeletal myoblasts, cardiocytes, or any progenitor cell driven down a muscle lineage) appear to be a better first choice. However, contractile potential is not the only consideration; the local cardiac milieu must also be considered. For example, in poorly perfused myocardium, transplanted cardiomyocytes perish,[9] whereas myoblasts and undifferentiated bone marrow cells appear to survive in higher numbers. Thus, cardiocytes are not an option unless coadministration of angiogenic cells or surgical and/or interventional revascularization is considered. To complete the assessment, in the decompensated, hypertrophied heart, cells that are able to stabilize scar would likely be of benefit.

Mesenchymal bone marrow cells, fibroblasts, and skeletal myoblasts (all mesoderm-derived progenitors) improve diastolic function and reduce wall stress,[10] whereas bone marrow mononuclear cells, peripheral blood or bone marrow endothelial progenitor cells, and umbilical cord blood cells have not demonstrated this potential to date. Thus, in attempts to *prevent* negative remodeling, any mesodermal progenitor could be considered, whereas once severe dilatation has occurred, only cell types capable of reverse remodeling (e.g., myoblasts) may be of ultimate benefit. These theoretical considerations are just that, however. Ultimate proof of any cell superiority will require side-by-side comparisons of cells in similar disease states.

Systole vs diastole

Initial preclinical comparisons of cells used to treat the ischemic failing heart (in rabbits) are summarized in Figure 8.2. Early comparisons of systolic parameters (regional stroke work) suggest that directly injected myoblasts offer the greatest positive improvement, followed by bone marrow stromal cells, and then by mononuclear cells—all of which are superior to fibroblast or sham treatment. Interestingly, in all cells evaluated, including fibroblasts, diastolic compliance improved several weeks prior to any improvement in systolic function (data not shown), but an improvement in compliance did not necessarily

Table 8.1 Cell therapy trials in patients with HF: comparison of clinical studies using myoblasts and bone marrow-derived cells for heart failure

Refs	*Cell type*[2]	*No. of patients treated*	Delivery[1]	LVEF (%)	Dose	Results
27	SKMB	10	Transepicardial, without CABG of treated region.	24±4	$8.7 \pm 1.9 \times 10^8$	Global LVEF increased.
42	SKMB	11	Transepicardial, with CABG of treated region.	36±8	$1.9 \pm 1.2 \times 10^8$	Global LVEF, regional wall motion, and viability increased.
43	SKMB	10	Transepicardial, with CABG of treated region.	25+40	$0.4–5.0 \times 10^7$	Global LVEF and regional wall motion increased.
30	SKMB	20	Transepicardial, without CABG of treated region.	28±3	$3.0 \pm 0.2 \times 10^8$	Global LVEF, regional wall motion, and viability increased.
21	SKMB	5	Transendocardial, guided by electromechanical mapping.	36±11	$2.0 \pm 1.1 \times 10^8$	Global LVEF and regional wall motion increased.
22	SKMB	9	Transcoronary-venous.	30–49	$17–106 \times 10^6$	Global LVEF improved in 6 of 9 cases.
4,15	CD133+	12	Transepicardial, without CABG of treated region.	36±11	$1–2.8 \times 10^6$	Global LVEF increased and LVEDV decreased.
5,44	CPC BMMNC	30 CPC 29 MNC	Intracoronary.	40±11	$1.7 \pm 0.8 \times 10^8$ $2.3 \pm 1.2 \times 10^7$	Global LVEF increased and LVEDV decreased in both cell-treated groups.
45	BMMNC	5	Transepicardial, during CABG.		$0.3–2.2 \times 10^9$	Perfusion increased in 3 of 5 patients.
16	BMMNC	8	Transendocardial, guided by electromechanical mapping.	58±11	40 ml BM	Regional wall motion and perfusion increased and angina reduced.
46	BM	10	Transendocardial, guided by electromechanical mapping.	47±10	$7.8 \pm 6.6 \times 10^7$	Perfusion increased and angina reduced.
20,47	BMMNC	14	Transendocardial, guided by electromechanical mapping.	30±6	$3.0 \pm 0.4 \times 10^7$	Global LVEF, regional wall motion, and perfusion increased, and angina and NYHA class reduced.

Currently, myoblasts show greater potential to treat late-stage disease due to their myogenic potential and contractility. In late-stage disease, bone marrow-derived stem cells have shown mainly angiogenic potential, with less potential to differentiate into myogenic cells when in scar tissue

BM, bone marrow; BMMNC, bone marrow mononuclear cell; CABG, coronary artery bypass grafting; CPC, cardiac-derived stem cell; LVEDV, left ventricular end-diastolic volume; LVEF, left ventricular ejection fraction; NYHA, New York Heart Association; SKMB, skeletal myoblast.

Table 8.2 Targets for cell-based cardiac repair in 2006

	Clinical target	*Cell type*	*Delivery*	*Timing*
Heart failure	Reverse remodel LV	SKMB, MSC, SMC	Epicardial, endocardial, transcoronary, or transvenous	Late (>1 month and up to 10 years after initial injury)
	Improve LV perfusion	MSC, MNC, EPC, VPC, cells + GF		
	Improve LV function	SKMB, CSC, MSC, cells + GF		
Acute myocardial infarction	Minimize acute myocardial loss	MNC, EPC	Intracoronary, transcoronary, or transvenous	Early (<2 weeks after initial injury)
	Improve LV perfusion	MSC, MNC, EPC, VPC		
	Improve LV function	MSC, CSC		

CSC, cardiac-derived stem cell; EPC, endothelial progenitor cell; GF, growth factors; LV, left ventricle; MNC, mononuclear cell; MSC, mesenchymal stem cell; SKMB, skeletal myoblast; SMC, smooth muscle cell; VPC, vascular progenitor cell.

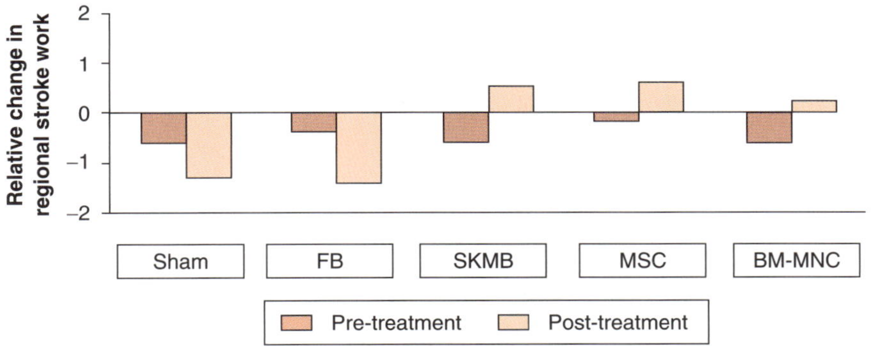

Figure 8.2 *Relative comparison of autologous cell types in restoring systolic function to the injured remodeled failing heart. The relative change in regional stroke work is illustrated before and after treatment in rabbits that received approximately 3×10^7 autologous cells 4–6 weeks after 1 cm cryoinjury of the left ventricle. Sham (vehicle)- and dermal fibroblast (FB)-treated animals showed a worsening of regional stroke work over the treatment period. Bone marrow mononuclear cells (BM-MNC), stromal cells (mesenchymal stem cells, MSC), and skeletal myoblasts (SKMB) increasingly improved regional stroke work. Histologic analysis of the treated animals showed increased angiogenesis in the MNC-, MSC-, and SKMB-treated groups compared with the sham- and FB-treated groups. Myogenesis as evidenced by combined sarcomeric myosin, actin, and desmin staining was demonstrated only in the SKMB and MSC groups.*

translate into a systolic benefit. These data suggest that cell transplantation may offer new hope in treating diastolic dysfunction[11] and further suggest that consideration of the functional goal should be a component of the cell type decision process. Comprehensively discussing and comparing the advantages and disadvantages of each cell type is beyond the scope of this chapter; however, more in-depth discussions have recently been published.[12,13]

Choosing a Delivery Method

With the rapid move of cell-based cardiac repair to clinical application, defining an optimal delivery method becomes a second important task. Facing the heterogeneous patient population suffering from cardiovascular disease again requires different delivery routes to be considered. Many early studies relied on precise surgical delivery of cells to allow direct visualization of the injured region.[14–16] The clear drawback of open-chest surgical delivery is the need for a largely invasive procedure that limits the potential patient population due to the perioperative risk. Recent attempts to minimize invasiveness by developing thoracoscopic techniques[17] and robotically assisted cell transplantation[18] may be promising options for patients with greatly reduced left ventricular function. Alternatively, percutaneous cell delivery has emerged[19] and has been used clinically to deliver cells endoventricularly,[20,21] transvenously,[22] or directly into the coronary arterial or venous circulation.[23] Again, specific cell characteristics influence the route of administration. Larger cells, including most mesodermal progenitors, likely impose the risk of cellular embolization after intracoronary injection.[19,24] Furthermore, after intravenous administration, the majority of these larger cells may be lost either to lung or to spleen and thus not be available for direct cardiac repair. However, this is applicable not only to larger cell types; with any cell after systemic delivery, homing becomes an important issue. If the homing signal is not sufficient—as is likely the case with chronic disease—the majority of progenitor cells are extracted in the lung, spleen,[25,26] or elsewhere (perhaps tumors) where a homing signal does exist. Thus, ultimately, both the clinical situation and cell type will direct the choice of delivery method. An acute injury may allow systemic cell administration of progenitor cells that can home from the periphery to the target lesion; the chronic setting of a remodeled, failing heart may call for very targeted direct injection. In summary, as cell-based cardiac repair moves to clinical application, each cell type is associated with both positive and negative outcomes. And although several generic cell delivery issues have arisen, the majority of cell-safety issues appear to be cell type-specific. Generic issues primarily revolve around cell size and route of administration.

Cells: the Negative

Specific negative outcomes have been associated with specific cells. A serious deleterious outcome to date associated primarily with myoblasts is the development of cardiac electrical instability for what appears to be a transient period after cell delivery. These early reports of electrical instability in patients after receipt of autologous skeletal myoblasts have raised serious concerns about the safety of these cells as a treatment in the injured heart. Patients who received myoblasts in the earliest clinical studies[21,27] were extremely ill with an expected high potential for adverse electrical events. In fact, many of the patients included in the early trials met the MADIT-II criteria, which were presented after those trials began and suggested that all patients who met the criteria be treated with automatic implantable cardioverter–defibrillators (AICDs). As a result, in more recent clinical studies, many investigators have enrolled only patients who have received AICDs and/or low dose anti-arrhythmic agents prophylactically. This has reduced the reported incidence of adverse events significantly. In the MAGIC trial, as reported at the American Heart Association meeting in November 2004, the incidence of electrical instability in patients post myoblast delivery was 10%, which is lower than the initial 40% reported by the same group. Whether this is due to better selection of patients in the second study, coadministration of anti-arrhythmic agents, or an improved cell safety profile remains to be determined. Our group has shown that the location of cell injection may affect the electrical impact of the cells.[28] Furthermore, Dib et al[29] have not reported an increased incidence of electrical instability after myoblast administration, nor have Chachques et al[30] in preclinical studies. However, these investigators observed differing percentages of myoblasts in the final product, differing doses, and differing delivery methods. Understanding whether this reported safety difference truly reflects the cell preparation, the dosage, the delivery, or some as-yet undefined issue is crucial to fully understanding the risk–benefit ratio of skeletal myoblasts for cardiac repair. Clearly, this is an area where collaborative approaches involving side-by-side comparisons of a supposedly similar product could greatly benefit the field. As it stands, randomized controlled trials underway at present are our only way to address these safety concerns and prove efficacy.

To develop a well-defined therapeutic tool, we need to understand the mechanism of endogenous and exogenous cell-based repair. Within the last 10 years, a myriad of preclinical and first-in-man clinical studies have suggested that cell therapy has a positive effect on cardiac and vascular repair.[31] In most studies, the tested cell types were found to be effective—even in the absence of evidence of robust cell engraftment. This unexpected outcome shows how little we actually understand at present about the underlying mechanism(s) of cell-mediated repair. We attribute much repair to direct participation of the transplanted cells in angiogenesis or myogenesis; but in truth, despite promising clinical outcomes, relatively few clinical data exist to support this contention. Instead, underlying neurohumoral changes altering wall stress, recruitment of endogenous stem/progenitor cells, rescue of injured cardiocytes, and limited degrees of angiogenesis and myogenesis are likely involved. Direct cell–cell interaction,[32] fusion of progenitor cells with cardiomyocytes,[33] transdifferentiation of progenitor cells,[34] and dedifferentiation of cardiomyocytes[35] have all also been discussed as potential mediators of the observed outcomes. The degree to which progenitor cells engraft in the injured heart, contribute to perfusion, and actively contract will not be discernible until noninvasive cell tracking becomes feasible. The current focus is on the development of magnetic resonance imaging (MRI)[36,37] and positron emission tomography imaging of labeled cells as preclinical tools. Unfortunately, no long-term clinically applicable tools currently exist.

Cells vs Growth Factors

Inherent in the idea of autologous cell therapy is the acceptance that autologous cells, if administered at the right dose into the correct location, are capable of repair. In other words, endogenous repair should be feasible if the appropriate endogenous cells can be mobilized to the site of injury. This suggests that disease, then, is a failure of endogenous progenitor cell-mediated repair. This idea has led to the use of granulocyte colony-stimulating factor (G-CSF)[38,39] and granulocyte–macrophage (GM)-CSF for mobilization of endogenous progenitor cells for cardiac repair, either as an adjunct to, or a substitute for, delivering exogenous cells. Unfortunately, this broad-based cell mobilization approach has forced us to face several areas where our knowledge is lacking. First, in patients who, after an acute myocardial infarction, underwent stenting and received G-CSF, a high incidence of in-stent restenosis was noted, suggesting that mobilized cells homed not just to the desired site at the ischemic cardiac lesion but also to an undesired site within the vascular bed.[38] More recently, Hill et al[39] reported that patients treated with G-CSF to promote myocardial revascularization and relief of ischemia, showed elevated levels of C-reactive protein; in 2 out of 16 patients, serious adverse events (non-ST-segment-elevation myocardial infarction and death) occurred. Taken together, these unanticipated outcomes illustrate the potential risks of cell therapy: approaches where we cannot control the cell number, delivery location, or cell type.

The Future: Prevention and Early Treatment

The ultimate knowledge gained about cell-based repair should shed new light on the development and progression of cardiovascular disease and enable us to formulate even earlier targets for cell therapy. For example, cell-based restoration of vessel patency and/or regeneration of functional vasculature before ischemic injury occurs could provide a new arena for cell transplantation. Recent data suggest that atherosclerosis may progress in part due to a decreased endogenous repair potential and a decrease in progenitor cell numbers.[6,40] Repeated intravenous injection of bone marrow from young ApoE-null mice prevented further progression of atherosclerotic lesions in aging ApoE-null mice. Injected cells differentiated into endothelial cells and engrafted in atherosclerotic lesions of recipient animals. Comparison of bone marrow cell fluorescence-activated cell sorting (FACS) profiles showed a specific depletion of intermediate vascular progenitor cells ($CD31^+CD45^+$), without parallel changes in more primitive stem cells (Sca-1^+, c-Kit^+, or $CD34^+$) or mature vascular cells (VEGFR-2^+). This depletion most likely accounted for the age-related loss of vascular repair capacity. More recent preliminary data from our group, suggesting that atherosclerotic changes are to some extent reversible, give hope that cell-mediated vascular repair may be an achievable goal in the prevention of ischemic heart disease. In a recent analysis, investigators modeled the potential health effects of bone marrow-derived endothelial progenitor cell therapy using data from the 1950–1996 follow-up of the Framingham Heart Study. To model cardiovascular disease mortality, progenitor cell therapy was applied at age 30, with the effect assumed to be a 10-year delay in atherosclerosis progression. According to this study, progenitor cell therapy might increase the life expectancy in the population as much as would the complete elimination of cancer (in females, an additional 3.67 vs 3.37 years; in males, an additional 5.94 vs 2.86 years, respectively).[41]

Summary

In summary, cell-based cardiovascular repair offers unprecedented potential to treat the underlying injuries associated with cardiovascular disease and ultimately perhaps to reverse the disease process. However, achieving the promise of this field demands that, while we recognize its potential, we also recognize our limits. Choosing the right cell, at the right time, for the right patient must become a scientific discipline. Conducting clinical trials that let us make those choices is critical. Learning from our predecessors in the gene therapy field is crucial. By doing so, we will have our first real opportunity to repair the injured human heart and thus improve the lives of millions worldwide.

References

1. Cohn JN, Francis GS. Cardiac failure: a revised paradigm. J Card Fail 1995;1:261–6.
2. Taylor DA, Atkins BZ, Hungspreugs P, et al. Regenerating functional myocardium: improved performance after skeletal myoblast transplantation. Nat Med 1998;4:929–33.
3. Wollert KC, Drexler H. Clinical applications of stem cells for the heart. Circ Res 2005;96:151–63.
4. Stamm C, Westphal B, Klein HD, et al. Autologous bone-marrow stem-cell transplantation for myocardial regeneration. Lancet 2003;361:45–6.
5. Schachinger V, Assmus B, Honold J, et al. Transplantation of Progenitor Cells and Regeneration Enhancement in Acute Myocardial Infarction (TOPCARE-AMI). Circulation 2002;106: 3009–17.
6. Rauscher FM, Goldschmidt-Clermont PJ, Davis BH, et al. Aging, progenitor cell exhaustion, and atherosclerosis. Circulation 2003;108:457–63.
7. Itescu S, Kocher AA, Schuster MD. Myocardial neovascularization by adult bone marrow-derived angioblasts: strategies for improvement of cardiomyocyte function. Heart Fail Rev 2003; 8:253–8.
8. Jiang Y, Jahagirdar BN, Reinhardt RL, et al. Pluripotency of mesenchymal stem cells derived from adult marrow. Nature 2002;418: 41–9.
9. Reinlib L, Field L. Cell transplantation as future therapy for cardiovascular disease?: A workshop of the National Heart, Lung, and Blood Institute. Circulation 2000;101:E182–7.
10. Thompson RB, Emani SM, Davis BH, et al. Comparison of intracardiac cell transplantation: autologous skeletal myoblasts versus bone marrow cells. Circulation 2003;108(Suppl 1):II264–71.
11. Atkins BZ, Hueman MT, Meuchel J, et al. Cellular cardiomyoplasty improves diastolic properties of injured heart. J Surg Res 1999;85:234–42.
12. Ott HC, McCue J, Taylor DA. Cell-based cardiovascular repair: the hurdles and the opportunities. Basic Res Cardiol 2005;99:1–14.
13. Bonaros N, Bernecker O, Ott H, Schlechta B, Kocher AA. Cell and gene therapy for ischemic heart disease. Minerva Cardioangiol 2005;53:265–73.
14. Menasche P, Hagege AA, Desnos M. Myoblast transplantation for heart failure. Lancet 2001; 357:279–80.
15. Stamm C, Kleine HD, Westphal B, et al. CABG and bone marrow stem cell transplantation after

myocardial infarction. Thorac Cardiovasc Surg 2004;52:152–8.
16. Tse HF, Kwong YL, Chan JK, et al. Angiogenesis in ischaemic myocardium by intramyocardial autologous bone marrow mononuclear cell implantation. Lancet 2003;361:47–9.
17. Thompson RB, Parsa CJ, van den Bos EJ, et al. Video-assisted thoracoscopic transplantation of myoblasts into the heart. Ann Thorac Surg 2004;78:303–7.
18. Ott HC, Brechten J, Swinger C, et al. Robotic minimally invasive cardiac cell transplantation for heart failure. JTCVS 2006; in press.
19. Taylor DA, Silvestry SC, Bishop SP, et al. Delivery of primary autologous skeletal myoblasts into rabbit heart by coronary infusion: a potential approach to myocardial repair. Proc Assoc Am Physicians 1997;109:245–53.
20. Perin EC, Dohmann HF, Borojevic R, et al. Transendocardial, autologous bone marrow cell transplantation for severe, chronic ischemic heart failure. Circulation 2003;107:2294–302.
21. Smits PC, van Geuns RJ, Poldermans D, et al. Catheter-based intramyocardial injection of autologous skeletal myoblasts as a primary treatment of ischemic heart failure: clinical experience with six-month follow-up. J Am Coll Cardiol 2003;42: 2063–9.
22. Siminiak T, Fiszer D, Jerzykowska O, et al. Percutaneous trans-coronary-venous transplantation of autologous skeletal myoblasts in the treatment of post-infarction myocardial contractility impairment: the POZNAN trial. Eur Heart J 2005;26:1188–95.
23. Strauer BE, Brehm M, Zeus T, et al. [Intracoronary, human autologous stem cell transplantation for myocardial regeneration following myocardial infarction]. Dtsch Med Wochenschr 2001;126:932–8.
24. Vulliet PR, Greeley M, Halloran SM, MacDonald KA, Kittleson MD. Intra-coronary arterial injection of mesenchymal stromal cells and microinfarction in dogs. Lancet 2004;363:783–4.
25. Aicher A, Brenner W, Zuhayra M, et al. Assessment of the tissue distribution of transplanted human endothelial progenitor cells by radioactive labeling. Circulation 2003;107:2134–9.
26. Barbash IM, Chouraqui P, Baron J, et al. Systemic delivery of bone marrow-derived mesenchymal stem cells to the infarcted myocardium: feasibility, cell migration, and body distribution. Circulation 2003;108:863–8.
27. Menasché P, Hagege AA, Vilquin JT. Autologous skeletal myoblast transplantation for severe postinfarction left ventricular dysfunction. J Am Coll Cardiol 2003;41:1078–83.
28. Soliman AH. Assessment of electrical instability after autologous myoblast transplantation in a rabbit infarct model. Circulation 2003;108:IV-547.
29. Dib N, Campbell A, Jacoby DB, et al. Safety and feasibility of autologous myoblast transplantation in patients with ischemic cardiomyopathy: four-year follow-up. Circulation 2005;112:1748–55.
30. Chachques JC, Herreros J, Trainini J, et al. Autologous human serum for cell culture avoids the implantation of cardioverter-defibrillators in cellular cardiomyoplasty. Int J Cardiol 2004; 95(Suppl 1):S29–33.
31. Bonaros N, Yang S, Ott H, Kocher A. Cell therapy for ischemic heart disease. Panminerva Med 2004; 46:13–23.
32. Koyanagi M, Brandes RP, Haendeler J, Zeiher AM, Dimmeler S. Cell-to-cell connection of endothelial progenitor cells with cardiac myocytes by nanotubes: a novel mechanism for cell fate changes? Circ Res 2005;96:1039–41.
33. Driesen RB, Dispersyn GD, Verheyen FK, et al Partial cell fusion: a newly recognized type of communication between dedifferentiating cardiomyocytes and fibroblasts. Cardiovasc Res 2005;68:37–46.
34. Yoon J, Shim WJ, Ro YM, Lim DS. Trans-differentiation of mesenchymal stem cells into cardiomyocytes by direct cell-to-cell contact with neonatal cardiomyocyte but not adult cardiomyocytes. Ann Hematol 2005;84:715–21.
35. Matsuura K, Wada H, Nagai T, et al. Cardiomyocytes fuse with surrounding noncardiomyocytes and reenter the cell cycle. J Cell Biol 2004;167:351–63.
36. van den Bos EJ, Wagner A, Mahrholdt H, et al. Improved efficacy of stem cell labeling for magnetic resonance imaging studies by the use of cationic liposomes. Cell Transplant 2003;12:743–56.
37. Bengel FM, Schachinger V, Dimmeler S. Cell-based therapies and imaging in cardiology. Eur J Nucl Med Mol Imaging 2005;32(Sup2):S404–16.
38. Kang HJ, Kim HS, Zhang SY, et al. Effects of intracoronary infusion of peripheral blood stem-cells mobilised with granulocyte-colony stimulating factor on left ventricular systolic function and restenosis after coronary stenting in myocardial infarction: the MAGIC cell randomised clinical trial. Lancet 2004;363:751–6.
39. Hill JM, Syed MA, Arai AE, et al. Outcomes and risks of granulocyte colony-stimulating factor in patients with coronary artery disease. J Am Coll Cardiol 2005;46:1643–8.
40. Schmidt-Lucke C, Rossig L, Fichtlscherer S, et al. Reduced number of circulating endothelial progenitor cells predicts future cardiovascular events: proof of concept for the clinical importance of endogenous vascular repair. Circulation 2005;111:2981–7.
41. Kravchenko J, Goldschmidt-Clermont PJ, Powell T, et al. Endothelial progenitor cell therapy for atherosclerosis: the philosopher's stone for an aging population? Sci Aging Knowledge Environ 2005;25:18.

42. Herreros J, Prosper F, Perez A, et al. Autologous intramyocardial injection of cultured skeletal muscle-derived stem cells in patients with non-acute myocardial infarction. Eur Heart J 2003;24: 2012–20.
43. Siminiak T, Kalmucki P, Kurpisz M. Autologous skeletal myoblast transplantation for the treatment of postinfarction myocardial injury: phase I clinical study with 12 months of follow-up. Am Heart J 2004;148:531–7.
44. Schachinger V, Assmus B, Britten MB, et al. Transplantation of progenitor cells and regeneration enhancement in acute myocardial infarction: final one-year results of the TOPCARE-AMI trial. J Am Coll Cardiol 2004;44:1690–9.
45. Hamano K, Nishida M, Hirata K, et al. Local implantation of autologous bone marrow cells for therapeutic angiogenesis in patients with ischemic heart disease: clinical trial and preliminary results. Jpn Circ J 2001;65:845–7.
46. Fuchs S, Satler LF, Kornowski R, et al. Catheter-based autologous bone marrow myocardial injection in no-option patients with advanced coronary artery disease: a feasibility study. J Am Coll Cardiol 2003;41:1721–4.
47. Perin EC, Dohmann HF, Borojevic R, et al. Improved exercise capacity and ischemia 6 and 12 months after transendocardial injection of autologous bone marrow mononuclear cells for ischemic cardiomyopathy. Circulation 2004;110:II-213–18.

chapter 9

Overview of the Clinical Applications of Stem Cells in Ischemic Heart Disease

Shaun R Opie and Nabil Dib

Introduction

Myocardial infarction is a leading cause of mortality in the USA, accounting for approximately 600 deaths per day.[1] Nearly 865 000 new and recurrent cases are diagnosed every year, and this number is expected to increase as the baby boomer population ages. Myocardial infarction results in damaged myocardium caused by occlusion of the coronary arteries from thrombus or from atherosclerotic plaque buildup. It can ultimately lead to congestive heart failure, as a result of the remodeling, which compromises survival and quality of life. With the exception of heart transplantation, which is limited by a severe shortage of donors and issues related to rejection, the currently available therapies for coronary artery disease, medication and revascularization, are unable to replace damaged or diseased tissue.

Renewed interest in regenerating diseased tissue by stem cell transplantation has arisen as a result of the development of sophisticated cell culture techniques and the identification of molecular pathways that direct stem cell differentiation into specific cell types. Stem cells have two fundamental properties: the ability to self-renew, so that a replenishable source of cells is continually available for cultivation, and the ability to differentiate into at least one alternative cell type. The concept behind stem cell therapy is that healthy cells can be isolated from one part of the body and be implanted into a damaged region for the purpose of tissue repair. Myocardial infarction is particularly amenable to stem cell therapy, since, following myocardial injury, very few of the remaining cardiac myocytes enter the mitotic cycle. As a result, replacement of dead or necrotic cells does not occur at a clinically acceptable rate. Additionally, myogenic precursors exist throughout the skeletal musculature, are relatively easy to procure, and can be physically implanted into damaged heart tissue.

Congestive Heart Failure and Left Ventricular Dysfunction

A myocardial infarction is usually the result of atherosclerotic plaque rupture and thrombus formation in the coronary vessels, blocking essential blood flow to the myocardium. In the absence of coronary blood flow, cardiomyocytes die, and the ability of the heart to contract becomes impaired. Consequently the reduced ventricular ejection fraction can ultimately lead to congestive heart failure. The pathophysiology that follows an infarction is well described and occurs in overlapping phases over several weeks, months, and even years. Initially, there is a massive loss of cardiac myocytes due to acute, severe ischemia. Within the healing infarct region, cells secrete pro-inflammatory cytokines that recruit macrophages and leukocytes. Over several weeks, ischemia-resistant fibroblasts eventually replace the dead myocytes, leading to areas of fibrosis that do not contribute to heart function. In an attempt to compensate for the decrease in heart function, the ventricular tissue undergoes pathophysiologic changes such as cardiomyocyte hypertrophy and matrix changes, to increase the output stroke volume in a process called remodeling. However, none of the compensatory mechanisms regenerates contractile tissue or prevents remodeling.

Cell Types and Culture Process for Myocardial Repair

Various precursor cells have been proposed for myocardial regeneration, including embryonic stem cells, bone marrow mesenchymal cells, peripheral blood stem cells, cardiac myocytes, and skeletal muscle stem cells.[2] The cell type best suited for this purpose is not known, but, given the complexity of the heart structure and the diversity of cell types, the most appropriate cell will likely be determined by the clinical substrate. In part, this is because each cell type has its own specific requirements for survival and proliferation, and the final cell phenotype is likely to be different among cells. Cardiomyocytes are difficult to obtain in sufficient numbers for implantation purposes, and a ventricular biopsy is an impractical solution. The use of embryonic stem cells has considerable ethical implications that are likely to remain unresolved for the near future. For the purposes of this chapter, we will focus on the cell types that are most likely to be clinical options in the future: myoblasts, bone marrow stem cells, and peripheral blood stem cells.

Autologous skeletal myoblasts

Myoblasts, also called muscle satellite cells, are small mononuclear cells located between the basal lamina and the sarcolemma on the periphery of the mature skeletal muscle fiber.[3] Following muscle injury, myoblasts are activated by biochemical signals to initiate active division and differentiate into fusion competent cells. An example of a myoblast culture and of fusion is shown in Figure 9.1. Myotube formation occurs by a process in which a group of individual myoblasts aggregate through cell membrane fusion to form a single large multinucleated cell. The myotubes are the basic building blocks of skeletal muscle, and when several myotubes align in the same direction, they become functional myofibers.

The basic outline for myoblast isolation and growth is as follows. Under strict sterile conditions, using local anesthesia, a biopsy specimen between 0.5 and 5 g is obtained from the quadriceps muscle. The specimen is placed in a glucose-containing medium and immediately transported to a tissue culture facility. Once inside a pre-irradiated laminar flow hood stocked with supplies, the container holding the biopsy specimen is opened and the muscle sample removed. With sterile scissors or scalpels, the biopsy is cut into small (approximately 1 mm^3) pieces. These pieces are placed into an enzymatic solution, often consisting of trypsin and collagenase, that will digest extracellular matrix and connective tissue in order to release individual cells. After the digestive process is complete, the enzymes are inactivated, and the cells are extensively washed to remove red blood cells and debris. The cells are then resuspended in a rich medium containing growth factors and necessary nutrients and are seeded onto a cell culture dish. The cells are transferred to a 37°C incubator and grown in high humidity until they reach approximately 70–80% confluency. Myoblast cultures must be carefully monitored and split before reaching confluency, as otherwise they have a tendency to convert into fibroblasts that are not of therapeutic benefit. It will take 4–6 weeks to grow 500 million cells.

Bone marrow-derived cells

Bone marrow stem cells (BMSCs) have received considerable attention since researchers first observed that they can selectively differentiate into myoblasts and endothelial progenitor cells and regenerate infarcted myocardium.[4–6] Both the

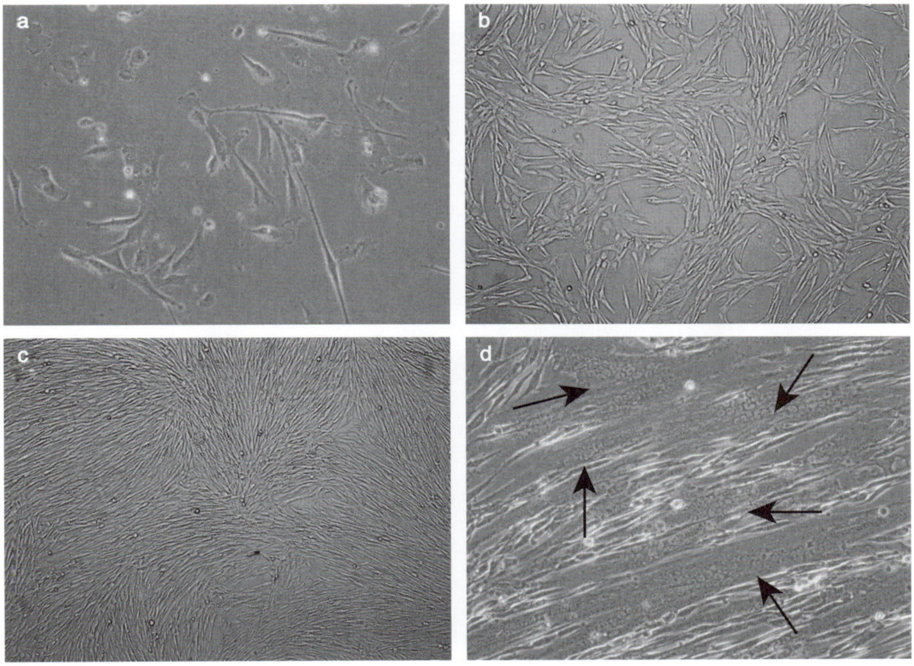

Figure 9.1 Myoblast growth and morphologic characteristics after preplating: (a) at 3 days; (b) at 5 days; (c) at 7 days. (d) Myoblast fusion is induced by switching from a medium with a high serum concentration to one with a low serum concentration. Arrows indicate aggregates of nuclei inside a large myotube. (a, d, 10 × Magnification; b, c, 4 × magnification).

mesenchymal fraction and the hematopoietic fraction contain endothelial progenitor cells able to differentiate into endothelial cells and contribute to neovascularization by forming nascent blood vessels.[4]

The basic outline for BMSC isolation is as follows. Typically, the bone marrow cells are mobilized prior to isolation by the administration of granulocyte colony-stimulating factor (G-CSF) per standard clinical protocol. Mobilization increases the overall yield of cells thought to have the characteristic differentiation requirements. BMSCs are collected by taking an aspirate from the iliac crest of the patient under local anesthesia. Alternatively, if direct injections are to be performed, bone marrow can be isolated from the sternal cavity when a surgeon gains direct access to the mediastinum. Bone marrow is composed of a heterogeneous mixture of cell types, of which only a small proportion is thought to be myogenic or angiogenic precursors.[7–9] The mononuclear subfraction can be isolated by Ficoll density centrifugation and filtered through a 100-μm nylon mesh to remove cell aggregates or bone spicules. Cells are washed several times in phosphate-buffered saline (PBS) and can either be reinjected directly or expanded in an endothelial cell-specific culture medium. Although BMSCs are promising candidates for cell transplantation, the invasiveness of bone marrow collection may ultimately limit its clinical application.

Peripheral blood-derived cells

Bone marrow produces many different cell types that are released into the blood stream after maturation. From peripheral blood, Asahara et al[10] isolated an endothelial progenitor cell with properties identical to those isolated from bone marrow. The identification of endothelial precursor cells from

Table 9.1 Clinical experience with stem cell transplantation

Ref	*Sample size*	*Mode of delivery*	*Associated procedure*	*Follow-up (months)*	*No. of cells injected*	*Donor cell*	*Results*	*Complications*
18	1	Direct injection	CABG	5	800×10^6	ASM	Increased LVEF (21% to 30%), increased segmental contractility (0% to 40%), increased PET viability	None
14	1	Direct injection	CABG	17	800×10^6	ASM	Histologic confirmation of myotube development and survival	None
16	12	Direct injection	CABG	3	$100–300 \times 10^6$	ASM	Improved LVEF (36% to 54%), improved regional WMSI (2.64 to 1.64), increased PET viability	None
19	10	Direct injection	CABG	11	$500–1100 \times 10^6$	ASM	Improved NYHA score (2.7 to 1.6), improved LVEF (24% to 32%)	1 noncardiac death, 4 SVT
21	5	Catheter injection	None	6	800×10^6	ASM	Increased LVEF (36% to 45%), regional wall thickening in transplant zones, increased contraction velocities	1 ICD implanted for NSVT
20	5	Direct injection	LVAD	2–7	300×10^6	ASM	Histologic confirmation of engraftment and angiogenesis, myotube development	1 death, 2 atrial fibrillation, 2 ventricular tachycardia
12	18	Direct injection	CABG	17	$10–300 \times 10^6$	ASM	Increased LVEF (25% to 34%), decreased EDV and ESV, histologic confirmation of engraftment and myotube development, improved PET viability	1 death, 5 NVST
15	5	Direct injection	CABG	12	$50–100 \times 10^6$	BMMC	Improved SPECT perfusion	None
7	10	Catheter infusion	PTCA and stent	3	28×10^6	BMMC	Decreased infarct size, increased WMV (2.0 to 4.0), improved SPECT perfusion, increased stroke volume (49 to 56 ml/min), decreased EDV (158 to 143 ml), decreased ESV (82 to 67 ml)	None

	2–4	25.5×10^6 injection	BMMCIncreased LVEF (20% to 29%), decreased				1 death, EDV (213 to 181 ml), decreased ESV (174 to 133 ml), improved mechanical movement, improved SPECT perfusion, improved NYHA score (2.21 to 1.28)	1 pulmonary edema
22	6	Direct injection	CABG	3–10	$1.2–3.3\times10^6$	BMMC	Improved SPECT perfusion, increased LVEF	2 supraventricular arrhythmia, 1 pneumonia infection, 1 LIMA bleeding, 2 pericardial effusion, 1 cholecystitis
23	8	Catheter injection	None	3	NR	BMMC	Reduction of weekly anginal episodes (26.5 to 10.1), decreased nitroglycerin consumption, increased wall thickness, increased wall motion	None
8	20	Catheter infusion	Stent	4	245×10^6	BMMC and PBSC	Increased global LVEF (51.6% to 60.1%), improved regional WMSI (1.4 to 1.19), decreased ESV (56.1 to 42.2 ml), increased PET viability, increased CFR	1 myocardial infarction unrelated to cell transplantation protocol
13	14	Direct injection	CABG	10	$>1000\times10^6$	PBSC	Under dobutamine stress: increased regional and global left ventricular function (47% to 55%), increased CI (2.7 to 4.3). Improved regional WMSI	None
17	20	Catheter infusion	Stent	6	1000×10^6	PBSC	Increased treadmill exercise time (450 to 578 s), increased LVEF (48.7% to 55.1%), improved SPECT perfusion	High rates of in-stent restenosis in patients with G-CSF mobilization

ASM, autologous skeletal myoblast; BMMC, bone marrow mononuclear cell; CABG, coronary artery bypass grafting; CFR, coronary flow reserve; CI, cardiac index; EDV, end-diastolic volume; ESV, end-systolic volume; G-CSF, granulocyte colony-stimulating factor; ICD, implantable cardioverter–defibrillator; LIMA, left internal mammary artery; LVAD, left ventricular assist device; LVEF, left ventricular ejection fraction; NR, not reported; NSVT, nonsustained ventricular tachycardia; NYHA, New York Heart Association; PBSC, peripheral blood stem cell; PET, positron emission tomography; PTCA, percutaneous transluminal coronary angioplasty; SPECT, single photon emission computed tomography; SVT, sustained ventricular tachycardia; WMSI, wall motion score index; WMV, wall movement velocity peripheral blood may abrogate the necessity of iliac crest bone marrow aspiration. Although the yield of cells is lower from peripheral blood than from bone marrow isolation, mobilization of these cells by cytokine therapy increases their yield to a level similar to that of BMSCs.[11]

The cell type chosen for transplantation will likely depend on the disease and desired clinical effect. Bone marrow cells or peripheral blood endothelial progenitor cells may be best suited for acute coronary syndromes and ischemic disease, since they are able to induce angiogenesis or directly participate in the formation of a nascent vascular network. Myoblasts may be best suited for myocardial infarction and chronic heart failure, in which regeneration of contractile tissue is desired. For either cell type, procurement of autologous cells with reimplantation is the preferred treatment choice, since immunosuppression is not required to prevent graft rejection. This requires that an individualized batch of cells be cultured for each transplant recipient, a process that is expensive and necessitates sophisticated good-manufacturing-practice (GMP) cell culture facilities staffed with highly trained individuals. Commercial developers of cell therapy are likely to prefer an allogeneic approach, because large numbers of cells can be grown and stored for "off-the-shelf" use. This approach appears to require at least short-term immunosuppressive therapy.

Clinical Trials of Cell Transplantation for Myocardial Infarction

At present, neither autologous skeletal myoblast nor bone marrow stem cell transplantation for cardiac tissue regeneration is approved by the US Food and Drug Administration (FDA). Since the cells used in transplantation are classified as investigational new drugs (INDs), US institutions conducting this type of human research must apply to the FDA and receive permission prior to treating any patients. This investigative process is time-consuming and expensive and demands rigorous scientific evaluation from both the investigator and the FDA in order to assure patient safety.

A summary of the reported phase I and phase II human cell transplantation clinical trials is given in Table 9.1.[7–9,12–23] Although the selection requirements differ among institutions, in general, the inclusion criteria require a reduced left ventricular ejection fraction (LVEF $<35\%$), ventricular wall hypokinesis or akinesis, and nonviable infarct-induced scar tissue. Most protocols were designed as small, nonrandomized trials to show the safety and feasibility, rather than the efficacy, of cell transplantation.

Three cell types have been examined: autologous skeletal myoblasts, bone marrow mesenchymal cells, and peripheral blood stem cells. It is remarkable that, despite different delivery methods, cell types, culturing protocols, and investigators, all centers have reported at least one positive functional benefit, the majority describing multiple, global benefits. Although some of the studies included adverse events, none of these could be directly attributed to cell transplantation. Taken together, these data suggest that cell transplantation, regardless of the cell type, is relatively safe and may benefit heart function. However, a randomized trial will be required to determine improvement of cardiac performance.

Methods of Cell Delivery

Direct epicardial injection during open-chest bypass surgery was first used to transplant stem cells into the damaged myocardium.[24] The main advantage of this approach is that the surgeon can visually confirm the region of myocardial infarction, due to its appearance and contractile characteristics, and can target the injections appropriately. However, since a significant number of the patients who could potentially benefit from cell transplantation are unable to tolerate anesthesia or surgery, a less invasive method is highly desirable. In an effort to include these patients, catheter-based delivery technology has been incorporated into stem cell protocols.

Angiographically guided catheter infusion of cells and plasmid DNA into the coronary arteries

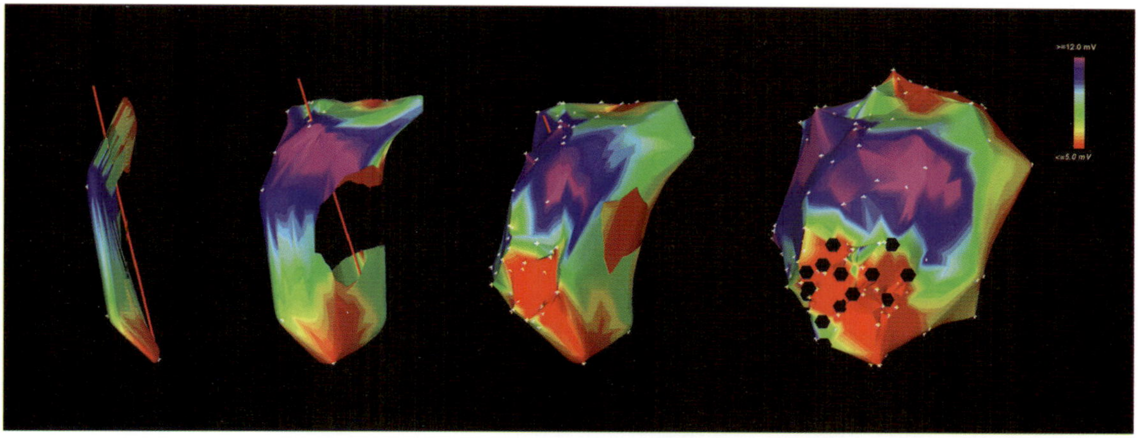

Figure 9.2 *Endoventricular cell delivery. Time-sequence graphical reconstruction of the left ventricle by NOGA mapping. As the mapping process proceeds (left to right), coordinate readings are taken and the image is updated in real time. A complete mapped ventricle is on the right. The color scale bar indicates voltage. On the final image (right), red areas at the apex of the ventricle have low voltage and demarcate the region of myocardial infarction. Black dots identify the locations of the myoblasts that were injected in the region of myocardial infarction using the MyoStar catheter.*

has been achieved and requires only a cardiac catheterization laboratory, with no need for additional training or equipment.[7,25] There are insufficient data to determine whether bioretention of the cells is limited to proximal branches of the coronary vessels or whether systemic diffusion can occur. Also, the possibility that microinfarcts or microstrokes might be created through capillary blockage is of concern and warrants further investigation.

The ideal endovascular approach would allow precise catheter deployment into diseased tissue, with high viability and retention of the delivered cells. The technique must be safe, reproducible, economical, and relatively easy to perform and must meet regulatory standards. Currently, no system fulfills these requirements. A new generation of catheters with innovative features that enable endocardial injections is currently awaiting FDA approval. Several catheters for use in the USA include the MyoCath (Bioheart, Inc., Santa Rosa, CA), the TransAccess MicroLume Delivery System (Transvascular, Menlo Park, CA), the Stiletto (Boston-Scientific, Inc., Natick, MA), and the Myostar (Biosense-Webster-Cordis, Diamond Bar, CA). These catheters have in common a 7–9 French coaxial sheath, a small-gauge needle on the distal end, and a syringe adaptor on the proximal end.

The Biosense-Webster-Cordis (BWC) system has been used successfully by many investigators in the preclinical setting to examine the electromechanical properties of the heart in large animal models. Additionally, a small number of investigational research protocols have been granted permission for human use. The BWC system consists of a locator pad having three coils that emit a low-energy magnetic field; a stationary reference catheter with a magnetic field sensor; separate mapping and injection catheters with a magnetic field sensor; and a computer processor. When the mapping catheter is in contact with the endocardium, two electrodes on the distal tip permit measurement of a voltage across a short segment of endocardium. The system is also able to determine the position of the catheter tip in three-dimensional space, so that data taken during these measurements can generate in real time a three-dimensional color-coded voltage map reconstruction of the left ventricle (LV) that clearly demarcates the area of myocardial infarction (Figure 9.2). When the LV map is complete, the mapping catheter is exchanged for a modified mapping catheter. This

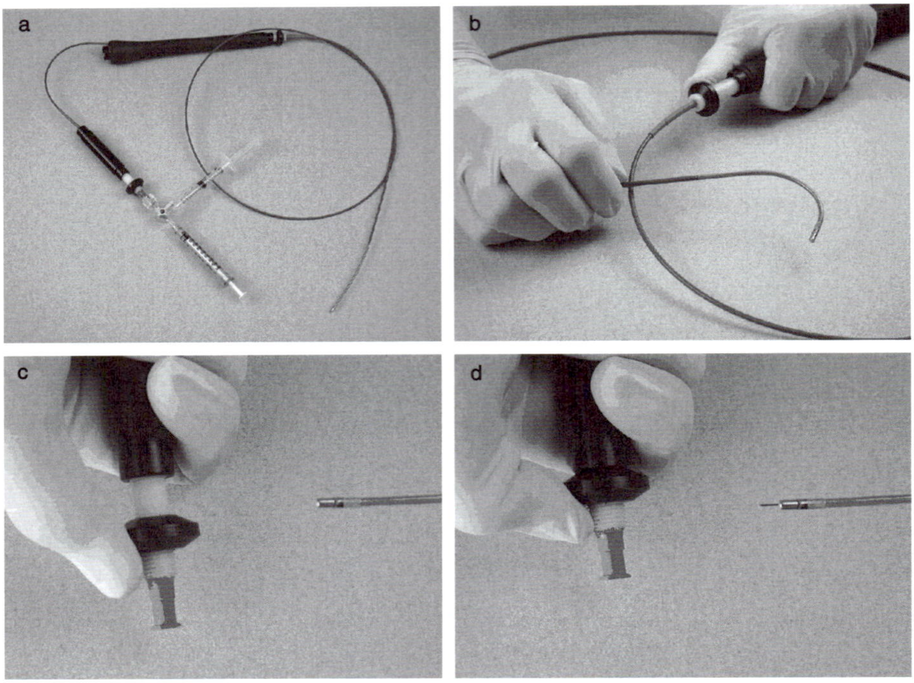

Figure 9.3 *Biosense-Webster MyoStarTM catheter. (a) The set-up includes a PTFE-coated nitinol catheter, a handle on the proximal end for catheter manipulation, and a second handle on the distal end for needle advancement and retraction. The second handle is attached to a Leur Lock adapter with two syringes. (b) The operator can "steer" the tip of the catheter to navigate in the left ventricle, a requirement for taking electromechanical voltage readings and for safe navigation through the vasculature and ventricle. (c, d) Injection needle advancement and retraction.*

hollow, steerable catheter has a 27-gauge nitinol needle on the distal tip that can be advanced or retracted by the operator, as well as a three-way Luer Lock adapter on the proximal end so that tuberculin syringes can be fitted to load samples into the lumen of the needle (Figure 9.3). Using the computer-generated image as a roadmap, the operator can perform endocardial injections in real time and mark their position marked throughout the procedure (Figure 9.2).

Endoventricular injection catheters have a commendable safety record. There are few reports in the literature of myocardial rupture from overly aggressive catheter manipulation or from injection. Rare instances of sustained ventricular tachycardia occur but are primarily related to catheter manipulation in patients with a previous myocardial infarction and severely reduced left ventricular function. Premature ventricular contractions (PVCs) and other short (< 10 s) arrhythmias are relatively common due to physical stimulation of the endocardium during mapping or injection. These usually resolve quickly without the need for cardiac defibrillation. Endoventricular injection carries the risk of pericardial effusion or cell leakage back into the circulatory system. Postmortem visualization of marker gene expression in noninjected normal tissue suggests that complete retention is unlikely to occur during the injection process. The consequence of leakage may be as simple as cell loss or as serious as distal embolization. Quantitative studies regarding the bioretention and biodistribution of injected substances will need to be performed to better understand these issues.

Monitoring Cell Delivery, Transplant Survival, and Biologic Effects

Determining the fate of the transplanted cells will be vital to understanding the success and efficacy of cell transplantation. One of the most significant obstacles to stem cell therapy for myocardial regeneration is the rapid disappearance of cells following transplantation. Although data from human trials have directly demonstrated that myoblasts are not damaged by injection and engraft successfully, semiquantitative studies suggest that at 17.5 months post transplantation, less than 1% of transplanted myoblasts survive and differentiate into myosin-expressing myotubes.[14,20,26] Unfortunately, similar cell survival studies have not yet been reported for bone marrow or peripheral blood stem cells.

Although obtaining a biopsy is the most direct method to demonstrate cell engraftment and to determine the differentiation status of the transplanted cells, patients are generally unwilling to undergo an invasive procedure for information that will not provide them any functional benefit. Accordingly, improved imaging methods able to evaluate cell transplants that are noninvasive and nontoxic have been assigned high priority status with both clinicians and scientific funding agencies in the USA. At this time, the imaging modalities available are used to assess ventricular function, ventricular volume and dimensions, myocardial perfusion, and myocardial metabolism. Noninvasive methods currently used to image heart function and viability include echocardiography, radiofluoroscopy, cineangiography, magnetic resonance imaging (MRI), single photon emission computed tomography (SPECT), and positron emission tomography (PET). The choice of imaging is dependent on multiple factors, including resolution, patient safety, ease, time required, and cost.

Echocardiography is relatively inexpensive, can be performed with ease, and provides structural and real-time wall movement assessment of heart and directional blood flow. However, its resolution is low because it relies on low-energy sound waves to penetrate tissue. Echocardiography has been used to direct catheter movement, and can also be used to demonstrate the increase in wall thickness after cell injection.[25] Radiofluoroscopy and cineangiography equipment is standard in all cardiac catheterization laboratories, and these methods are used to guide catheters safely throughout the arterial vasculature. They provide similar information about ventricular wall motion and the ventricular ejection fraction at a higher resolution. They have been used for catheter guidance, but, like echocardiography, have not gained widespread clinical acceptance for facilitating percutaneous endoventricular injections.[27,28]

Advances in MRI technology have resulted in improved image acquisition and display times, excellent tissue contrast, and radiation-free procedures. MRI provides the highest-resolution images available and also yields clear anatomic landmarks that are independent of the observer. The image resolution is dependent on the magnetic field strength and the image acquisition time, greater T values and longer exposure times providing higher resolution. Although MRI cannot provide the same real-time analysis of ventricular wall motion and ejection fraction as echocardiography, it has been used to guide endoventricular injections.[29] The densities of injected cells and of the surrounding myocardium are similar, so it can be difficult to distinguish between transplant and normal tissue. Paramagnetic contrast agents may help determine the location of an injection.[30] The development of a nontoxic, biocompatible, FDA-approved, exogenous contrast agent that is not adsorbed or metabolized would be extremely beneficial to cell transplantation. The major limitation of MRI is that many of the patients who require myoblasts have an automated implantable cardioverter defibrillator (AICD) and a pacemaker.

Quantitative scintigraphic assessment with SPECT and PET relies upon the cellular uptake of a specific radioactive tracer and is able to analyze the metabolic activity and perfusion of heart muscle in addition to supplying functional data about the ejection fraction, wall motion, and wall thickening.[31] The ability to analyze the

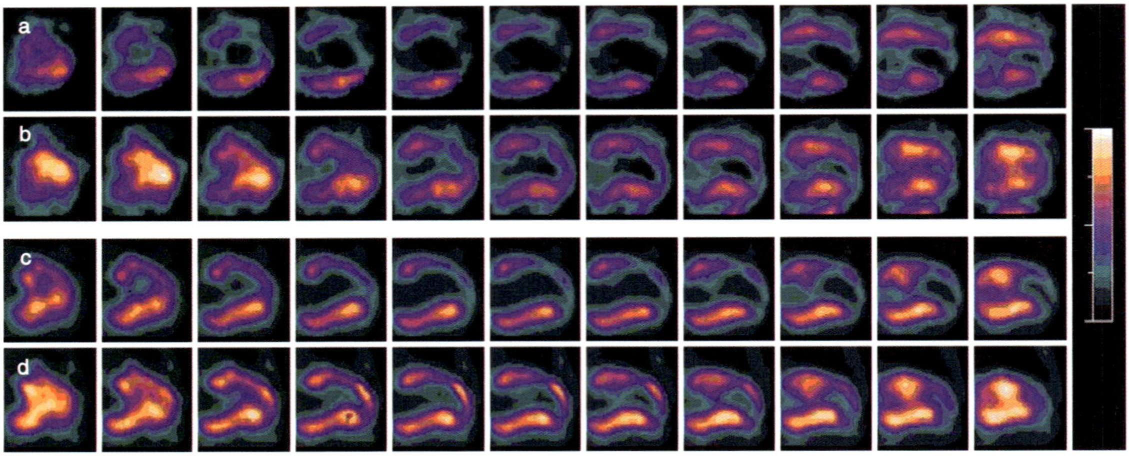

Figure 9.4 Quantitative positron emission tomography (PET) and single photon emission computed tomography (SPECT) scanning. Serial PET and SPECT scan images of the ventricular walls (vertical long-axis view) in a CABG patient receiving myoblast transplantation. SPECT (a, b) and PET (c, d) images were obtained at baseline (a, c) and 6 months (b, d) following skeletal myoblast transplantation. Improved viability is seen by the increased yellow/orange regions.

metabolism enables discrimination between ischemic, infarcted, and hibernating myocardium while analyzing perfusion (Figure 9.4). Because these imaging modalities are able to indirectly assess the survival of transplanted cells and also provide functional data, the large majority of published trials have included one of these. In the majority of human studies of transplantation of myoblasts or bone marrow stem cells, SPECT or PET has shown increased viability and/or perfusion in regions of the myocardium that have received cells.[7–9,15–17,22,24] This finding is of crucial significance to the clinical potential of this therapy.

The isotope tracers commonly used for nuclear imaging include [^{18}F]fluorodeoxyglucose (FDG) for PET and thallium-201 and technetium-99m-sestamibi for SPECT. They are taken up intracellularly by specific transporters or receptors on the exterior of the cell. Pretreating cells with a labeled tracer during the final stage of expansion might assist immediate post-transplantation imaging and tracking of the distribution of radiolabeled cells in vivo until the tracer decays. An alternative approach would be to genetically engineer a batch of cells to express a novel receptor or metabolic process that other cells in the heart do not possess. Selective tracer uptake by the "marker gene" would facilitate viability assessments of the transplanted cells and has the potential for daughter cell labeling and long-term tracking.

Obstacles to Successful Cell Transplantation

Although cell transplantation has received tremendous scientific and media attention lately, many questions remain about what is necessary for long-term survival and function. The pathophysiologic changes that occur within the infarct region are temporally regulated and complex. The known regulators include cytokine release, leukocyte activation and associated inflammatory responses, tissue apoptosis and necrosis, and cell infiltration. No studies have systematically examined the most appropriate time for either bone marrow or myoblast transplantation. In acute cases, success is most likely if the transplantation is performed after the inflammatory process subsides but prior to scar tissue formation. From a clinical perspective, it would be beneficial to be able to include patients with old myocardial scarring for whom there are no other options.

Few quantitative studies have directly examined the survival of cells transplanted into the myocardium. Preclinical studies suggest that the magnitude of myocardial regeneration is related to the cell dose. Although it is presumed that successful engraftment will benefit the patient, a theoretical concern is aberrant differentiation into a detrimental cell type. This is more likely to be the case for bone marrow stem cells, which have shown the ability to differentiate into adipocytes, osteocytes, and chondrocytes.[32] Recent reports in conflict with previous data suggest that bone marrow progenitor cells may not acquire a cardiac phenotype but may instead adopt a mature hematopoietic phenotype.[33,34] These data suggest that in addition to the local tissue environment, regulators of cell differentiation exist that could affect the eventual phenotype and survival of delivered stem cells.

Cardiac muscle expresses gap junction proteins that facilitate the rapid conduction of electrical stimuli required for efficient myocardial contraction. Whether stem cell transplants remain electrically insulated from the surrounding myocardium or whether the gap junction protein connexin 43 is expressed at biologically significant levels remains the subject of scientific debate.

Conclusions

Stem cell transplantation has the potential to provide an alternative therapeutic option to patients with myocardial infarction and congestive heart failure. The type of cell best suited for transplantation has not yet been determined; however, several candidates have emerged, each with its own biologic characteristics that may apply to the specific need of the individual patient. Although surgical delivery was first used to transplant cells, engineering advances in catheter technologies will provide a safer, relatively noninvasive method to deliver the cell product. Improved imaging techniques and additional cellular and biochemical knowledge will be crucial to providing a better understanding of the clinical outcome following transplantation. Although many questions still remain unanswered about cell transplantation for myocardial infarction, the convergence of cell processing, bioengineering, and clinical medicine offers the hope of new therapies to treat this disease.

References

1. American Heart Association. Heart Disease and Stroke Statistics – 2004 Update. http://www.americanheart.org/downloadable/heart/HS_State_02.pdf 2004.
2. Menasche P. Skeletal myoblast transplantation for cardiac repair. Expert Rev Cardiovasc Ther 2004;2:21–8.
3. Mauro A. Satellite cell of skeletal muscle fibers. J Biophys Biochem Cytol 1961;9:493–5.
4. Prockop DJ. Marrow stromal cells as stem cells for nonhematopoietic tissues. Science 1997;276:71–4.
5. Orlic D, Kajstura J, Chimenti S, et al. Bone marrow cells regenerate infarcted myocardium. Nature 2001;410:701–5.
6. Bossolasco P, Corti S, Strazzer S, et al. Skeletal muscle differentiation potential of human adult bone marrow cells. Exp Cell Res 2004;295:66–78.
7. Strauer BE, Brehm M, Zeus T, et al. Repair of infarcted myocardium by autologous intracoronary mononuclear bone marrow cell transplantation in humans. Circulation 2002;106:1913–18.
8. Assmus B, Schachinger V, Teupe C, et al. Transplantation of Progenitor Cells and Regeneration Enhancement in Acute Myocardial Infarction (TOPCARE-AMI). Circulation 2002;106:3009–17.
9. Perin EC, Dohmann HF, Borojevic R, et al. Transendocardial, autologous bone marrow cell transplantation for severe, chronic ischemic heart failure. Circulation 2003;107:2294–302.
10. Asahara T, Murohara T, Sullivan A, et al. Isolation of putative progenitor endothelial cells for angiogenesis. Science 1997;275:964–7.
11. Takahashi T, Kalka C, Masuda H, et al. Ischemia- and cytokine-induced mobilization of bone marrow-derived endothelial progenitor cells for neovascularization. Nat Med 1999;5:434–8.
12. Dib N, McCarthy P, Campbell A, et al. Feasibility and safety of autologous myoblast transplantation in patients with ischemic cardiomyopathy. Cell Transplant 2004;14(1):11–19.
13. Galinanes M, Loubani M, Davies J, Chin D, Pasi J, Bell PR. Autotransplantation of unmanipulated bone marrow into scarred myocardium is safe and enhances cardiac function in humans. Cell Transplant 2004;13:7–13.
14. Hagege AA, Carrion C, Menasche P, et al. Viability and differentiation of autologous skeletal myoblast

grafts in ischaemic cardiomyopathy. Lancet 2003; 361:491–2.
15. Hamano K, Nishida M, Hirata K, et al. Local implantation of autologous bone marrow cells for therapeutic angiogenesis in patients with ischemic heart disease: clinical trial and preliminary results. Jpn Circ J 2001;65:845–7.
16. Herreros J, Prosper F, Perez A, et al. Autologous intramyocardial injection of cultured skeletal muscle-derived stem cells in patients with non-acute myocardial infarction. Eur Heart J 2003;24: 2012–20.
17. Kang HJ, Kim HS, Zhang SY, et al. Effects of intracoronary infusion of peripheral blood stem-cells mobilised with granulocyte-colony stimulating factor on left ventricular systolic function and restenosis after coronary stenting in myocardial infarction: the MAGIC cell randomised clinical trial. Lancet 2004;363:751–6.
18. Menasche P, Vilquin JT, Desnos M. Early results of autologous skeletal myoblast transplantation in patients with severe ischemic heart failure. Circulation 2001;104(Suppl II):II-598.
19. Menasche P, Hagege AA, Vilquin JT, et al. Autologous skeletal myoblast transplantation for severe postinfarction left ventricular dysfunction. J Am Coll Cardiol 2003;41:1078–83.
20. Pagani FD, DerSimonian H, Zawadzka A, et al. Autologous skeletal myoblasts transplanted to ischemia-damaged myocardium in humans. Histological analysis of cell survival and differentiation. J Am Coll Cardiol 2003;41:879–88.
21. Smits PC, van Geuns RJ, Poldermans D, et al. Catheter-based intramyocardial injection of autologous skeletal myoblasts as a primary treatment of ischemic heart failure: clinical experience with six-month follow-up. J Am Coll Cardiol 2003;42: 2063–9.
22. Stamm C, Westphal B, Kleine HD, et al. Autologous bone-marrow stem-cell transplantation for myocardial regeneration. Lancet 2003;361:45–6.
23. Tse HF, Kwong YL, Chan JK, Lo G, Ho CL, Lau CP. Angiogenesis in ischaemic myocardium by intramyocardial autologous bone marrow mononuclear cell implantation. Lancet 2003;361:47–9.
24. Menasche P, Hagege AA, Scorsin M, et al. Myoblast transplantation for heart failure. Lancet 2001;357: 279–80.
25. Park SW, Gwon HC, Jeong JO, et al. Intracardiac echocardiographic guidance and monitoring during percutaneous endomyocardial gene injection in porcine heart. Hum Gene Ther 2001;12: 893–903.
26. Oron U, Halevy O, Yaakobi T, et al. Technical delivery of myogenic cells through an endocardial injection catheter for myocardial cell implantation. Int J Cardiovasc Intervent 2000;3:227–230.
27. Sanborn TA, Hackett NR, Lee LY, et al. Percutaneous endocardial transfer and expression of genes to the myocardium utilizing fluoroscopic guidance. Catheter Cardiovasc Interv 2001;52:260–6.
28. Sanborn TA. Catheter-based therapeutic angiogenesis: fluoroscopic versus electromechanical mapping and guidance. J Invasive Cardiol 2001; 13:328–9.
29. Garot J, Unterseeh T, Teiger E, et al. Magnetic resonance imaging of targeted catheter-based implantation of myogenic precursor cells into infarcted left ventricular myocardium. J Am Coll Cardiol 2003;41:1841–6.
30. Lederman RJ, Guttman MA, Peters DC, et al. Catheter-based endomyocardial injection with real-time magnetic resonance imaging. Circulation 2002;105:1282–4.
31. Soufer R, Dey HM, Ng CK, Zaret BL. Comparison of sestamibi single-photon emission computed tomography with positron emission tomography for estimating left ventricular myocardial viability. Am J Cardiol 1995;75:1214–19.
32. Pittenger MF, Mackay AM, Beck SC, et al. Multilineage potential of adult human mesenchymal stem cells. Science 1999;284:143–7.
33. Balsam LB, Wagers AJ, Christensen JL, Kofidis T, Weissman IL, Robbins RC. Haematopoietic stem cells adopt mature haematopoietic fates in ischaemic myocardium. Nature 2004;428:668–73.
34. Murry CE, Soonpaa MH, Reinecke H, et al. Haematopoietic stem cells do not transdifferentiate into cardiac myocytes in myocardial infarcts. Nature 2004;428:664–8.

chapter 10

Patients with End-Stage Ischemic Heart Failure: a Growing Target Population for Cardiac Stem Cell Therapy

Pilar Jimenez-Quevedo, Ricardo Sanz, and Javier Lopez

Introduction

About 22% of men and 46% of women with myocardial infarctions will be disabled by congestive heart failure (CHF) within 6 years after the infarction.[1] Currently, 4.6 million Americans have CHF, and 550 000 new cases are added annually.[2] This is the only type of cardiovascular disease whose prevalence, incidence, and mortality have generally increased over the past 25 years. With the aging of the Western population and the decline in mortality related to other types of cardiovascular disease, CHF can be expected to take an even greater toll on public health.

This chapter concentrates on patients with end-stage CHF who are not candidates for standard therapies, and it discusses the alternative strategies that have been developed during the last few decades.

"No-Option" Patients

Percutaneous coronary intervention (PCI) and coronary artery bypass grafting (CABG) are effective at relieving symptoms and improving outcomes in patients with CAD. Despite advances in medical treatment and revascularization, some patients with symptomatic CAD are no longer candidates for percutaneous or surgical revascularization. These "no-option" patients may account for up to 12% of those referred for diagnostic catheterization.[3] Their number is growing, mainly because life expectancy is increasing, even in patients with advanced disease. Many of these patients have already undergone multiple PCIs or previous surgical revascularization, and thus are not candidates for additional procedures. Other conditions that result in "no-option" status include diffuse CAD (Figure 10.1), small distal vessels, recurrent in-stent restenosis, chronic total occlusion (Figure 10.2), and comorbidities that preclude any conventional revascularization technique.

However, "no-option" patients are a heterogeneous group. Myocardial viability identifies two different clinical and prognostic patterns in this population. The first group includes patients with a substantial amount of viable myocardium, in whom angina is the predominant symptom. In these patients, improved myocardial perfusion may relieve symptoms, improve the left ventricular ejection fraction (LVEF), reverse ventricular remodeling,[4] and increase survival.[5] Conversely, the second group includes patients with limited or no myocardial viability, in whom heart failure symptoms predominate. This group has a poorer response to increased myocardial perfusion.[6]

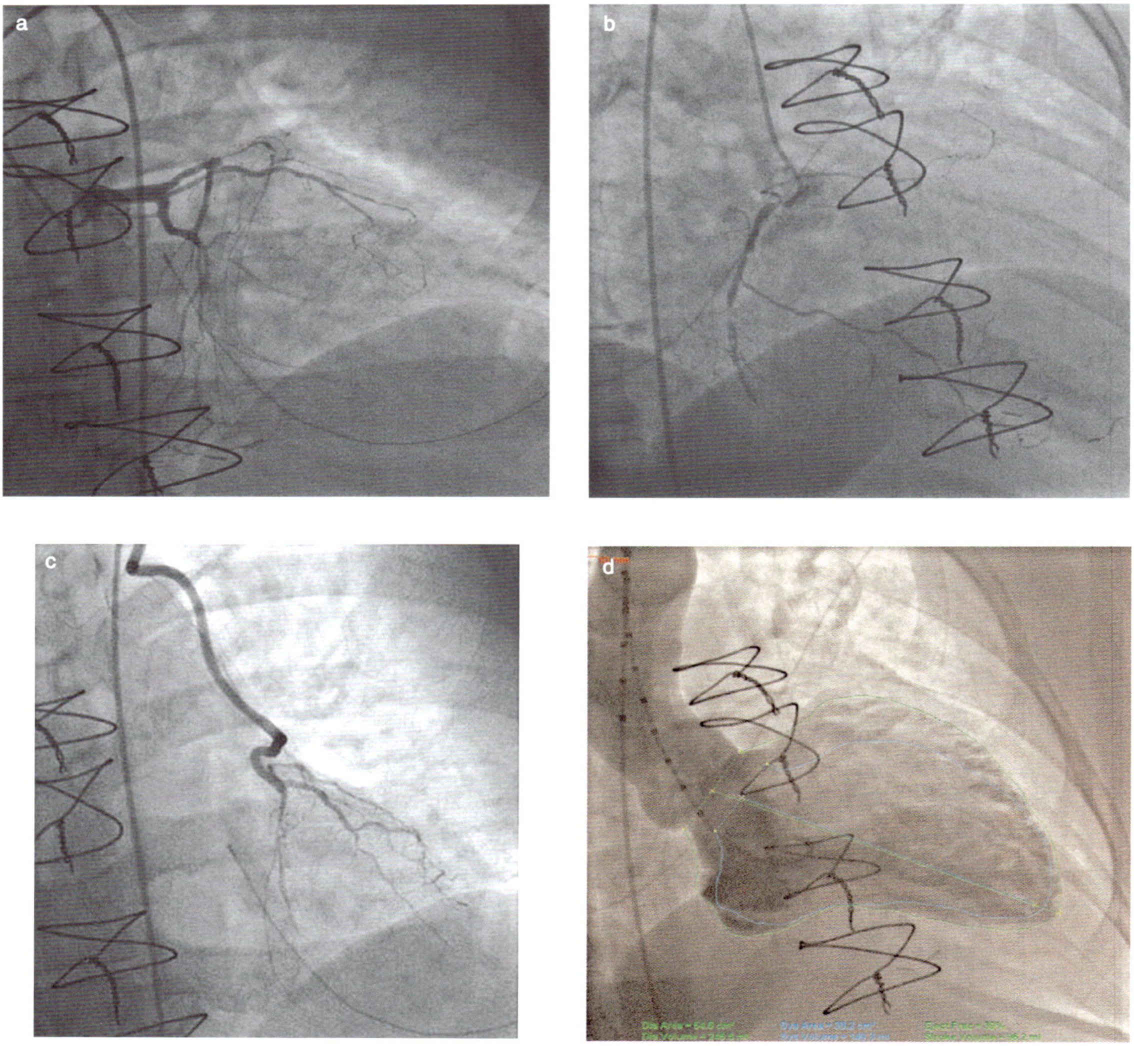

Figure 10.1 *Coronary angiography showing the coronary anatomy of a patient without the option for myocardial revascularization with surgery or angioplasty. (a) Left coronary tree, with occluded left anterior descending (LAD) and circumflex arteries. (b) Occlusion of the mid segment of the right coronary artery. (c) The left internal mammary artery graft to the LAD is patent, but the distal part of the native LAD is diffusely diseased and occluded. (d) Left ventriculogram analysis showing an ejection fraction of 39%.*

Establishing the "no-option" status requires a multidisciplinary approach, which should include cardiologists and cardiac surgeons. It is important to ensure that all conventional medical therapies are applied at the maximally tolerated dose. These therapies include antianginal agents (β-blockers, calcium-channel blockers, and nitrates), antiplatelet agents, angiotensin-converting enzyme (ACE) inhibitors, statins, and diuretics. In addition, the patient's lifestyle must be modified, and secondary causes of angina such as anemia and uncontrolled hypertension

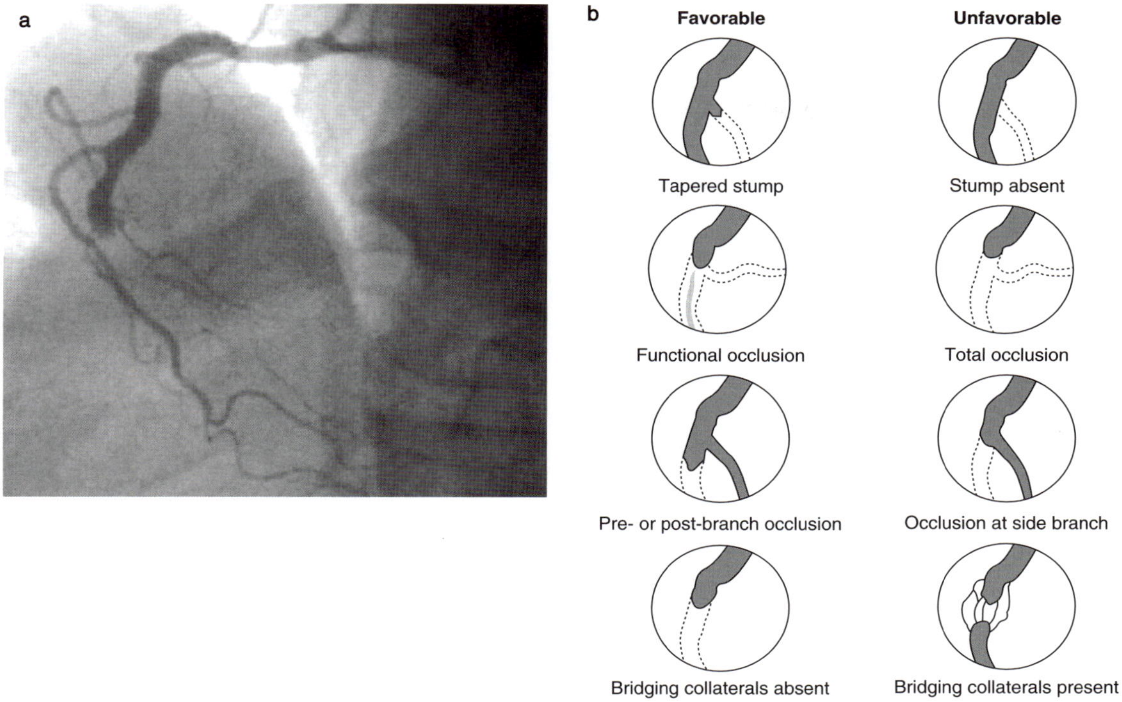

Figure 10.2 (a) Chronic total occlusion of the mid segment of the right coronary artery. (b) Anatomic patterns predicting success of percutaneous treatment of a chronic total occlusion. Adapted from Freed M. Chronic total occlusion. In: Freed M, Grineds C, Safian R (eds). The New Manual of Interventional Cardiology, Birmingham, MI: Physician's Press, 1996.

must be excluded. Despite optimal conventional therapy, many patients continue to have not only severe symptoms that limit their quality of life but also a poor long-term clinical outcome with an increased incidence of myocardial infarction and mortality.[7]

Adaptation After Myocardial Ischemia: Development of Collateral Circulation

When vascular obstruction in either circulatory system is so extensive that direct revascularization cannot be undertaken successfully, the heart spontaneously develops new collateral blood vessels to supply the ischemic area. The severity of residual ischemia will largely depend on the ability to create these new vessels.[8]

The coronary collateral circulation is an anastomotic vascular network that interconnects the three major epicardial coronary arteries and plays a protective role in the different clinical presentations of ischemic heart disease (Figure 10.3). Thus, in patients with a myocardial infarction, collaterals limit infarct size, preserve viability, and reduce long-term mortality;[9–12] in stable coronary artery disease,[13] they are associated with fewer cases of angina. Collaterals protect against perioperative myocardial infarction and ischemia during off-pump cardiac surgery and decrease the rate of adverse events after PCI.[14]

Previous human studies have shown that newly developing collaterals become visible on angiograms within a maximum of 10 days after persistent acute occlusion.[15] However, the exact timing of collateral development in humans remains uncertain, as the collateral status before

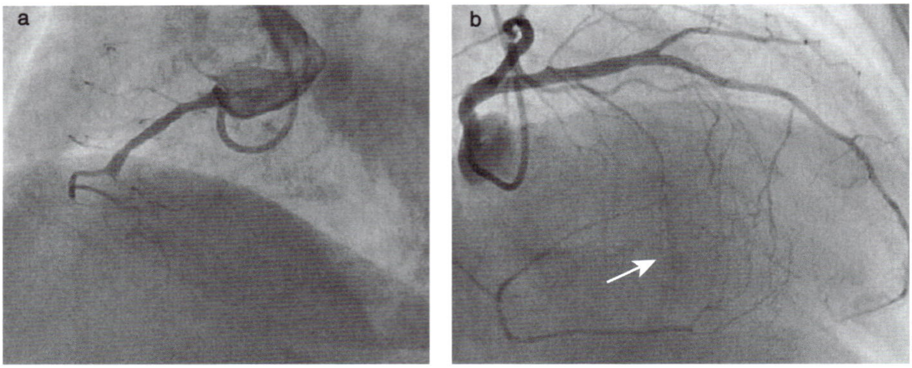

Figure 10.3 Collateral circulation in a patient with chronic total occlusion. (a) Chronic total occlusion at the mid segment of the right coronary artery. (b) Collateral circulation from the left anterior descending artery (arrow).

a coronary occlusion occurs is not known. In studies of an animal model of hind-limb occlusion,[16] collateral circulation started within 24 hours, becoming almost complete after 1 week. Other studies have shown that full functional maturation takes 8–12 weeks.[17,18]

Two methods have been described for assessing collateral circulation in humans:

- In the quantitative method, which is the only direct approach to collateral assessment, flow velocity and pressure are measured distal to an occlusion. Collateral function is quantified by calculating a collateral flow index on the basis of pressure recordings[19] or Doppler recordings.
- In the nonquantitative method, which uses angiography and is based on the Rentrop Classification (Table 10.1) a threshold value >1 indicates the presence of collateral circulation.[20] Although the quantitative method is an approximation of collateral functions, it has a higher spatial resolution than does the nonquantitative method.[21]

Table 10.1 The Rentrop Classification[a]

Grade	*Definition*
0	No visible filling of any collateral channel
1	Filling of the side branches of the occluded artery; no dye reaches the epicardial segment
2	Partial filling of the epicardial vessel
3	Complete filling of the epicardial vessel by collateral vessels

[a]Adapted from Rentrop KP et al. J Am Coll Cardiol 1985;5: 587–92[20] with permission from the American College of Cardiology Foundation.

Understanding how collateral blood vessels form has been one of the most challenging objectives of the past decade. Unraveling these mechanisms would offer therapeutic options for ameliorating or perhaps even curing today's leading causes of mortality. Growth of collateral vessels involves two different processes – angiogenesis and arteriogenesis – designed to supply blood flow in subtended tissues in the presence of arterial occlusion (Table 10.2). In arteriogenesis, a preexisting arteriole of the resistance-vessel class matures into an artery of the conductance-vessel class, whereas, in angiogenesis, new capillaries arise from a preexisting capillary.[22]

The development of collaterals after sudden or slowly progressing stenosis of coronary arteries depends on the endothelium and inflammatory cells, which lead to the interaction of locally

Table 10.2 Differences between angiogenesis and arteriogenesis

	Angiogenesis	*Arteriogenesis*
Source	Preexisting capillaries	Preexisting arterioles
Trigger	Ischemia	Shear stress
Increases blood flow maximally	1.5- to 1.7-fold increase	10- to 20-fold increase
Compensates for an occluded artery	No	Yes

Table 10.3 Alternative medical treatment in "no-option" patients

Drug	*Mechanism of action*
Partial inhibitor of fatty acid oxidation	Inhibits fatty acid metabolism and promotes glycolysis, making the heart more energy-efficient
Potassium-channel activator	Dilates arteries and veins
Endothelin receptor blocker	Causes vasodilatation
Ivabradine	Inhibits a specific sinus node pacemaker, thus reducing the heart rate
Testosterone	Causes coronary vasodilatation and increases blood hemoglobin levels
Thrombolytic therapy	Dissolves thrombus and improves blood viscosity, increasing coronary blood flow
Adenosine	Causes vasodilatation
Heparin	May accelerate collateral vessel formation

generated growth factors and cytokines.[23,24] In addition, recent studies have shown that normal adults have a small number of circulating endothelial progenitor cells in their peripheral blood. In response to cytokine stimulation and an ischemic insult, these cells mobilize from bone marrow, home to the ischemic tissue, and contribute to neovascularization and angiogenesis. On the other hand, factors that may negatively affect the angiogenesis process include advanced age,[8] the presence of diabetes mellitus,[25–27] and impaired renal function.[28]

New Strategies for Teatment

Nonconventional pharmacotherapy

A diverse group of drugs with documented anti-ischemic effects may potentially play a role as alternative medical treatments in "no-option" patients. These drugs include metabolic myocardial modulators,[29–36] potassium-channel activators,[37] endothelin receptor blockers,[38,39] ivabradine,[40] testosterone,[41,42] intravenous thrombolytic agents, adenosine, and heparin (Table 10.3). To date, however, there has been no evidence that they benefit the "no-option" population, and certain safety issues need to be resolved before they can be considered for standard therapy.

Transmyocardial laser revascularization

Transmyocardial laser revascularization (TMLR) uses laser ablation to create transmural channels in the ischemic myocardium in order to restore myocardial perfusion. The physiologic premise behind the application of TMLR is based on the work of investigators who were seeking to emulate the reptilian circulation in the mammalian heart by creating conduits for blood to flow from the ventricular cavity into the myocardium.

The mechanism of action of TMLR is still uncertain. The laser may destroy sympathetic nerve endings, thus resulting in a form of sympathectomy,[43] it may improve myocardial perfusion secondary to angiogenesis,[44] or it may simply have a placebo effect. At present, two types of lasers are being evaluated in the treatment of refractory angina: the carbon dioxide (CO_2) and the holmium:yttrium aluminium garnet (Ho:YAG) lasers. Animal experiments have shown that both lasers produce histologic effects after 6 weeks but that thermoacoustic damage is greater with the Ho:YAG device.[45]

Several randomized trials evaluating surgical TMLR in "no-option" versus medically treated patients have shown symptomatic improvement after TMLR. In the first study, Schofield et al[46] randomly assigned 188 patients to either TMLR or medical treatment. At 1 year, the TMLR patients had better angina scores and less need for anti-anginal medications but no improvement in exercise capacity. Frazier et al[47] randomized 192 patients to receive either TMLR or medical therapy. At 12 months, the TMLR group had a significant improvement in angina class, quality-of-life scores, and cardiac perfusion, as assessed by single-photon emission computed tomography (SPECT). Similarly, Burkhoff et al[48] reported better total exercise tolerance and quality of life at 1 year but no intergroup differences in myocardial perfusion or ejection fraction. Only one trial has shown that TMLR has survival benefits. Allen et al[49] demonstrated that patients randomized to undergo TMLR versus medical treatment had a significantly increased Kaplan–Meier survival rate. Interestingly, however, neither group had an improvement in myocardial perfusion. Finally, a meta-analysis of seven randomized trials, involving TMLR in 1053 patients, showed that TMLR significantly improved the angina class but not the survival rate.[50] In all of these trials, post-TMLR complications were almost always cardiac, and included myocardial infarction, left ventricular failure, atrial fibrillation, and ventricular arrhythmias. The perioperative mortality rate has ranged from 3% to 5% in most reports, but rates as high as 12% have been described.

Recently, percutaneous TMLR has been advocated to reduce the perioperative mortality of surgical TMLR. The results after percutaneous TMLR are similar to those seen in open-chest studies.[51]

In conclusion, TMLR causes clinical improvement but does not increase survival. Moreover, it is impossible to judge how large a role the placebo effect plays, as symptomatic benefits do not always correlate with objective findings (improved LVEF or myocardial perfusion). Therefore, measurable physiologic benefits will have to be demonstrated, beyond any placebo effect, before TMLR can become an established option for treating coronary artery disease.

Enhanced external counterpulsation

Enhanced external counterpulsation (EECP) uses three sets of cuffs to compress the vascular beds of the leg and thigh in a sequential manner timed to the patient's electrocardiogram (ECG). The cuffs are wrapped around the patient's legs and, using compressed air, sequential pressure (300 mmHg) is applied from the lower legs to the lower and upper thighs during early diastole to propel blood back to the heart. This technique increases the mean arterial blood pressure, the retrograde aortic blood flow during diastole causing diastolic augmentation,[52] and coronary perfusion.[53] In a multicenter randomized controlled trial (MUST-EECP),[54] 139 patients with angina and documented ischemia on treadmill testing were randomized to receive 35 hours of active counterpulsation (300 mmHg of cuff pressure) or inactive counterpulsation (75 mmHg of cuff pressure) for 4–7 weeks. The active group had a significant decrease in angina episodes and nitroglycerin usage. Moreover, the time to $\geq$1 mm ST-segment depression also increased in the active group compared with the inactive group. Other registries have shown the same results: most of the patients (including diabetic patients) treated with EECP have experienced a significant reduction in angina and improvement in quality of life[55,56] that have persisted for more than 2 years.[57,58] Despite reports of clinical improvement, more clinical data are required before EECP can be recommended as standard therapy.[59]

Neurostimulation

Neurostimulation methods attempt to palliate angina by interrupting or modulating the afferent neural signals through which pain is perceived. There are two modalities of neurostimulation: transcutaneous electrical nerve stimulation (TENS) and spinal cord stimulation (SCS).

Based on the "gate-control theory," TENS provides transcutaneous stimulation at large, high-frequency, non-nociceptive myelinated type A fibers. It also inhibits the neural impulse through smaller unmyelinated type C fibers, reducing the activation of central pain receptors. In addition, TENS reduces sympathetic discharge, leading to a decrease in the cardiac workload and myocardial oxygen demand.[60] In studies with TENS, increased exercise capacity and reduced ischemia have been noted on the exercise ECG, along with decreased angina and reduced nitrate use.[61]

In SCS, the epidural space is punctured at the level of the 4th or 6th thoracic vertebra, and an electrode is introduced to the level of the T_1–T_2 dorsal epidural space. An electrode stimulator is then placed subcutaneously in the upper left side of the abdomen. Stimulation of this electrode suppresses the capacity of intrinsic cardiac sympathetic neurons to generate activity during myocardial ischemia, thereby decreasing pain[62] and redistributing myocardial blood flow from nonischemic to ischemic areas.[63] Initial studies documented a reduction in angina, an increase in exercise capacity, and a reduction in the degree of ST-segment depression at a given workload.[64] Later, Hautvast et al[65] showed decreased ischemic ECG changes during ambulatory 48-hour monitoring in patients with refractory angina. Greco et al[66] reported a significant decrease in New York Heart Association (NYHA) functional class without any effect on mortality. Spinal cord stimulation does not induce adverse effects in patients with transient ischemia,[67] who retain their capacity to sense angina during an increased workload.[68] This method prevents hospital admissions without leading to silent infarctions and also reduces the mean duration of hospitalization.[69]

The only randomized trial of SCS, the Electrical Stimulation versus Coronary Bypass Surgery (ESBY) trial,[70] showed that SCS is equivalent to CABG in terms of symptom relief. However, the CABG group had a better exercise capacity and less ST-segment depression at maximum and comparable workloads. It also had a higher 6-month mortality and more cerebrovascular events. Therefore, the researchers concluded that SCS is an alternative to CABG in patients at high operative risk.

In summary, symptoms and ischemia seem to improve with either TENS or SCS, but the SCS data are more convincing. On the other hand, neither of these methods has any effect on survival, myocardial infarction, left ventricular function, or the need for repeat revascularization. Concerns about neurostimulation include the invasive nature of SCS and cutaneous side effects of TENS, as well as a strong placebo effect.[71] In fact, the 2002 American College of Cardiology/ American Heart Association guidelines on the treatment of chronic stable angina[59] state that more data are needed about intermediate and long-term outcomes before neurostimulation can be accepted as a standard treatment for refractory angina.

Percutaneous in situ coronary venous arterialization

These approaches supply blood to the ischemic myocardium retrogradely through the venous system. Percutaneous in situ coronary venous arterialization (PICVA) redirects arterial blood flow from the occluded artery into an adjacent coronary vein, thereby arterializing the vein and retroperfusing the ischemic myocardium. Percutaneous in situ coronary artery bypass (PICAB) is a variant of PICVA in which arterial blood flow is redirected from a diseased artery to an adjacent coronary vein, and is then rerouted back to the original artery, to a position beyond the lesion.[71,72] Although still at an experimental stage, these technologies currently offer a feasible alternative for "no-option" patients with refractory angina and may have great potential for the future.

Gene therapy

To treat refractory angina, gene transfer technology with growth factors has been proposed to induce angiogenesis and arteriogenesis.

The following substances have been shown to stimulate these processes: vascular endothelial growth factor (VEGF), fibroblast growth factor (FGF), platelet-derived growth factor (PDGF), platelet-activating factor (PAF), angioproteins, cytokines such as interleukins, master switch genes, hypoxia-inducible factor 1α (HIF-1α), and nitric oxide (NO).

By increasing the rate of endothelial cell proliferation, VEGF improves myocardial perfusion and the angina functional class. This growth factor has been used intramuscularly as plasmid-encoded VEGF and with adenoviral vectors. All patients have reported symptomatic improvement with no evidence of systemic or cardiac toxicity.[73–75]

FGF also increases the rate of endothelial cell proliferation. Basic FGF (bFGF), delivered in sustained-release microcapsules, improved patient perception of angina.[76] Recombinant FGF, studied via the intracoronary and intravenous routes, improved SPECT perfusion abnormalities.[77] The first randomized, double-blinded, placebo-controlled trial of gene therapy was performed with intracoronary delivery of recombinant adenovirus 5 FGF-4.[78] The treatment group had a greater improvement in exercise duration than did the placebo group, but the latter group had a marked improvement from baseline, demonstrating an important placebo effect.

Because of the lack of randomized trials, the true efficacy of gene therapy cannot be definitively evaluated. Researchers still do not know whether the improvements in myocardial perfusion can be attributed to angiogenesis.[71] In addition, the safest, most effective delivery strategy for inducing angiogenesis in ischemic myocardium is uncertain and needs further study.[72] Potential complications include aberrant vascular proliferation, increased vascular permeability leading to edema, triggering of unrecognized neoplasms, proatherogenic effects, and induction of immune or inflammatory responses.[72]

Stem Cell Therapy

Stem cell transplantation is a promising area for the treatment of end-stage heart disease.[79] Several cell types have been suggested as potential sources for tissue grafts, including skeletal myoblasts, fibroblasts, endothelial progenitor cells, smooth muscle cells, mesenchymal cells, and embryonic cells. Increasing evidence from preclinical and clinical studies suggests that cell therapy may improve myocardial perfusion and LVEF.

Human hearts have a minimal regenerative capacity after traumas such as a myocardial infarction. Therefore, so far, therapy for end-stage ischemic cardiomyopathy has been based on the improvement of myocardial perfusion. Now, with the advent of stem cell therapy and the possibility of cardiac regeneration, the "no-option" concept should be extended to include patients with end-stage heart failure, myocardial nonviability, and nonischemic cardiomyopathy who are not candidates for cardiac transplantation.

References

1. American Heart Association. Heart Disease and Stroke Statistics – 2005 Update. Dallas: American Heart Association, 2005:2–16.
2. Cooper R, Cutler J, Desvigne-Nickens P, et al. Trends and disparities in coronary heart disease, stroke, and other cardiovascular diseases in the United States: findings of the national conference on cardiovascular disease prevention. Circulation 2000;102:3137–47.
3. Mukherjee D, Bhatt DL, Roe MT, Patel V, Ellis SG. Direct myocardial revascularization and angiogenesis – how many patients might be eligible? Am J Cardiol 1999;84:598–600.
4. Rizzello V, Poldermans D, Boersma E, et al. Opposite patterns of left ventricular remodeling after coronary revascularization in patients with ischemic cardiomyopathy: role of myocardial viability. Circulation 2004;110:2383–8.
5. Di Carli MF, Maddahi J, Rokhsar S, et al. Long-term survival of patients with coronary artery disease and left ventricular dysfunction: implications for the role of myocardial viability assessment in management decisions. J Thorac Cardiovasc Surg 1998;116:997–1004.
6. Rizzello V, Poldermans D, Biagini E, et al. Relation of improvement in left ventricular ejection fraction versus improvement in heart failure symptoms after coronary revascularization in patients with ischemic cardiomyopathy. Am J Cardiol 2005;96:386–9.
7. Mukherjee D, Comella K, Bhatt DL, Roe MT, Patel V, Ellis SG. Clinical outcome of a cohort of

patients eligible for therapeutic angiogenesis or transmyocardial revascularization. Am Heart J 2001;142:72–4.
8. Rivard A, Fabre JE, Silver M, et al. Age-dependent impairment of angiogenesis. Circulation 1999; 99:111–20.
9. Habib GB, Heibig J, Forman SA, et al. Influence of coronary collateral vessels on myocardial infarct size in humans: results of phase I Thrombolysis In Myocardial Infarction (TIMI) trial: the TIMI Investigators. Circulation 1991;83:739–46.
10. Charney R, Cohen M. The role of the coronary collateral circulation in limiting myocardial ischemia and infarct size. Am Heart J 1993;126: 937–45.
11. Sabia PJ, Powers ER, Ragosta M, Sarembock IJ, Burwell LR, Kaul S. An association between collateral blood flow and myocardial viability in patients with recent myocardial infarction. N Engl J Med 1992;327:1825–31.
12. Antoniucci D, Valenti R, Moschi G, et al. Relation between preintervention angiographic evidence of coronary collateral circulation and clinical and angiographic outcomes after primary angioplasty or stenting for acute myocardial infarction. Am J Cardiol 2002;89:121–5.
13. Cohen M, Rentrop KP. Limitation of myocardial ischemia by collateral circulation during sudden controlled coronary artery occlusion in human subjects: a prospective study. Circulation 1986;74: 469–76.
14. Nathoe HM, Buskens E, Jansen EW, et al. Role of coronary collaterals in off-pump and on-pump coronary bypass surgery. Circulation 2004;110: 1738–42.
15. Schwartz H, Leiboff RH, Bren GB, et al. Temporal evolution of the human coronary collateral circulation after myocardial infarction. J Am Coll Cardiol 1984;4:1088–93.
16. Herzog S, Sager H, Khmelevski E, Deylig A, Ito WD. Collateral arteries grow from preexisting anastomoses in the rat hindlimb. Am J Physiol Heart Circ Physiol 2002;283:H2012–20.
17. Gorge G, Schmidt T, Ito BR, Pantely GA, Schaper W. Microvascular and collateral adaptation in swine hearts following progressive coronary artery stenosis. Basic Res Cardiol 1989;84:524–35.
18. Boatwright RB, Williams DO, Rugh KS, et al. Distribution of coronary collateral blood flow at different levels of collateral growth in conscious ponies. Am J Physiol 1992;263:H1145–53.
19. Seiler C, Fleisch M, Garachemani A, et al. Coronary collateral quantitation in patients with coronary artery disease using intravascular flow velocity or pressure measurements. J Am Coll Cardiol 1998;32:1272–9.
20. Rentrop KP, Cohen M, Blanke H, Phillips RA. Changes in collateral channel filling immediately after controlled coronary artery occlusion by an angioplasty balloon in human subjects. J Am Coll Cardiol 1985;5:587–92.
21. L'Abbate A, Sambuceti G, Haunso S, Schneider-Eicke J. Methods for evaluating coronary microvasculature in humans. Eur Heart J 1999;20: 1300–13.
22. Schaper W, Scholz D. Factors regulating arteriogenesis. Arterioscler Thromb Vasc Biol 2003;23: 1143–51.
23. Van Royen N, Piek JJ, Schaper W, Bode C, Buschmann I. Arteriogenesis: mechanisms and modulation of collateral artery development. J Nucl Cardiol 2001;8:687–93.
24. Helisch A, Schaper W. Arteriogenesis: The development and growth of collateral arteries. Microcirculation 2003;10:83–97.
25. Duh E, Aielo LP. Vascular endothelial growth factor and diabetes: the agonist versus antagonist paradox. Diabetes 1999;48:1899–906.
26. Waltenberger J. Impaired collateral vessel development in diabetes: potential cellular mechanisms and therapeutic implications. Cardiovasc Res 2001; 49:554–60.
27. Chou E, Suzuma I, Way KJ, et al. Decreased cardiac expression of vascular endothelial growth factor and its receptors in insulin-resistant and diabetic states: a possible explanation for impaired collateral formation in cardiac tissue. Circulation 2002; 105:373–9.
28. Chiarelli F, Cipollone F, Mohn A, et al. Circulating monocyte chemoattractant protein-1 and early development of nephropathy in type 1 diabetes. Diabetes Care 2002;25:1829–34.
29. Cole PL, Beamer AD, McGowan N, et al. Efficacy and safety of perhexiline maleate in refractory angina. A double-blind placebo-controlled clinical trial of a novel antianginal agent. Circulation 1990;81:1260–70.
30. Stewart S, Voss DW, Northey DL, et al. Relationship between plasma perhexiline concentration and symptomatic status during short-term perhexiline therapy. Ther Drug Monit 1996;18:635–9.
31. Szwed H, Sadowski Z, Elikowski W, et al. Combination treatment in stable effort angina using trimetazidine and metoprolol: results of a randomized, double-blind, multicentre study (TRIMPOL II). TRIMetazidine in POLand. Eur Heart J 2001; 22:2267–74.
32. Marzilli M, Klein WW. Efficacy and tolerability of trimetazidine in stable angina: a meta-analysis of randomized, double-blind, controlled trials. Coron Artery Dis 2003;14:171–9.
33. Effect of 48-h intravenous trimetazidine on short- and long-term outcomes of patients with acute myocardial infarction, with and without thrombolytic therapy: a double-blind, placebo-controlled, randomized trial. The EMIP-FR Group.

European Myocardial Infarction Project – Free Radicals. Eur Heart J 2000;21:1537–46.
34. Guler N, Eryonucu B, Gunes A, et al. Effects of trimetazidine on submaximal exercise test in patients with acute myocardial infarction. Cardiovasc Drugs Ther 2003;17:371–4.
35. Wolff AA. The MARISA Investigators and CV Therapeutics. MARISA: Monotherapy Assessment of Ranolazine in Stable Angina. J Am Coll Cardiol 2000;35:408A.
36. Chaitman BR, Pepine CJ, Parker JO, et al. Effects of ranolazine with atenolol, amlodipine, or diltiazem on exercise tolerance and angina frequency in patients with severe chronic angina: a randomized controlled trial. JAMA 2004;291:309–16.
37. IONA Study group. Effect of nicorandil on coronary events in patients with stable angina: the Impact Of Nicorandil in Angina (IONA) randomised trial. Lancet 2002;359:1269–75.
38. Wenzel RR, Fleisch M, Shaw S, et al. Hemodynamic and coronary effects of the endothelin antagonist bosentan in patients with coronary artery disease. Circulation 1998;98:2235–40.
39. Kyriakides ZS, Kremastinos DT, Kolettis TM, Tasouli A, Antoniadis A, Webb DJ. Acute endothelin-A receptor antagonism prevents normal reduction of myocardial ischemia on repeated balloon inflations during angioplasty. Circulation 2000;102:1937–43.
40. Borer JS, Fox K, Jaillon P, Lerebours G; Ivabradine Investigators Group. Antianginal and antiischemic effects of ivabradine, an I(f) inhibitor, in stable angina: a randomized, double-blind, multicentered, placebo-controlled trial. Circulation 2003;107: 817–23.
41. Rosano GM, Leonardo F, Pagnotta P, et al. Acute anti-ischemic effect of testosterone in men with coronary artery disease. Circulation 1999;99:1666–70.
42. English KM, Steeds RP, Jones TH, Diver MJ, Channer KS. Low-dose transdermal testosterone therapy improves angina threshold in men with chronic stable angina: a randomized, double-blind, placebo-controlled study. Circulation 2000;102: 1906–11.
43. Kwong KF, Kanellopoulos GK, Nickols JC, et al. Transmyocardial laser treatment denervates canine myocardium. J Thorac Cardiovasc Surg 1997;114: 883–9.
44. Roethy W, Yamamoto N, Burkhoff D. An examination of potential mechanisms underlying transmyocardial laser revascularization induced increases in myocardial blood flow. Semin Thorac Cardiovasc Surg 1999;11:24–8.
45. Fisher PE, Khomoto T, DeRosa CM, Spotnitz HM, Smith CR, Burkhoff D. Histologic analysis of transmyocardial channels: comparison of CO_2 and holmium:YAG lasers. Ann Thorac Surg 1997;64: 466–72.
46. Schofield PM, Sharples LD, Caine N, et al. Transmyocardial laser revascularisation in patients with refractory angina: a randomised controlled trial. Lancet 1999;353:519–24.
47. Frazier OH, March RJ, Horvath KA. Transmyocardial revascularization with a carbon dioxide laser in patients with end-stage coronary artery disease. N Engl J Med 1999;341:1021–8.
48. Burkhoff D, Schmidt S, Schulman SP, et al. Transmyocardial laser revascularisation compared with continued medical therapy for treatment of refractory angina pectoris: a prospective randomised trial. ATLANTIC Investigators. Angina Treatments – Lasers and Normal Therapies in Comparison. Lancet 1999;354:885–90.
49. Allen KB, Dowling RD, Angell WW, et al. Transmyocardial revascularization: 5-year follow-up of a prospective, randomized multicenter trial. Ann Thorac Surg 2004;77:1228–34.
50. Liao L, Sarria-Santamera A, Matchar DB, et al. Meta-analysis of survival and relief of angina pectoris after transmyocardial revascularization. Am J Cardiol 2005;95:1243–5.
51. Oesterle SN, Sanborn TA, Ali N, et al. Percutaneous transmyocardial laser revascularisation for severe angina: the PACIFIC randomised trial. Potential Class Improvement From Intramyocardial Channels. Lancet 2000;356:1705–10.
52. Sinvhal RM, Gowda RM, Khan IA. Enhanced external counterpulsation for refractory angina pectoris. Heart 2003;89:830–3.
53. Michaels AD, Accad M, Ports TA, Grossman W. Left ventricular systolic unloading and augmentation of intracoronary pressure and Doppler flow during enhanced external counterpulsation. Circulation 2002;106:1237–42.
54. Arora RR, Chou TM, Jain D, et al. The Multicenter Study of Enhanced External Counterpulsation (MUST-EECP): effect of EECP on exercise-induced myocardial ischemia and anginal episodes. J Am Coll Cardiol 1999;33:1833–40.
55. Lawson WE, Hui JC, Lang G. Treatment benefit in the enhanced external counterpulsation consortium. Cardiology 2000;94:31–5.
56. Linnemeier G, Rutter MK, Barsness G, Kennard ED, Nesto RW; IEPR Investigators. Enhanced external counterpulsation for the relief of angina in patients with diabetes: safety, efficacy and 1-year clinical outcomes. Am Heart J 2003;146:453–8.
57. Lawson WE, Hui JC, Cohn PF. Long-term prognosis of patients with angina treated with enhanced external counterpulsation: five-year follow-up study. Clin Cardiol 2000;23:254–8.
58. Michaels AD, Linnemeier G, Soran O, Kelsey SF, Kennard ED. Two-year outcomes after enhanced external counterpulsation for stable angina pectoris (from the International EECP Patient Registry [IEPR]). Am J Cardiol 2004;93:461–4.

59. Gibbons RJ, Abrams J, Chatterjee K, et al. American College of Cardiology; American Heart Association Task Force on Practice Guidelines. Committee on the Management of Patients With Chronic Stable Angina. ACC/AHA 2002 guideline update for the management of patients with chronic stable angina – summary article: a report of the American College of Cardiology/American Heart Association Task Force on Practice Guidelines (Committee on the Management of Patients With Chronic Stable Angina). Circulation 2003; 107:149–58.
60. Mannheimer C, Carlsson CA, Emanuelson H, et al. The effects of transcutaneous electrical stimulation in patients with severe angina pectoris. Circulation 1985;71:308–16.
61. Hautvast RWM, Brouwer J, DeJonste MJL, Lie KI. Effect of spinal cord stimulation on heart rate variability and myocardial ischemia in patients with chronic intractable angina pectoris: a prospective ambulatory electrocardiographic study. Clin Cardiol 1998;21:33–8.
62. Foreman RD, Linderoth B, Ardell JL, et al. Modulation of intrinsic cardiac neurons by spinal cord stimulation: implications for its therapeutic use in angina pectoris. Cardiovasc Res 2000;47:367–75.
63. Murray S, Collins PD, James MA. Neurostimulation treatment for angina pectoris. Heart 2000; 83:217–20.
64. Mannheimer C, Augustinsson LE, Carlsson CA, et al. Epidural spinal electrical stimulation in severe angina pectoris. Br Heart J 1988;49:46–61.
65. Hautvast RW, DeJongste MJ, Staal MJ, et al. Spinal cord stimulation in chronic intractable angina pectoris: a randomized, controlled efficacy study. Am Heart J 1998;137:1114–20.
66. Greco S, Auriti A, Fiume D, et al. Spinal cord stimulation for the treatment of refractory angina pectoris: a two-year follow up. Pacing Clin Electrophysiol 1999;22:26–32.
67. Sanderson JE, Brooksby P, Waterhouse D, Palmer RB, Neubauer K. Epidural spinal electrical stimulation for severe angina: a study of its effects on symptoms, exercise tolerance and degree of ischemia. Eur Heart J 1992;13:628–33.
68. Mannheimer C, Eliasson T, Andersson B, et al. Effects of spinal cord stimulation in angina pectoris induced by pacing and possible mechanisms of action. BMJ 1993;307:477–80.
69. Murray S, Carson KG, Ewings PD, Collins PD, James MA. Spinal cord stimulation significantly decreases the need for acute hospital admission for chest pain in patients with refractory angina pectoris. Heart 1999;82:89–92.
70. Mannheimer C, Eliasson T, Augustinsson LE, et al. Electrical stimulation versus coronary artery bypass surgery in severe angina pectoris: the ESBY study. Circulation 1998;37:1157–63.
71. Kim MC, Kini A, Sharma SK. Refractory angina pectoris: mechanism and therapeutic options. J Am Coll Cardiol 2002;39:923–34.
72. Gowda RM, Khan IA, Punukollu G, Vasavada BC, Nair CK. Treatment of refractory angina pectoris. Int J Cardiol 2005;101:1–7.
73. Baumgartner I, Pieczek A, Manor O, et al. Constitutive expression of ph VEGF 165 after intramuscular gene transfer promotes collateral vessel development in patients with critical limb ischemia. Circulation 1998;97:1114–23.
74. Losordo DW, Vale PR, Symes JF, et al. Gene therapy for myocardial angiogenesis: initial clinical results with direct myocardial injection of ph VEGF 165 as sole therapy for myocardial ischemia. Circulation 1998;98:2800–4.
75. Rosengart TK, Lee LY, Patel SR, et al. Angiogenesis gene therapy: phase I assessment of direct intramyocardial administration of an adenovirus vector expressing VEGF121 cDNA to individuals with clinically significant severe coronary artery disease. Circulation 1999;100:468–74.
76. Laham RJ, Sellke FW, Edelman ER, et al. Local perivascular delivery of basic fibroblast growth factor in patients undergoing coronary bypass surgery: results of a phase I randomized, double-blind, placebo-controlled trial. Circulation 1999; 100:1865–71.
77. Udelson JE, Dilsizian J, Laham RJ, et al. Therapeutic angiogenesis with recombinant fibroblast growth factor-2 improves stress and rest myocardial perfusion abnormalities in patients with severe patients with stable angina pectoris. Circulation 2000;102:1605–10.
78. Grines CL, Watkins MW, Helmer G, et al. Angiogenic Gene Therapy (AGENT) trial in patients with stable angina pectoris. Circulation 2002;105: 1291–7.
79. Perin EC, Silva GV. Stem cell therapy for cardiac diseases. Curr Opin Hematol 2004;11:399–403.

chapter 11

Stem Cell Delivery Modalities

Guilherme V Silva, Emerson C Perin, Amanda C Heinl-Green, Jonathan Clague, and Eric W Alton

Introduction

Recent advances in the understanding of stem cell biology have underscored the great clinical potential of cardiac stem cell therapy. The discovery that human adults retain the capacity for cardiac repair and vasculogenesis has broadened the horizon for the treatment of ischemic heart disease. However, the challenges facing cardiac stem cell therapy are multiple: What is the ideal stem cell? How many cells should be given? And, specific to the present discussion, how should those cells be given?

The current understanding of stem cell biology and kinetics gives us important clues as to how we should deliver stem cells. Obviously, the efficacy of therapeutic stem cells will depend in part on their successful delivery. Stem cells have been delivered indirectly through peripheral and coronary veins (transvascular delivery) and coronary arteries (intracoronary delivery). Alternatively, they have been delivered directly by way of intramyocardial injections via surgical, transendocardial, or transvenous approaches. Another potential delivery strategy is mobilization of stem cells from the bone marrow by means of cytokine therapy with or without peripheral harvesting. This chapter will address the most commonly utilized cell delivery strategies and the experimental and clinical evidence in support of each one.

Stem Cell Delivery: The Ideal Method

The main objective of any cell delivery modality is to achieve the ideal concentration of viable stem cells needed for repairing the myocardial region of interest. To that end, the ideal modality should have the following characteristics:

- *Safety*. Any cell delivery modality should have minimal procedure-related complications. The incidence of those complications should be well studied, and potential measures for avoiding unnecessary procedure-related morbidity should be implemented.
- *Ease of use and cost*. The ideal cell delivery modality should employ technology that can be easily understood and performed by practitioners. In addition, its cost–benefit ratio should be within range of the ratios for other, more traditional therapies for ischemic heart disease.
- *Widespread clinical utility*. The ideal cell delivery modality should be applicable across a wide range of clinical scenarios (e.g., chronic and acute myocardial ischemia, systolic and diastolic ischemic heart failure).
- *Targeting*. Cell delivery strategies must take into account different clinical settings and local milieus, since stem cells are believed to perform differently in response to different local signals. Therefore, placing stem cells precisely in an adequate cardiac environment should influence outcomes.
- *Product retention*. Notwithstanding the importance of local signaling, the cardiac environment may also help determine the extent of cell retention. The ideal delivery strategy should result in high rates of stem cell retention in the targeted myocardial segments.

Stem Cell Mobilization

After an acute myocardial infarction (AMI), mobilization of progenitor cells from the bone marrow has been shown to occur in humans, suggesting a "natural" attempt at cardiac repair.[1] In theory, therapeutic mobilization of bone marrow progenitor cells after an AMI would amplify the existing healing response. Because of its simplicity, mobilization of stem cells is an attractive delivery strategy.[2,3] This approach would not only obviate the need for invasive harvesting or delivery procedures but also take advantage of the clinical procedures already established for the use of progenitor cell-mobilizing granulocyte colony-stimulating factor (G-CSF) in treating hematologic disorders. However, safety concerns associated with "off-label" applications of G-CSF have been raised, given the possibility of adverse events in a different patient population and the theoretical possibility of tumorigenesis. In the recent MAGIC trial from South Korea,[4] an increased restenosis rate was thought to be related to the increased availability of inflammatory cells to recently injured but healing coronary arteries at stented sites. This finding is not surprising, since coronary artery disease, to a certain extent, is known to be a consequence of localized inflammation. It also highlights one of the potential drawbacks of stem cell mobilization—namely, the creation of a proinflammatory state that promotes the progression of atherosclerosis.

Transvascular Cell Delivery

Peripheral (intravenous) infusion

Peripheral (intravenous) infusion of stem cells as performed in bone marrow transplantation would be a very convenient—not to mention simple, widely available, and inexpensive—way of delivering therapeutic stem cells to myocardial targets. A study in a mouse model has confirmed that bone marrow cells infused into the peripheral circulation do indeed home in on peri-infarct areas.[2] However, the number of cells that reach the affected area is very small, and the technique would be most applicable only after an AMI, as it would rely on physiologic homing signals alone. Moreover, since peripherally infused stem cells home in on acutely infarcted areas only when injected within a few days after an AMI, this delivery strategy would be much less suitable for treating chronic myocardial ischemia.

The major drawback to using an intravenous route of cell delivery is the possibility that the therapeutic cells could become trapped in the microvasculature of the lungs, liver, and lymphoid tissues. This theoretical limitation of systemic transvenous delivery of stem cells has been confirmed experimentally. In a study by Toma et al,[5] human mesenchymal stem cells (MSCs) were injected into the left ventricular (LV) cavity of experimental mice; 4 days later, an estimated 0.44% of the injected cells remained in the myocardium, and the rest of the cells had localized to the spleen, liver, and lungs. Other studies using the systemic delivery approach have produced similar results, with very low local cell retention rates (<5%).[6,7] Thus, the transvenous delivery route appears unlikely to achieve the local cell concentration needed to produce a significant therapeutic benefit.

Retrograde coronary venous delivery

Although probably the least well studied vessels in the myocardial anatomy, the coronary sinus and coronary venous network have historically been used for a variety of therapeutic purposes and offer the advantage of a percutaneous approach. Retrograde synchronized diastolic coronary perfusion via the myocardial capillaries has been used to oxygenate acutely ischemic myocardium in patients with AMIs and unstable angina, patients in cardiogenic shock, and patients undergoing high-risk percutaneous transluminal coronary angioplasty (PTCA).[8] However, because of the complexity of this technique, it has never come into widespread clinical use. Pharmacologic agents such as antiarrhythmic drugs and fibrinolytic agents[9] have been delivered via the coronary sinus in cases when the arterial system was severely restricted. Cardiac surgeons have also used the coronary venous system to administer cardioplegic solution during surgical procedures.[10] Compared with coronary arterial delivery, coronary venous delivery allows substantially more contact time, which in turn enhances regional delivery, tissue binding, and the myocardial concentration of the therapeutic product being delivered.[11] It also can be performed in "no-option" patients who have total coronary artery occlusions. This makes it a promising delivery route for cell therapy.

Coronary venous delivery techniques

Two methodologies have been described for the delivery of products via the coronary venous system. Low-pressure delivery aims to increase the amount of time that the therapeutic product is in contact with the vessels without disrupting the venous endothelium.[11–13] High-pressure delivery aims to create a biologic reservoir of product by disrupting the tight endothelial junctions of the venocapillary vasculature and mechanically driving cells across them into the myocardial interstitium.[14–16] Both techniques involve catheterization of the subclavian or femoral artery, cannulation of the coronary sinus, and cannulation of a subselective coronary vein.

A number of studies of coronary venous delivery have been undertaken in porcine models. Early feasibility studies indicated that total occlusion of coronary veins for up to 30 minutes does not result in myocardial ischemia, arrhythmias, chest pain, or systolic dysfunction.[14] Injections of diatrizoate or Evans blue dye into the anterior intraventricular vein resulted in staining of the anterior LV wall, apex, and intraventricular septum. Dye injection into the posterior intraventricular vein resulted in staining of the inferior LV wall, posterior septum, and posterior walls of the left and right ventricles. Four minutes after dye injection, 50% of the maximal signal clearance had occurred; 30 minutes after injection, 20% of the initial signal intensity was still present. It is unlikely that these time courses and percentages also apply to cell retention.

Boekstegers and co-workers[11] have conducted a number of studies in porcine models of ischemia. In one, they demonstrated that adenoviral gene transfer via pressure-regulated retrograde coronary venous delivery to ischemic tissues led to increased transfection efficiency when compared with antegrade intracoronary delivery; in the absence of ischemia, there was no difference. In a chronic myocardial ischemia model, they found that retrograde, as opposed to antegrade, infusion of basic fibroblast growth factor (bFGF, also known as FGF-2) significantly improved regional perfusion and myocardial function.[13] Hou et al[15] used a high-pressure retrograde coronary venous approach to deliver a plasmid encoding developmentally regulated endothelial locus- 1 (Del-1) in a porcine model. This resulted in efficient widespread regional distribution of Del-1. Fearon et al[17] compared the delivery of bFGF via high-pressure retrograde venous and intracoronary routes in a porcine model of chronic myocardial ischemia. They found that significantly more bFGF was retained in the LV after retrograde venous delivery.

All of these porcine studies are inherently limited by the fact that the porcine coronary venous system differs substantially from the human system.[18] The main tributary of the porcine coronary sinus, the left azygos vein, is not present in humans. In addition, porcine coronary vessels tend to be larger in caliber, more collateralized, and less tortuous. Thus, the catheter systems designed for effective stem cell delivery in pigs may not be appropriate for clinical use in humans.

Although the data from large animal (i.e., porcine) studies appear to support the use of retrograde coronary venous delivery, no controlled clinical trials have yet been undertaken. Murad-Netto et al[12] published the first case report of autologous bone marrow $CD34^+$ cell infusion via the coronary veins in a patient 14 days after an AMI. No complications were noted, and the patient was discharged 48 hours after treatment.

A group at the National Heart and Lung Institute and at the Royal Brompton Hospital in London is undertaking a randomized placebo-controlled trial of retrograde coronary venous delivery of bone marrow mononuclear cells in patients with ischemic heart failure not amenable to conventional revascularization techniques (E Alton, personal communication). This will be preceded by a pilot study in which a subpopulation of cells will be labeled with indium-111 so that their distribution and time course of residence in the myocardium can be assessed.

A number of key variables associated with this technique need to be addressed. The optimal delivery pressure, volume, and infusion time are yet to be defined. At present, high-pressure delivery, which aims to cause endothelial disruption and thus allow interstitial delivery without rupturing the epicardial veins or dissecting the coronary sinus, relies on manual control reinforced by fluoroscopic feedback from myocardial blushing. Also, it remains to be established whether biologic activity will be greater within a small area containing a high concentration of cells or within a larger area containing a lower or an equal concentration of cells. As a consequence, the number of veins to be targeted has not been established. Technical difficulties associated with cannulating tortuous coronary sinus tributaries may also mean that certain areas of the myocardium may not be accessible. Despite these drawbacks, the retrograde venous route is promising.

Intracoronary Delivery

Intracoronary infusion has been the most popular mode of stem cell delivery in the clinical setting, especially after an AMI. Intracoronary stem cell delivery 4–9 days after an AMI has a good clinical safety profile (Table 11.1).[19–25] The technique is similar to that used for coronary angioplasty, which involves over-the-wire positioning of an angioplasty balloon in a coronary artery (Figure 11.1). Coronary blood flow is stopped for approximately 2–4 minutes while the stem cells are infused under pressure. This maximizes their contact with the microcirculation of the infarct-related artery, thereby increasing their homing time. Again, this delivery technique would be suitable only in the setting of acute ischemia, when adhesion molecules and cytokine signaling are temporarily upregulated. The size of the cells infused into a coronary artery may have possible deleterious implications. Larger cells such as MSCs or myoblasts may occlude the microcirculation. Vulliet et al[26] described the occurrence of AMIs and subacute myocardial microinfarctions after intracoronary arterial injection of bone marrow MSCs in dogs. These findings were particularly worrisome because they were obtained in healthy dogs with normal epicardial coronary arteries. Microcirculatory plugging is believed to have caused the microinfarctions. These results are concordant with our own findings concerning MSC intracoronary infusion in a canine model of acute ischemia (unpublished data) (Figure 11.2). In an experimental study of AMIs in which we directly compared intracoronary infusion and transendocardial injection of MSCs,[27] the only significant improvement in function (LV dimensions and ejection fraction, LVEF) occurred in the transendocardial injection group. In addition, as demonstrated by colocalization of the nuclear markers DAPI and DiI, therapeutically administered stem cells became part of vascular structures along the border zone of the infarct only in the transendocardial injection group. Beyond cell size, other potentially important factors to consider are the rate of stem cell infusion and the concentration of such cells, especially in patients who have suffered a recent myocardial injury. Unfortunately, even though the intracoronary delivery route is widely used, there is no strong experimental evidence for its safety or efficacy compared with that of other delivery approaches (see below).

The intracoronary delivery route does have the advantages of being simple, easy to use, and inexpensive. However, once the epicardial coronary arteries of patients with ischemic heart disease have become either severely stenosed or totally occluded, the use of this route might be limited. This is especially important to remember when patients have chronic ischemic heart failure, who will likely have undergone several previous revascularization procedures and have extensively diseased coronary arteries. These concerns notwithstanding, and, in light of the clinical experience so far, the intracoronary route remains the preferred route for therapeutic stem cell delivery in AMI.

Intramyocardial Injection

Intramyocardial injection has been performed in the clinical setting of chronic myocardial ischemia.

Table 11.1 Trials of intracoronary cell therapy in patients with acute myocardial infarctions (AMIs)

Study	No. of patients	Cell type	Dose	Days after AMI	Therapeutic effects: Improvement	Therapeutic effects: No change
Nonrandomized						
Strauer et al[24]	10 treated 10 controls[a]	ABMMNC	$2.8 \pm 2.2 \times 10^7$	5–9	Regional wall motion[b] Perfusion[b] ↓Infarct size	Global LVEF[b] LVEDV[b]
TOPCARE-AMI[19,20,23]	29 ABMMNC 30 CPC 11 controls[a]	ABMMNC CPC	$2.1 \pm 0.8 \times 10^8$ $1.6 \pm 1.2 \times 10^7$	5 ± 2	Regional wall motion[b] Global LVEF[b] ↓Infarct size[b] Coronary flow[b]	LVEDV[b]
Fernández-Avilés et al[22]	20 treated 13 controls[a]	ABMMNC	$7.8 \pm 4.1 \times 10^7$	14 ± 6	Regional wall motion[b] Global LVEF[b]	LVEDV[b]
Randomized						
BOOST[25]	30 treated 30 controls	NC	$2.5 \pm 0.9 \times 10^{10}$	6 ± 1	Regional wall motion Global LVEF	LVEDV Infarct size
Chen et al[21]	34 treated 35 controls	MSC	$4.8 \pm 6.0 \times 10^{10}$	18	Regional wall motion Global LVEF ↓Infarct size ↓LVEDV	

Values shown are mean ± standard deviation.
[a]Nonrandomized control groups.
[b]Effects reported only within cell therapy groups.
ABMMNC, autologous bone marrow-derived mononuclear cell; BOOST, Bone Marrow Transfer to Enhance ST Elevation Infarct Regeneration; CPC, circulating blood-derived progenitor cell; LVEDV, left ventricular end-diastolic volume; LVEF, left ventricular ejection fraction; MSC, mesenchymal stem cell; NC, bone marrow-derived nucleated cell; TOPCARE, Transplantation of Progenitor Cells and Regeneration Enhancement; ↓, decreased.
Adapted from Wollert KC, Drexler H. Clinical applications of stem cells for the heart. Circ Res 2005;96:151–63, with permission from Lippincott Williams & Wilkins.

It is the preferred delivery route in patients with chronic total occlusion of coronary arteries and in patients with chronic conditions (e.g., congestive heart failure) that involve weaker homing signals. In theory, intramyocardial injection should be the most suitable route for delivering larger cells such as skeletal myoblasts and MSCs, which are prone to microvascular "plugging." Intramyocardial injection can be performed via transepicardial, transendocardial, or transcoronary venous routes.

Transepicardial injection

Transepicardial injection of stem cells has been performed during open surgical revascularization procedures to deliver the cells to infarct border zones or areas of infarcted or scarred myocardium. Because a sternotomy is required, this approach is highly invasive and associated with surgical morbidity. However, in the setting of a planned open heart procedure, the ancillary delivery of cell therapy in this fashion can be easily justified.

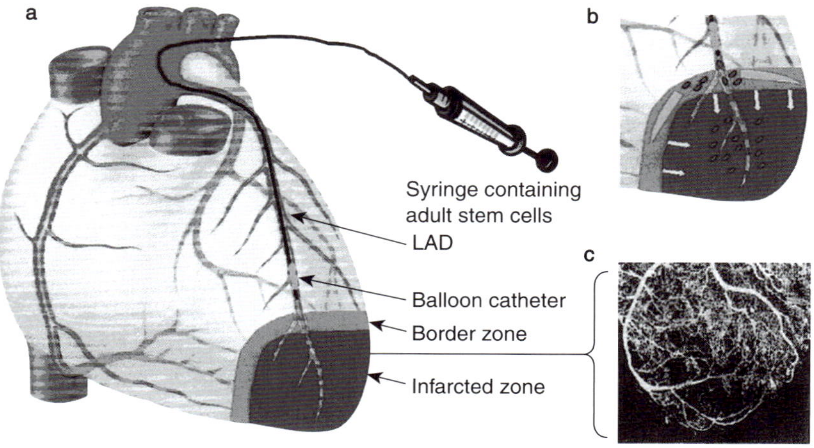

Figure 11.1 *Technique for cardiac stem cell transplantation in patients with myocardial infarctions. (a) Balloon catheterization of the infarct-related artery (left anterior descending, LAD) above the infarct border zone, followed by high-pressure infusion of stem cells into the artery. (b) Migration of stem cells (red dots) into the infarcted zone, possibly via infarct-related blood vessels (arrows). (c) Migration of cells into both the infarcted and border zones via existing blood flow within the infarcted zone. Reproduced from Strauer BE Circulation 2002;106:1913–18[24] with permission from Lippincott Williams and Wilkins.*

Interestingly, not all areas of the myocardium (e.g., the interventricular septum) can be reached via a direct external approach.

The main advantages of direct surgical injection are its proven safety in several preclinical and human trials[28–35] and its ease of use. However, it is costly and relies only on external inspection of the myocardium for optimal targeting. The surgeon can choose to inject stem cells into the border zone of an infarcted area or scar tissue on the basis of visual assessment, but such assessment may be limited. In addition, the safety of direct surgical injection in patients with a recent AMI has not been evaluated in clinical trials. Nevertheless, direct surgical injection might certainly have a role in the future of stem cell therapy. One can easily envision the cardiac surgeon, during coronary artery bypass grafting surgery, bypassing all areas which it is technically feasible to bypass and then concomitantly injecting stem cells into those areas containing totally occluded epicardial coronary arteries.

Transendocardial injection

Transendocardial injection is performed via a percutaneous femoral approach. An injection-needle catheter is advanced in retrograde fashion across the aortic valve and positioned against the endocardial surface. Stem cells are then injected directly into targeted areas of the LV wall. Three catheter systems are currently available for transendocardial cell delivery: the Stilleto (Boston Scientific, Natick, MA), the BioCardia (BioCardia, South San Francisco, CA), and the Myostar (Biosense-Webster, Diamond Bar, CA) (Figure 11.3).

In the clinical arena, the Stilleto is used under visual fluoroscopic guidance. A drawback inherent to this approach is the bidimensional orientation of the catheter. Even when biplane fluoroscopy is employed, there is still an inherent lack of pre cision associated with this method. Another drawback is the inability to characterize the underlying or target myocardium. This lack of precision and targeting may or may not be important, depending on the therapy being delivered. Cell therapy may be more dependent on the microenvironment than is gene therapy, and the results of injecting therapeutic cells inadvertently into healthy tissue may produce as-yet unknown differential effects. Nevertheless, this technology may be promising when used in

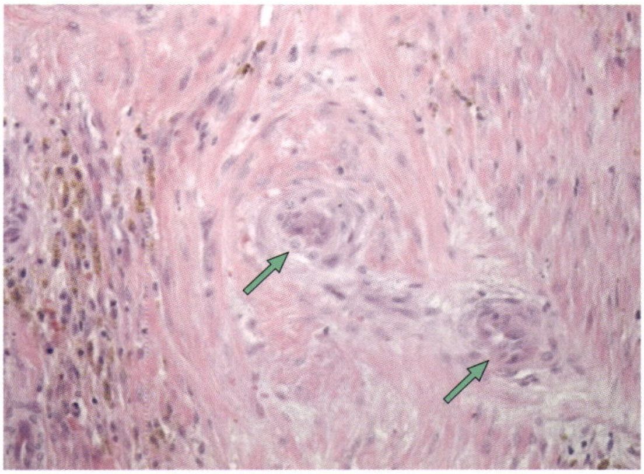

Figure 11.2 Photomicrograph of myocardium after intracoronary mesenchymal infusion (hematoxylin– eosin). Note the plugged arterioles (arrows).

association with imaging technologies such as magnetic resonance imaging (MRI) or when targeting of myocardial therapy is not necessary. To this end, in preclinical experiments, the Stilleto catheter has been coupled with real-time cardiac MRI, which permits online assessment of full-thickness myocardium and perfusion. Although still investigational and not currently practical in terms of clinical application, the simultaneous use of MRI offers three-dimensional spatial orientation. Few preclinical studies have been performed, and no safety data from human studies have been assessed.[36] Theoretically, the use of MRI also provides a unique opportunity to track the intramyocardial retention of therapeutic cells after direct injection. This will, however, require the labeling of cells with iron particles that can be detected in the beating heart.

The BioCardia delivery system uses a catheter whose deflectable tip includes a helical needle for infusion. Initial preclinical and clinical experience with this system has provided preliminary evidence of its safety and feasibility.[37,38] The BioCardia catheter does not offer any additional navigational or targeting capability beyond fluoroscopy. More extensive preclinical experience with this catheter is needed before human trials can begin.

The Myostar injection catheter takes advantage of nonfluoroscopic magnetic guidance.[39] Injections are targeted with the help of a three-dimensional LV "shell," or NOGA electromechanical map (EMM), representing the endocardial surface of the left ventricle (Figure 11.4). The shell is constructed by acquiring a series of points at multiple locations on the endocardial surface, which are gated to a surface electrocardiogram; the shell then serves as a virtual environment in which an icon representing the catheter tip can be navigated in real time. Ultralow magnetic fields (10^{-6}–10^{-5} T) are generated by a triangular magnetic pad positioned beneath the patient. The magnetic fields intersect with a sensor just proximal to the deflectable tip of a 7 Fr mapping catheter, which helps determine the real-time location and orientation of the catheter tip inside the left ventricle.

The NOGA system algorithmically calculates and analyzes the movement of the catheter tip or the location of an endocardial point throughout systole and diastole. That movement is then compared with the movement of neighboring points in an area of interest. The resulting value, called linear local shortening (LLS), is expressed as a percentage that represents the degree of mechanical function of the LV region at that endocardial point. Data are obtained only when the catheter tip is in stable contact with the endocardium. This contact is determined automatically. The mapping catheter also incorporates electrodes that measure endocardial electrical signals (unipolar or bipolar voltage).[39] Voltage values are assigned to each point acquired during LV mapping, and an electrical map is constructed concurrently with the mechanical map. Each data point has an LLS value and a voltage value. When the map is complete, all the data points are integrated by the NOGA workstation and displayed thereon. The points are presented in a three-dimensional color-coded reconstruction of the endocardial surface, as well as in 9- and 12-segment bull's-eye views that show average values for the LLS and voltage data in each myocardial segment (Figure 11.5). These maps can be spatially manipulated in real time on a Silicon Graphics workstation

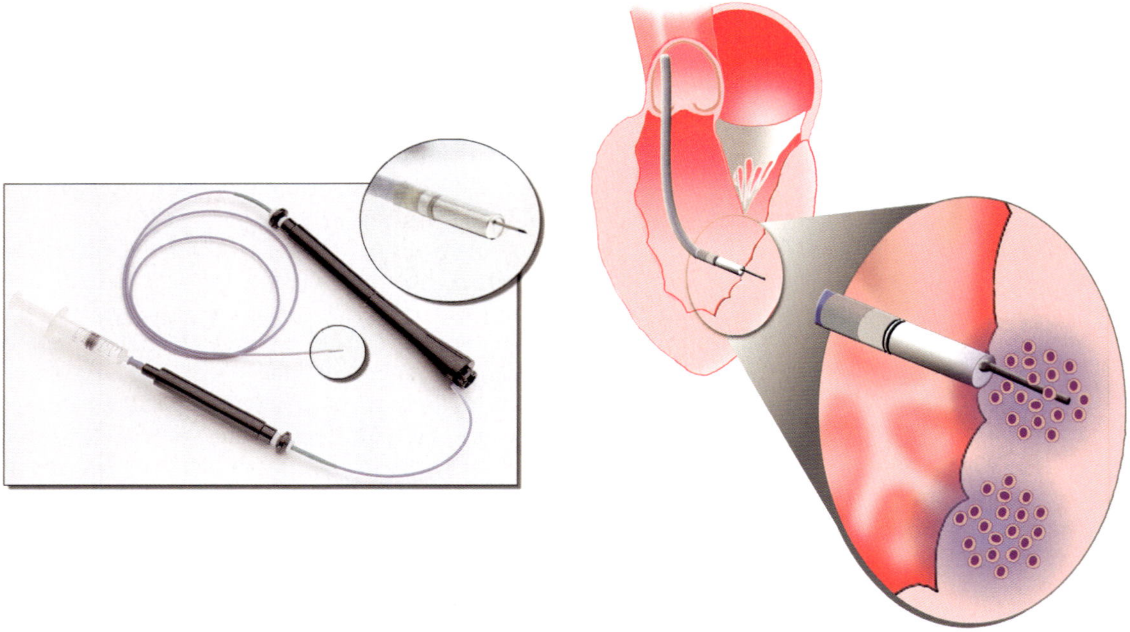

Figure 11.3 Left: The NOGA Myostar® injection catheter, with the needle in the extended position. Right: Injection catheter advanced into the left ventricle through the aortic valve. The catheter tip is placed against the endocardial surface (insert) with the needle extended into the myocardium and delivering stem cells.

(Mountain View, CA). The three-dimensional representations acquired during the cardiac cycle can also be used to calculate the LV volume and LVEF.

Thus, the EMM provides a three-dimensional platform on which the catheter can navigate the LV and be oriented for transendocardial injections, as well as a diagnostic platform on which ischemic areas (i.e., those with low LLS and preserved unipolar voltage, UniV) can be distinguished from areas of infarct (i.e., those with low LLS and low UniV).[40] Moreover, the Myostar catheter allows assessment of myocardial viability at each specific injection site where the catheter touches the endocardial surface. The operator thus has the ability to target therapy to viable tissue (desirable in situations of chronic ischemia, where neoangiogenesis may play an important role) or nonviable tissue (where the target of cell therapy may be an area of scar tissue). Because of the patchy nature of myocardial involvement in human ischemic heart disease, the ability to distinguish underlying tissue characteristics is important when delivering stem cells.

The EMM technology has been widely tested in both animals and humans and has an excellent safety profile.[41–48] Kornowski et al[45] have studied the dynamics of transendocardial delivery using different needle extensions to inject 0.1 ml of methylene blue dye as a tracer in pigs. A total of 152 injections were performed, with needle extensions varying from 3 to 4 mm in length. Two myocardial regions were injected per animal, and injection sites were located after the animals were sacrificed acutely. Staining extended to a depth of 7.1 ± 2.1 mm (range 2–11 mm) and to a width of 2.3 ± 1.8 mm (range 1–9 mm). In 2.6% of cases (4 of 152), the injected dye stained the epicardial surface, suggesting pericardial extravasation; more importantly, three of those four injections were made in the apical area. No animal deaths, no instances of pericardial effusion or tamponade, and no episodes of sustained

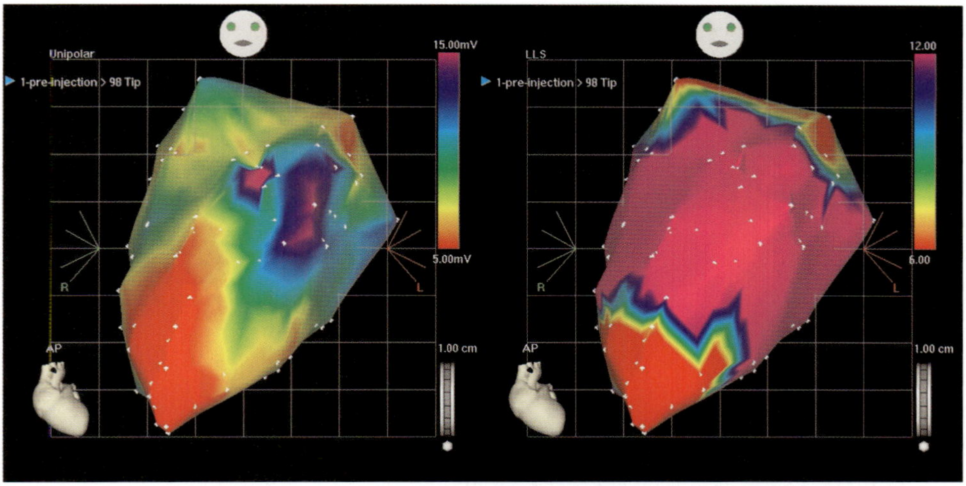

Figure 11.4 *Electromechanical mapping of the left ventricle performed with the NOGA® XP platform in an acute model of myocardial ischemia in a sheep (antero-apical myocardial infarction). Left: Unipolar voltage mapping (mV). The red area at the apex represents the infarcted myocardium Right: Linear local shortening mapping (%) confirms impaired contractility at the apical infarct.*

ventricular arrhythmia were associated with the transendocardial injections.

Transendocardial stem cell delivery guided by EMM has not been tested in the post-AMI setting in humans. However, in our experience at the Texas Heart Institute with a canine model of acute ischemia,[27] the safety profile of this delivery technique has been excellent, with no documented instances of injection-related pericardial effusion or malignant arrhythmia. Further assessment of the safety of transendocardial cell injection after AMI is warranted.

At the Texas Heart Institute, we have performed over 1000 preclinical myocardial injections with this system. This large preclinical experience has translated well into clinical trials. However, it is very important to note that the clinical safety profile of transendocardial delivery so far has entailed precise preinjection measurements of needle extension and a maximal needle-to-wall ratio.

We have pioneered the delivery of autologous mononuclear bone marrow cells to targeted viable or ischemic zones via the EMM-guided transendocardial route in patients with end-stage heart failure.[46,47] Other investigators have used the transendocardial route to target the delivery of skeletal myoblasts.[49,50] In light of (a) the need for stem cell targeting, (b) the need in some cases to inject cells into areas other than those supplied by patent coronary arteries, and (c) the current clinical experience, it is likely that the transendocardial route will become the first choice for cell delivery in treating patients with chronic myocardial ischemia.

Transcoronary venous direct injection

Transcoronary venous injection is performed with a catheter system that is placed percutaneously into the coronary sinus. Initial studies in swine models have confirmed the feasibility and safety of this approach.[51] This delivery method has also been used to deliver skeletal myoblasts to scarred myocardium in cardiomyopathy patients.[33] It utilizes intravascular ultrasound guidance, thus enabling the operator to extend a catheter and needle away from the pericardial space and coronary artery into the adjacent myocardium. To date, human feasibility studies have had a good safety profile. Unlike the transendocardial approach, in which cells are injected perpendicularly into the LV wall, the transcoronary venous approach

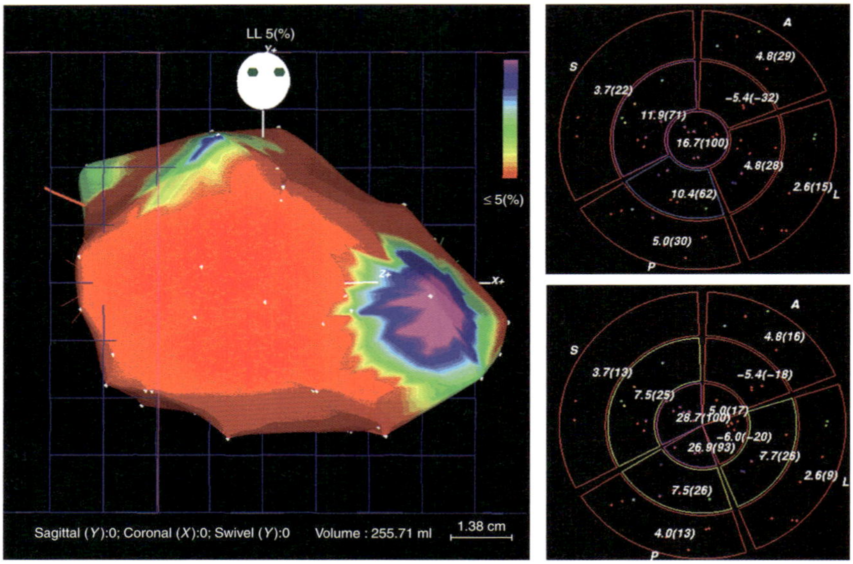

Figure 11.5 *Three-dimensional color-coded map of the endocardial surface, with bull's-eye views showing mean linear local shortening (LLS) and voltage values in each myocardial segment. From Leite RS, Silva GV, Dohman HFR, et al. Comparison of left ventricular electromechanical mapping with left ventricular angiography: defining practical standards for the analysis of NOGA maps. Tex Heart Inst J 2003;30:19-26, with permission.*

allows parallel cell injection, which will likely result in greater cell retention. The limitations of this technique are similar to those mentioned above with regard to coronary venous tortuosity and lack of site-specific targeting, as well as the fact that this is one of the most technically challenging percutaneous delivery modes available.

Conclusions

Stem cell delivery remains a major challenge in the development of cardiac stem cell therapy strategies. Technology is advancing at a fast pace, and newer imaging and automated software may soon make some of the above-described delivery techniques archaic. The incorporation of Microelectronic Mechanical Systems (MEMS) and nanotechnology will likely take much of the focus away from stem cell therapy delivery methods and allow for simpler and more intuitive interfaces for the clinical application of stem cell therapy in humans.

References

1. Shintani S, Murohara T, Ikeda H, et al. Mobilization of endothelial progenitor cells in patients with acute myocardial infarction. Circulation 2001;103:2776–9.
2. Lew WY. Mobilizing cells to the injured myocardium: a novel rescue strategy or an unwelcome intrusion? J Am Coll Cardiol 2004;44:1521–2.
3. Maekawa Y, Anzai T, Yoshikawa T, et al. Effect of granulocyte–macrophage colony-stimulating factor inducer on left ventricular remodeling after acute myocardial infarction. J Am Coll Cardiol 2004;44:1510–20.
4. Kang HJ, Kim HS, Zhang SY, et al. Effects of intracoronary infusion of peripheral blood stem-cells mobilised with granulocyte-colony stimulating factor on left ventricular systolic function and restenosis after coronary stenting in myocardial infarction: the MAGIC cell randomised clinical trial. Lancet 2004;363:751–6.
5. Toma C, Pittenger MF, Cahill KS, et al. Human mesenchymal stem cells differentiate to a cardiomyocyte phenotype in the adult murine heart. Circulation 2002;105:93–8.
6. Aicher A, Brenner W, Zuhayra M, et al. Assessment of the tissue distribution of transplanted human

endothelial progenitor cells by radioactive labeling. Circulation 2003;107:2134–9.

7. Barbash IM, Chouraqui P, Baron J, et al. Systemic delivery of bone marrow-derived mesenchymal stem cells to the infarcted myocardium: feasibility, cell migration, and body distribution. Circulation 2003;108:863–8.
8. Pohl T, Giehrl W, Reichart B, et al. Retroinfusion-supported stenting in high-risk patients for percutaneous intervention and bypass surgery: results of the prospective randomized Myoprotect I study. Catheter Cardiovasc Interv 2004;62:323–30.
9. Miyazaki A, Hatori N, Tadokoro H, et al. More rapid thrombolysis with coronary venous retroinfusion of streptokinase compared with intravenous administration. An experimental study in canines. Eur Heart J 1990;11:936–44.
10. Frater RW. Retrograde cardioplegia. J Heart Valve Dis 1999;8:118–19.
11. Boekstegers P, von Degenfeld G, Giehrl W, et al. Myocardial gene transfer by selective pressure-regulated retroinfusion of coronary veins. Gene Ther 2000;7:232–40.
12. Murad-Netto S, Moura R, Romeo LJ, et al. Stem cell therapy with retrograde coronary perfusion in acute myocardial infarction. A new technique. Arq Bras Cardiol 2004;83:352–4; 349–51.
13. von Degenfeld G, Raake P, Kupatt C, et al. Selective pressure-regulated retroinfusion of fibroblast growth factor-2 into the coronary vein enhances regional myocardial blood flow and function in pigs with chronic myocardial ischemia. J Am Coll Cardiol 2003;42:1120–8.
14. Herity NA, Lo ST, Oei F, et al. Selective regional myocardial infiltration by the percutaneous coronary venous route: a novel technique for local drug delivery. Catheter Cardiovasc Interv 2000;51: 358–63.
15. Hou D, MacLaughlin F, Thiesse M, et al. Widespread regional myocardial transfection by plasmid encoding Del-1 following retrograde coronary venous delivery. Catheter Cardiovasc Interv 2003;58:207–11.
16. Raake P, von Degenfeld G, Hinkel R, et al. Myocardial gene transfer by selective pressure-regulated retroinfusion of coronary veins: comparison with surgical and percutaneous intramyocardial gene delivery. J Am Coll Cardiol 2004;44:1124–9.
17. Fearon WF, Ikeno F, Bailey LR, et al. Evaluation of high-pressure retrograde coronary venous delivery of FGF-2 protein. Catheter Cardiovasc Interv 2004;61:422–8.
18. Ghoshal NG. Porcine heart and arteries. In: Getty R (ed). The Anatomy of Domestic Animals. Philadelphia: WB Saunders 1975:1306–12.
19. Assmus B, Schachinger V, Teupe C, et al. Transplantation of Progenitor Cells and Regeneration Enhancement in Acute Myocardial Infarction (TOPCARE-AMI). Circulation 2002;106:3009–17.
20. Britten MB, Abolmaali ND, Assmus B, et al. Infarct remodeling after intracoronary progenitor cell treatment in patients with acute myocardial infarction (TOPCARE-AMI): mechanistic insights from serial contrast-enhanced magnetic resonance imaging. Circulation 2003;108:2212–18.
21. Chen SL, Fang WW, Ye F, et al. Effect on left ventricular function of intracoronary transplantation of autologous bone marrow mesenchymal stem cell in patients with acute myocardial infarction. Am J Cardiol 2004;94:92–5.
22. Fernández-Avilés F, San Roman JA, García-Frade J, et al. Experimental and clinical regenerative capability of human bone marrow cells after myocardial infarction. Circ Res 2004;95:742–8.
23. Schachinger V, Assmus B, Britten MB, et al. Transplantation of progenitor cells and regeneration enhancement in acute myocardial infarction: final one-year results of the TOPCARE-AMI trial. J Am Coll Cardiol 2004;44:1690–9.
24. Strauer BE, Brehm M, Zeus T, et al. Repair of infarcted myocardium by autologous intracoronary mononuclear bone marrow cell transplantation in humans. Circulation 2002;106:1913–18.
25. Wollert KC, Meyer GP, Lotz J, et al. Intracoronary autologous bone-marrow cell transfer after myocardial infarction: the BOOST randomised controlled clinical trial. Lancet 2004;364:141–8.
26. Vulliet PR, Greeley M, Halloran SM, et al. Intracoronary arterial injection of mesenchymal stromal cells and microinfarction in dogs. Lancet 2004;363:783–4.
27. Perin EC, Silva GV, Assad JA, et al. Comparison between intracoronary infusion and direct transendocardial injection of mesenchymal stem cells in a dog acute ischemia model. J Am Coll Cardiol 2005;45(Suppl A):435A (Abst 856-3).
28. Hamano K, Nishida M, Hirata K, et al. Local implantation of autologous bone marrow cells for therapeutic angiogenesis in patients with ischemic heart disease: clinical trial and preliminary results. Jpn Circ J 2001;65:845–7.
29. Herreros J, Prosper F, Perez A, et al. Autologous intramyocardial injection of cultured skeletal muscle-derived stem cells in patients with non-acute myocardial infarction. Eur Heart J 2003;24:2012–20.
30. Menasche P, Hagege AA, Vilquin JT, et al. Autologous skeletal myoblast transplantation for severe postinfarction left ventricular dysfunction. J Am Coll Cardiol 2003;41:1078–83.
31. Orlic D, Kajstura J, Chimenti S, et al. Bone marrow cells regenerate infarcted myocardium. Nature 2001;410:701–5.

32. Silva GV, Litovsky S, Assad JA, et al. Mesenchymal stem cells differentiate into an endothelial phenotype, enhance vascular density, and improve heart function in a canine chronic ischemia model. Circulation 2005;111:150–6.
33. Siminiak T, Kalawski R, Fiszer D, et al. Autologous skeletal myoblast transplantation for the treatment of postinfarction myocardial injury: phase I clinical study with 12 months of follow-up. Am Heart J 2004;148:531–7.
34. Stamm C, Kleine HD, Westphal B, et al. CABG and bone marrow stem cell transplantation after myocardial infarction. Thorac Cardiovasc Surg 2004;52:152–8.
35. Stamm C, Westphal B, Kleine HD, et al. Autologous bone-marrow stem-cell transplantation for myocardial regeneration. Lancet 2003;361:45–6.
36. Hill JM, Dick AJ, Raman VK, et al. Serial cardiac magnetic resonance imaging of injected mesenchymal stem cells. Circulation 2003;108:1009–14.
37. Amado LC, St. John M, Saliaris AP, et al. Cardiac repair with mesenchymal stem cells following myocardial infarction in pigs. Circulation 110(Suppl):III-170–1 (Abst 815).
38. Amado LC, Saliaris AP, Schuleri KH, et al. Cardiac repair with intramyocardial injection of allogeneic mesenchymal stem cells after myocardial infarction. Proc Natl Acad Sci USA 2005;102:11474–9.
39. Sarmento-Leite R, Silva GV, Dohmann HF, et al. Comparison of left ventricular electromechanical mapping and left ventricular angiography: defining practical standards for analysis of NOGA maps. Tex Heart Inst J 2003;30:19–26.
40. Perin EC, Silva GV, Sarmento-Leite R, et al. Assessing myocardial viability and infarct transmurality with left ventricular electromechanical mapping in patients with stable coronary artery disease: validation by delayed-enhancement magnetic resonance imaging. Circulation 2002;106:957–61.
41. Fuchs S, Baffour R, Zhou YF, et al. Transendocardial delivery of autologous bone marrow enhances collateral perfusion and regional function in pigs with chronic experimental myocardial ischemia. J Am Coll Cardiol 2001;37:1726–32.
42. Fuchs S, Satler LF, Kornowski R, et al. Catheter-based autologous bone marrow myocardial injection in no-option patients with advanced coronary artery disease: a feasibility study. J Am Coll Cardiol 2003;41:1721–4.
43. Kawamoto A, Tkebuchava T, Yamaguchi J, et al. Intramyocardial transplantation of autologous endothelial progenitor cells for therapeutic neovascularization of myocardial ischemia. Circulation 2003;107:461–8.
44. Kornowski R, Fuchs S, Tio FO, et al. Evaluation of the acute and chronic safety of the biosense injection catheter system in porcine hearts. Catheter Cardiovasc Interv 1999;48:447–53; discussion 454–5.
45. Kornowski R, Leon MB, Fuchs S, et al. Electromagnetic guidance for catheter-based transendocardial injection: a platform for intramyocardial angiogenesis therapy. Results in normal and ischemic porcine models. J Am Coll Cardiol 2000; 35:1031–9.
46. Perin EC, Dohmann HF, Borojevic R, et al. Transendocardial, autologous bone marrow cell transplantation for severe, chronic ischemic heart failure. Circulation 2003;107:2294–302.
47. Perin EC, Dohmann HF, Borojevic R, et al. Improved exercise capacity and ischemia 6 and 12 months after transendocardial injection of autologous bone marrow mononuclear cells for ischemic cardiomyopathy. Circulation 2004;110:II213–18.
48. Tse HF, Kwong YL, Chan JK, et al. Angiogenesis in ischaemic myocardium by intramyocardial autologous bone marrow mononuclear cell implantation. Lancet 2003;361:47–9.
49. Agbulut O, Vandervelde S, Al Attar N, et al. Comparison of human skeletal myoblasts and bone marrow-derived $CD133^+$ progenitors for the repair of infarcted myocardium. J Am Coll Cardiol 2004;44:458–63.
50. Smits PC, van Geuns RJ, Poldermans D, et al. Catheter-based intramyocardial injection of autologous skeletal myoblasts as a primary treatment of ischemic heart failure: clinical experience with six-month follow-up. J Am Coll Cardiol 2003;42: 2063–9.
51. Thompson CA, Nasseri BA, Makower J, et al. Percutaneous transvenous cellular cardiomyoplasty. A novel nonsurgical approach for myocardial cell transplantation. J Am Coll Cardiol 2003; 41:1964–71.

chapter 12

Understanding the Basics of Clinical Imaging for Assessing Stem Cell Therapy in the Heart

Marco A Costa and Theodore A Bass

Introduction

Our understanding of stem cell biology has advanced considerably in the past few years. Cell transplantation has been proposed as a strategy to promote both neovascularization and cardiac tissue replacement.[1–10] There is increasing evidence that cell transplantation may improve the perfusion and contractile function of the ischemic myocardium. Whether this is achieved by replacing necrotic cardiomyocytes with new functional cells, by increasing the number of contractile elements in remnant viable cells, by improving myocardial perfusion as a result of local angiogenesis, or by a combination of these mechanisms remains to be elucidated.

Endpoints of cell therapy studies should determine the clinical effectiveness of such an approach, demonstrate an absence of adverse side effects such as development of atherosclerosis or cancer, and provide a mechanistic assessment of the therapeutic effect.[1] Documentation of in vivo angiogenesis is possible in experimental models by the use of high-resolution intravital microscopy techniques,[11] but such methods cannot be applied in humans. Early clinical experiments have utilized currently available, yet minimally validated, imaging modalities such as angiography, nonfluoroscopic electromechanical mapping, nuclear imaging [single photon emission computed tomography (SPECT) and positron emission tomography (PET)], echocardiography, or cardiac magnetic resonance imaging (MRI) (Table 12.1). However, these sophisticated imaging modalities still lack the spatial resolution of microscopy-based imaging applied in experimental models.[12] The resolution of MRI is about 500 μm, while that of PET and echocardiography is in the millimeters range.

Stem cell tracking is hampered by the lack of an imaging modality sensitive enough to detect a single cell or even groups of cells. Molecular labeling of transplanted cells or the use of contrast agents, which have not yet been approved for clinical application, considerably improves the ability of these imaging modalities to directly assess angiogenesis in experimental studies.[13–15] However, cellular labeling may lead to genetic mutations. In addition, dilution of the agent during cell division may decrease imaging detection.[13] In this chapter, we will discuss the value of currently available imaging modalities as surrogate endpoints for clinical trials involving cell transplantation therapy.

Angiography

The technique of coronary angiography, the gold standard method to define severity of atherosclerosis disease, is based on X-ray cine acquisition of the vascular lumen silhouette during passage of

Table 12.1 Value of imaging techniques to assess myocardial properties

Technique	*Viability*	*Function*		*Perfusion*
		Rest	*Stress*	
PET:				
FDG	++	Inv	Inv	–
$^{13}NH_3$	+	–	–	++
SPECT:				
^{201}Tl	++	–	–	++
^{99m}Tc	++	–	–	++
Echocardiography:				
Rest	+	++	–	–
Stress	++	–	++	–
Contrast	Inv	–	–	Inv
MRI:				
Rest	+	+++	–	–
Stress	++	–	++	–
Contrast	++	–	–	Inv
Angiography	+	++	0	0
EM mapping	Inv	Inv	Inv	–

PET, positron emission tomography; FDG, [^{18}F]fluorodeoxyglucose; MRI, magnetic resonance imaging; EM, electromechanical.
0, no value; +, some value but not first choice; ++, can be used as primary imaging modality; Inv, investigational.
Adapted from Underwood SR, et al. Eur Heart J 2004;25:815–36[47] by permission of the European Society of Cardiology.

iodine contrast. Coronary angiography and cardiac catheterization protocols are integral parts of stratification pathways for patients with congestive heart failure (CHF). Angiography provides valuable information regarding the etiology of CHF and the extension of coronary artery disease (CAD), which is essential for screening patients for cell transplant therapy, although no temporal or causal relationship can be obtained in the catheterization laboratory (Figure 12.1). The simplicity and worldwide availability of this imaging modality make it attractive for clinical trials. However, the invasive nature of angiography and its associated risks, albeit small, limit its application for serial follow-up assessments.

Angiography may be useful in identifying new collateral growth.[16,17] However, coronary angiography is a planar imaging modality and does not have the minimum spatial resolution (approximately 100 μm) to visualize and determine the development of microvessels (≤50 μm). Lack of standardization for volume, speed, and pressure of contrast injection, routinely performed manually, limits the proper quantification of collateral vasculature. In addition, distinction between preexisting and newly formed collaterals represents a challenge.

Gorge et al[18] initially observed the correlation between a dense blush on tomographic angiograms and the presence of numerous small vessels in response to ischemia in a porcine heart. Subsequently, the Zwolle Myocardial Infarction Study Group proposed a blush grading system to determine microvascular perfusion,

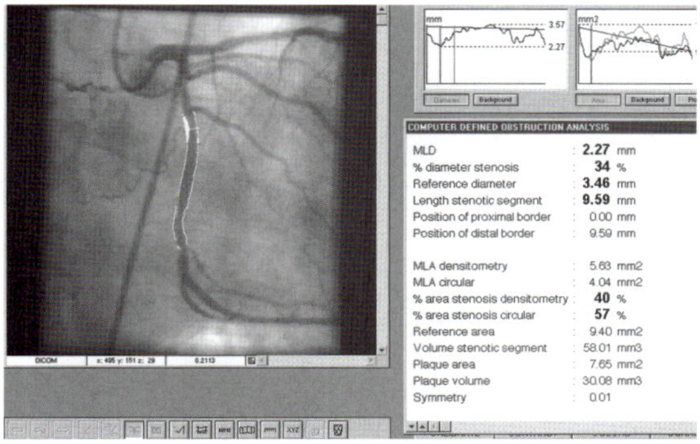

Figure 12.1 *Example of quantitative coronary angiography (QCA) of the left circumflex coronary artery showing 34% stenosis. Measurements are performed in at least two orthogonal projections. QCA can be performed in multiple vessels from a single angiogram and compared with serial matched images.*

which was found to be an important predictor of clinical outcomes after acute myocardial infarction.[19] A similar prognostic value for the blush score was observed by others.[20] The blush score is defined as follows:

Score
- 0 Minimal or no blush in the affected myocardium. Indicates lack of myocardial perfusion.
- 1 Contrast enters slowly but fails to exit the microvasculature for ≥30 s, suggesting severely impaired microvascular perfusion.
- 2 Delayed entry and exit of dye from the microvasculature, with persistence of dye for ≥3 cardiac cycles of the washout phase.
- 3 Normal microvascular perfusion—the blush clears normally and is either absent or only mildly/moderately persistent after three cardiac cycles of the washout phase.

Quantification of myocardial capillary "blush," with or without digital subtraction,[21] is somewhat subjective but can be easily performed in most clinical angiograms. However, the accuracy and reproducibility of this method are affected by variability in image acquisition protocols, including projections, volume of contrast injection, and duration of ciné recording.

Adventitial neovascularization has been shown to play a role in the formation of atherosclerotic plaques.[22,23] Angiogenic promoters such as vascular endothelial growth factor (VEGF), basic fibroblast growth factor (bFGF), and granulocyte colony-stimulating factor (G-CSF), applied alone or in combination with cell transplantation, have been associated with the development of neointimal hyperplasia or coronary disease in experimental and clinical studies, particularly when associated with coronary injury (i.e., angioplasty or stenting).[22–26] Thus, quantification of coronary atherosclerosis progression by serial quantitative coronary angiography represents an indispensable safety endpoint in angiogenesis clinical trials. Ideally, intravascular ultrasound (IVUS) assessment should be performed to determine the plaque burden and late changes in vessel wall morphology in the treated coronary territory.

Finally, the global and regional ejection fraction and regional wall motion of the infarcted zone can be assessed during cardiac catheterization by left ventriculography, which has played an important role in determining treatment effectiveness in early clinical trials of cell therapy.

Nonfluoroscopic Electromechanical Mapping

Left ventricular electromechanical mapping uses a nonfluoroscopic catheter navigation (NOGA) system with three-dimensional real-time reconstruction of the endocardial surface and provides simultaneous information on electrical and motion properties of the myocardium. NOGA allows the detection of myocardial viability online in the catheterization laboratory,[27] based on electrical activity (unipolar voltage potentials) and local endocardial shortening (Figure 12.2). Low unipolar voltage (<7 mV) has shown good correlation with nuclear and MRI imaging techniques to detect nonviable myocardium.[28–30] This technique is reproducible (Figure 12.2) and has been utilized for guidance of intramyocardial injection of bone marrow-derived cells or gene therapy,[4,31–33] as well as monitoring of therapeutic effects[4] in multiple angiogenesis trials. New catheter design and user-friendly software are expected to decrease the

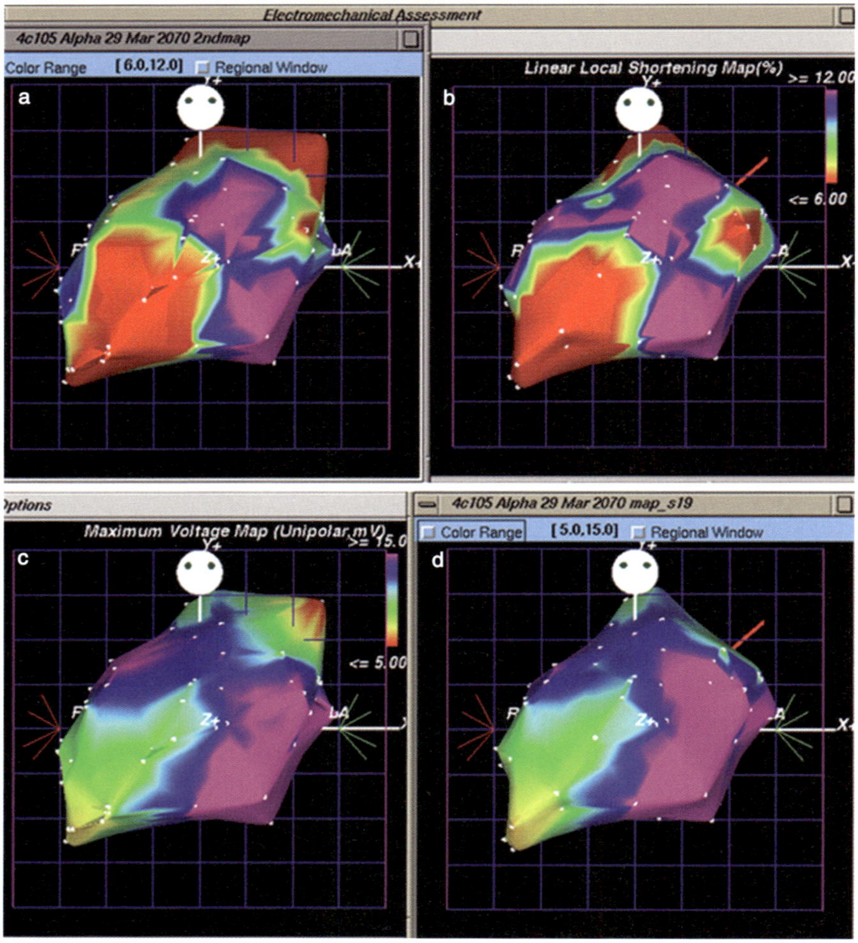

Figure 12.2 *Electromechanical mapping at two different time points (a, c and b, d, respectively) in the same heart, illustrating the reproducibility of the method. Both maps show the apical wall with very low linear local shortening (a, b) and low maximum unipolar voltage (c, d), indicating nonviable, infarcted myocardium.*

mapping time dramatically. A more detailed discussion of NOGA technology and techniques is given in Chapter 11.

Echocardiography

Echocardiographic examination has been an integral part of most angiogenesis protocols, because of its portability, availability, cost-effectiveness, and ability to provide quantification of global and regional wall motion, cardiac function, and systolic and diastolic volumes of cardiac chambers.[4] Advanced echocardiographic techniques with intravenous injection of contrast agents (microbubbles) as red cell tracers during ultrasound imaging provide the ability to quantify infarct size and interrogate the microcirculation. The tissue concentration of bubbles within the myocardium can be determined by videodensitometry.[34,35] The ultrasound beam destroys the microbubbles, and intermittent images are obtained during continuous

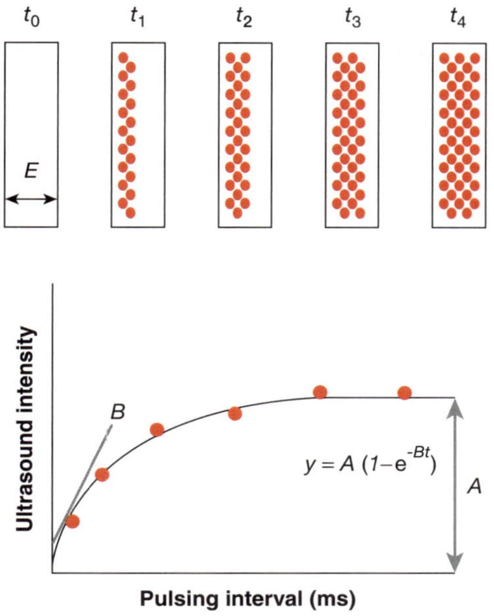

Figure 12.3 *Schematic illustration of the basics of myocardium contrast ultrasound image acquisition. Images are acquired intermittently because the ultrasound beam destroys the bubbles. At time* $t=0$*, no microbubbles are present. E represents the elevation (thickness) of the ultrasound beam. The first image, at* $t=t_1$*, detects some microbubbles in the myocardium – the longer the delay, the more bubbles replenish the beam, until it is completely filled, at* $t=t_4$*. The initial slope of the curve, B, represents the blood velocity, and the height of the plateau (maximum intensity), A, represents the blood volume. From Wei K, et al. Circulation 1998;97:473–83*[36] *by permission of Lippincott Williams & Wilkins.*

microbubble infusion. The time and intensity of replenishment of the ultrasound beam have been suggested to represent capillary red cell velocity (Figure 12.3).[36,37]

The use of myocardial contrast echocardiography as an angiogenesis endpoint has been proposed.[38,39] One study used second-generation microbubbles composed of a phospholipid bilayer shell and perfluoropropane with a mean size of 2.5 μm, which were injected intravenously (100 μl/min) in a chronic ischemic porcine model of autologous bone marrow cell transplantation. Contrast intensity was measured at two different phases: when the region of interest was filled by contrast and when 80% of the contrast was destroyed by a series of ultrasound beams. A myocardial contrast index derived from these measurements correlated well with capillary density measured by histology ($r=0.92$). Both histology and contrast echocardiography were able to demonstrate increased capillary formation 1 month after cell transplantation.[39] The possibility of intracoronary injection of contrast also provided a reliable perfusion index with good predictive value for ventricular remodeling post myocardial infarction.[37,40]

Echocardiography also has the potential to image single cells loaded with ultrasmall contrast agents. However, the acoustic shadow generated by the contrast agents closest to the ultrasound beam and the potential for contrast dilution secondary to cell division or transfer of contrast molecules to other cell types impose considerable limitations on this imaging approach. In general, the application of echocardiography in clinical trials is limited by poor visualization of some anatomic sites, suboptimal spatial resolution, and high operator dependence, particularly when more advanced techniques are used.

Nuclear Imaging

Radioactive agents such as thallium-201 (^{201}Tl), technetium-99m-labeled 2-methoxy-2-methylpropylisonitrile (^{99m}Tc-sestamibi), [^{13}N]ammonia and [^{18}F]fluorodeoxyglucose (FDG) have been routinely used as tracers of myocardial blood flow distribution, regional ventricular function, and cellular metabolism.[41,42] SPECT is a routine nuclear imaging technique[43] and has been applied in most angiogenesis clinical protocols.[4,6] Semi-quantitative SPECT imaging analyses have shown good sensitivity and specificity to determine regional myocardial blood flow and absolute ventricular volumes, ejection fraction, and wall motion thickening. Despite concerns about its poor spatial resolution, SPECT imaging has been able to detect improvement in myocardial blood flow in patients undergoing angiogenic gene or protein therapy.[44,45] The potassium analog ^{201}Tl is

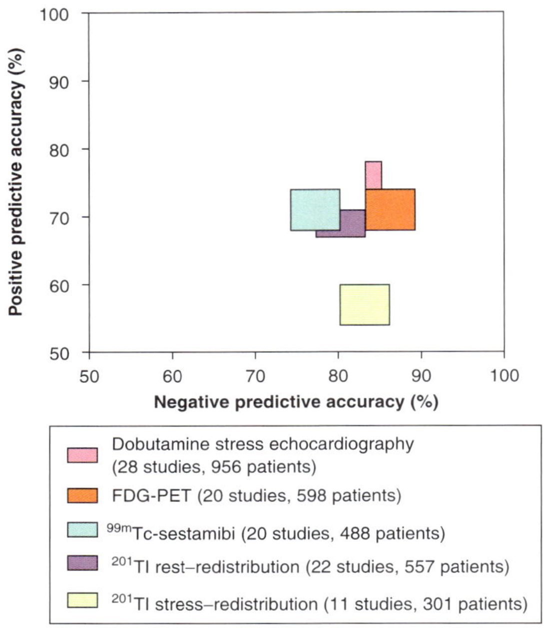

Figure 12.4 *Accuracy of nuclear and echocardiographic techniques to predict viable myocardium: data from a recent meta-analysis. The rectangles are centered on the weighted means, and the sizes of the rectangles indicate 95% confidence intervals. From Underwood SR, et al. Eur Heart J 2004;25:815–36[47] by permission of the European Society of Cardiology.*

actively transported into viable myocytes. The kinetics of uptake and exchange of ^{201}Tl with the systemic reservoir and, most importantly, its redistribution provide a measure of myocardial viability. This SPECT technique has shown sensitivities of up to 88% but a low specificity (49%) (Figure 12.4).[46]

Improved detection of regional blood flow can be achieved by PET using [^{13}N]ammonia. This is a perfusion tracer that is avidly extracted and retained in viable myocytes by incorporation into glutamine.[47] This tracer, combined with FDG, which is mainly a cell viability marker, provides the most sensitive PET technique (88% in a pooled analysis)[46] to determine myocardial viability[47] (Figure 12.4). Nonviable myocardium has a concordantly reduced uptake of both [^{13}N]ammonia and FDG, whereas a perfusion–metabolism mismatch is characteristic of viable myocardium. Because myocardial recovery represents one of the ultimate goals of cell transplant therapy, recent studies have utilized PET to demonstrate improved myocardial viability following cell transplantation.[6] However, angiogenesis clinical trials may require precise border detection for quantitative measurements and differentiation between endocardial and epicardial perfusion, which is not possible with most available scintigraphic techniques, including PET, because of their poor spatial resolution.

The use of radioligands targeted at membrane receptors uniquely expressed on tumor blood vessels represents a promising use of nuclear imaging to directly determine angiogenesis in vivo. Immunoscintigraphy has been able to detect ^{99m}Tc-labeled anti-CD105 monoclonal antibody in tumor endothelial cells of patients with renal cell carcinoma.[48] CD105 (endoglin) is a protein that serves as a modulator of transforming growth factor β (TGF-β) signaling and is abundantly expressed on angiogenic endothelial cells. Increased expression of $\alpha_v\beta_3$ integrin has also been observed in angiogenic vessels. A radiolabeled indium-111-labeled quinolone (^{111}In-RP748) for $\alpha_v\beta_3$ integrin has been used to detect angiogenesis in experimental models.[14] Similarly, MRI paramagnetic contrast agents using monoclonal antibodies targeted to endothelial $\alpha_v\beta_3$ integrin has been able to depict angiogenesis.[49]

Finally, nuclear imaging can be utilized to track the biodistribution of injected endothelial progenitor cells. ^{111}In-oxine (with a physical half-life of 2.8 days, γ-ray energies of 171 keV and 245 keV, and activity 37 MBq/ml) radiolabeled cells were detected predominantly in the liver and spleen within 96 hours after intravenous injection, while only 1–2% could be detected in the hearts of experimental rat models.[50] Although this study demonstrated preserved cell viability or function after radiolabeling in vitro, others have found impaired proliferation and differentiation of hematopoietic cells after ^{111}In-oxine labeling.[51] Further, leakage of ^{111}In from labeled cells and cellular viability in vivo remains a matter of

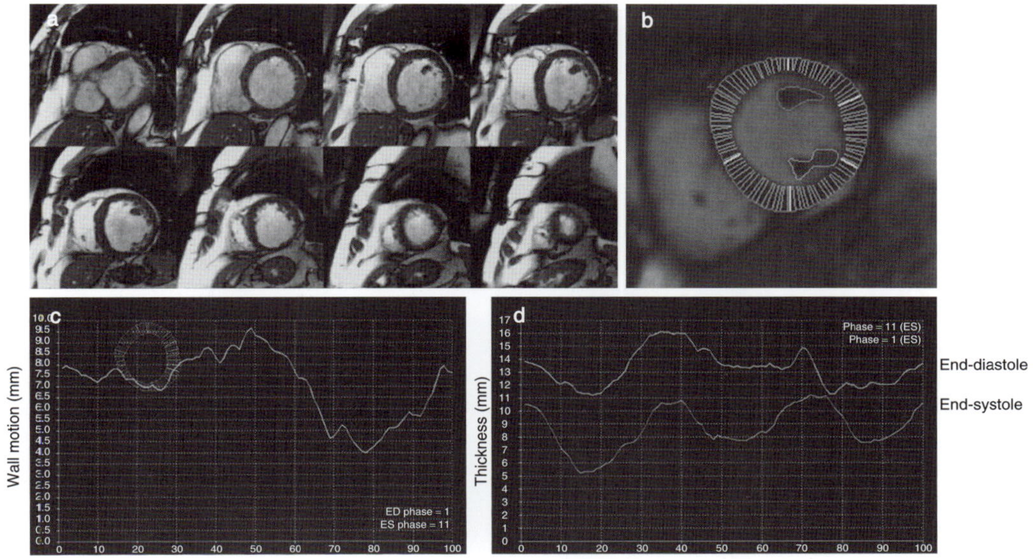

Figure 12.5 *(a) These image slices of the entire heart from base to apex illustrate the high resolution of cine MRI. (b) Contour detection of the endocardial and epicardial borders for quantitative measurements. Each slice can be divided into 5 regions representing different heart walls (thick white lines; i.e., anterior, lateral, and inferior walls, septum, etc). In addition, measurements are performed in 100 sections of the cross-sectional slices of the heart (thin lines). (c, d) Graphical display of the wall motion (c) and thickness (d) of each of the sections (100 data points arranged by slice number along the horizontal axis). In (d) the upper line displays the thickness at end-diastole and the lower line the thickness at end-systole.*

concern for the application of radiolabeling in clinical studies. The amounts of radioactive agents required to generate a detectable signal of angiogenesis in vivo likely exceed human toxic levels.

Magnetic Resonance Imaging

The field of cardiac MRI is maturing rapidly. Although cardiac MRI is less well established than the imaging technologies discussed above, it is likely to become the preferred imaging modality for clinical trials of cell therapy because of its ability to provide a comprehensive assessment of cardiac function, metabolism, and perfusion in a single, radiation-free examination.[52,53] MRI has a spatial resolution of $1.5 \times 2 \times 8$ mm, which is much higher than that of SPECT ($10 \times 10 \times 10$ mm). The resolution of MRI can reach 200 μm using high-field magnets (≥3 T) to increase the signal-to-noise ratio and reduce scanning time. Clinical 3T MRI scanners have now become available.[54] The limitations of MRI include its temporal resolution (20 and 50 ms) and the need for breath-holding with some acquisition sequences. It is a relative contraindication for claustrophobic patients and those with pacemakers and implantable cardioverter–defibrillators (ICDs), which represent an important element of the contemporary therapeutic paradigm for patients with more advanced CHF.

MRI is excellent to assess ventricular volumes, ejection fraction, myocardial mass, and regional wall motion (Figure 12.5).[47] Cine MRI provides better endocardial border definition than other methods, facilitating the detection of subtle changes in endocardial and transmural wall motion. High reproducibility, which is essential for longitudinal studies, has been demonstrated, with <5% variability between two observers for measurements of ejection fraction and end-diastolic and end-systolic volumes.[55] A myocardial wall thickness of <5.5 mm, as measured by

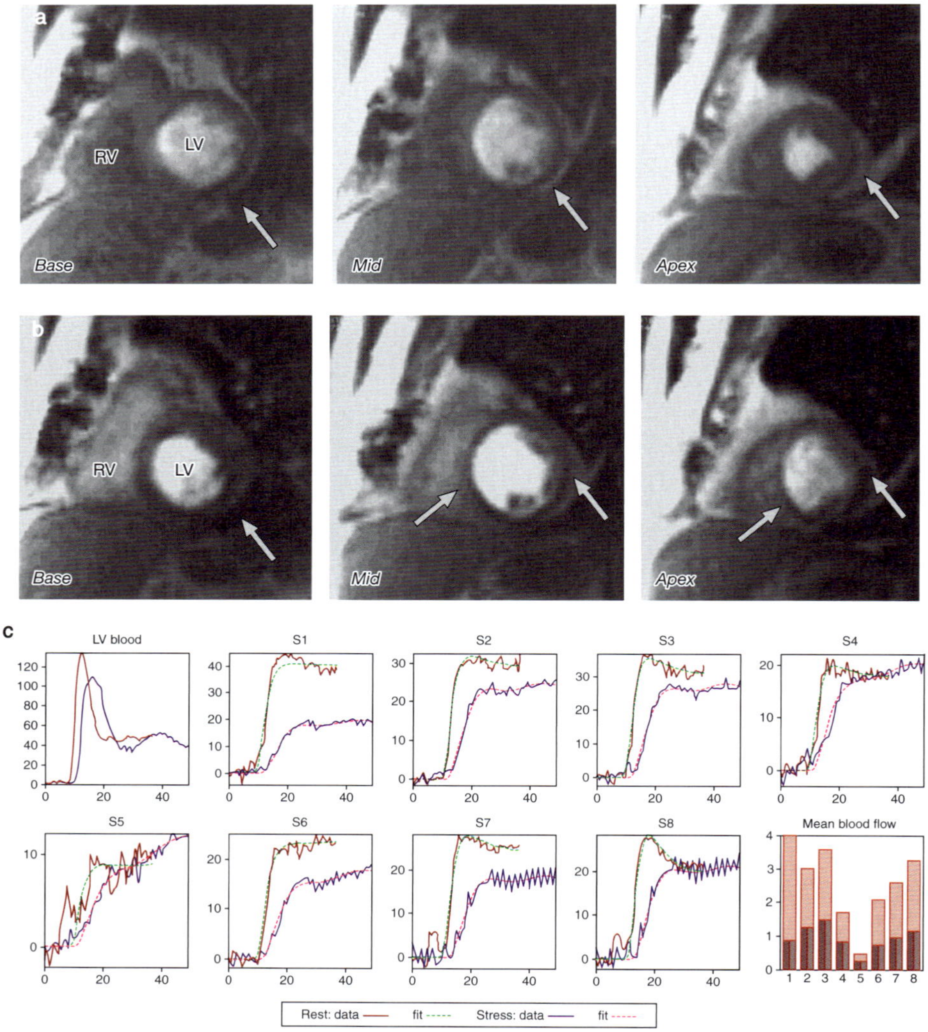

Figure 12.6 *First-pass gadolinium perfusion MRI images at rest (a) and during adenosine-induced stress (b). Slices of the base, mid ventricle, and apex display a perfusion defect (arrows) in the apical area at rest, which is expanded during stress involving the mid section of the ventricle (septum). (c) Typical signal intensity (SI)-over-time curves, both at rest (blue, raw data; red, fitted data) and under stress (thick red, raw data; green, fitted data). The first set of curves were derived from the left ventricular cavity and used for calibration of the gadolinium signal intensity. A fit (deconvolution) of the SI curves was used to provide the true myocardial perfusion flow and reserve. The bar chart depicts the difference between at-rest and stressed mean myocardial blood flow for each wall of the myocardium (8 divisions, similar to Figure 12.5). RV, right ventricle; LV, left ventricle. Courtesy of N Wilke and Alu Suiciac.*

MRI, has significantly reduced FDG uptake and has been proposed as a parameter to determine myocardial viability.[56] Thus, improved wall thickening has been used as an effectiveness endpoint of transmyocardial laser revascularization.[57]

Contrast-enhanced MRI using gadolinium-based contrast agents has been used to evaluate myocardial perfusion patterns and to quantify infarct size (Figure 12.6).[53,58–60] Gadolinium is primarily an extracellular agent and does not pass through normal cardiac myocyte membranes. Unlike intact myocardium, infarcted regions demonstrate significant hyperenhancement late after contrast administration. This phenomenon occurs in both acute and chronic infarction. The mechanism of delayed hyperenhancement in infarcted myocardium is not fully understood but appears to be related to interstitial edema and prolonged contrast washout.[53] The accuracy of high-resolution contrast-enhanced MRI to assess infarcted myocardium has shown very strong correlations with histology (r=0.94–0.99)[61,62] and other clinical parameters of location and extent of myocardial infarction.[63] Serial contrast-enhanced MRI demonstrated a 20% decrease in late hyperenhancement volume at 4 months after intramyocardial injection of bone marrow or circulating progenitor cells in the TOPCARE-AMI study.[64]

Assessment of microvascular perfusion is essential to determine angiogenic effectiveness. The passage of gadolinium through the myocardium can be plotted as signal intensity versus time (Figure 12.6),[65] which allows assessment of myocardial perfusion by appearance of first pass of contrast and washout rates on MRI. However, MRI measures contrast arrival not only at the capillaries but also at the interstitium. The superior spatial resolution of MRI allows regional quantification of transmural flow gradients and changes in subendocardial perfusion. Both relative and absolute blood flow can be quantified with good precision and reproducibility by first-pass MRI perfusion at rest and during hyperemia.[66] The inverse mean transit time calculated from the signal intensity–time curve shows a linear correlation with the absolute myocardial blood flow derived from radiolabeled microsphere data.[67] Quantitative first-pass MRI perfusion has shown improved regional myocardial perfusion after transmyocardial laser revascularization.[68] In addition, the myocardial perfusion reserve (MPR) can be estimated from the ratio of absolute myocardial blood flow during vasodilatation and at baseline, in units identical to those used for invasive measurements with labeled microspheres. A deconvolution technique to fit the time–intensity curves and provide an adjusted or "true" myocardial blood flow measurement has been validated[69] and extensively utilized by Wilke et al[60,67,70] at the Cardiovascular Imaging Core Laboratories, University of Florida Shands–Jacksonville. Serial MRI assessments of both myocardial function and perfusion are currently being used at the Texas Heart Institute, Houston, to determine the effectiveness of adult bone marrow cell transplantation in patients with severe cardiomyopathy.

Techniques using antibody-conjugated paramagnetic contrast agents to directly map angiogenesis in vivo have been developed in various laboratories. The use of superparamagnetic ion oxide (SPIO)-labeled progenitor cells has been proposed as a means of tracking transplanted cells. Electron microscopy showed uptake of the iron oxide particles, with their encasement within membrane-bound organelles.[71] Cell viability and proliferation were not affected in SPIO-labeled cells, and these labeled cells could be detected by high-resolution MRI.[71] The US Food and Drug Administration (FDA) has approved SPIO formulations for clinical use, although not in the context of mesenchymal cell labeling. There have been other reports of in vivo 1.5 T MRI of mesenchymal cells labeled with iron fluorophore particles, which did not alter the cellular proliferation and differentiation capacity. MRI was able to detect as few as 105 labeled cells at the injection sites.[15] Challenges associated with cellular labeling (discussed above) and the lack of clinically approved contrast agents will likely delay the application of such techniques in clinical trials. Weber et al[72] have exploited the magnetic properties of the antibody-coated beads that are commonly used for isolation of progenitor cells in clinical protocols to directly image intramyocardially injected cells using 8.5 and 3 T MRI scanners in a preliminary ex vivo experiment. Myocardium containing $CD34^+$ cells was identified as a low-intensity region on T2-weighted images, which correlated well with fluorescence microscopy. This relatively simple approach is appealing because it does not require changes in the procedure for progenitor cell isolation and can be applied to freshly isolated cells. However, the feasibility of in vivo cellular imaging using clinically available MRI scanners has yet to be demonstrated.

Conclusions

In summary, contemporary clinical trials testing cell transplant therapy could certainly benefit from a multimodality imaging approach, because currently there is no single imaging technique that can provide all of the information necessary to monitor this multifaceted therapy. The lack of comparative studies and standardization of most imaging techniques further complicates the selection of proper endpoints in angiogenesis clinical trials. In response to the need for a true double-blinded large angiogenesis study, clinical research protocols should incorporate objective, quantitative data assessments performed by independent analysts unaware of the treatment assignments, as subtle changes in myocardial function or perfusion may be overlooked by inexperienced or biased image interpreters.

References

1. Simons M, Bonow RO, Chronos NA, et al. Clinical trials in coronary angiogenesis: issues, problems, consensus: an expert panel summary. Circulation 2000;102:E73–86.
2. Menasche P, Hagege AA, Vilquin JT, et al. Autologous skeletal myoblast transplantation for severe postinfarction left ventricular dysfunction. J Am Coll Cardiol 2003;41:1078–83.
3. Smits PC, van Geuns RJ, Poldermans D, et al. Catheter-based intramyocardial injection of autologous skeletal myoblasts as a primary treatment of ischemic heart failure: clinical experience with six-month follow-up. J Am Coll Cardiol 2003;42:2063–9.
4. Perin EC, Dohmann HF, Borojevic R, et al. Transendocardial, autologous bone marrow cell transplantation for severe, chronic ischemic heart failure. Circulation 2003;107:2294–302.
5. Strauer BE, Brehm M, Zeus T, et al. Repair of infarcted myocardium by autologous intracoronary mononuclear bone marrow cell transplantation in humans. Circulation 2002;106:1913–18.
6. Assmus B, Schachinger V, Teupe C, et al. Transplantation of Progenitor Cells and Regeneration Enhancement in Acute Myocardial Infarction (TOPCARE-AMI). Circulation 2002;106:3009–17.
7. Stamm C, Westphal B, Kleine HD, et al. Autologous bone-marrow stem-cell transplantation for myocardial regeneration. Lancet 2003;361:45–6.
8. Fuchs S, Satler LF, Kornowski R, et al. Catheter-based autologous bone marrow myocardial injection in no-option patients with advanced coronary artery disease: a feasibility study. J Am Coll Cardiol 2003;41:1721–4.
9. Herreros J, Prosper F, Perez A, et al. Autologous intramyocardial injection of cultured skeletal muscle-derived stem cells in patients with non-acute myocardial infarction. Eur Heart J 2003;24:2012–20.
10. Caplice NM, Gersh BJ. Stem cells to repair the heart: a clinical perspective. Circ Res 2003;92:6–8.
11. Brown EB, Campbell RB, Tsuzuki Y, et al. In vivo measurement of gene expression, angiogenesis and physiological function in tumors using multiphoton laser scanning microscopy. Nat Med 2001;7:864–8.
12. McDonald DM, Choyke PL. Imaging of angiogenesis: from microscope to clinic. Nat Med 2003;9:713–25.
13. Frangioni JV, Hajjar RJ. In vivo tracking of stem cells for clinical trials in cardiovascular disease. Circulation 2004;110:3378–83.
14. Meoli DF, Sadeghi MM, Krassilnikova S, et al. Noninvasive imaging of myocardial angiogenesis following experimental myocardial infarction. J Clin Invest 2004;113:1684–91.
15. Hill JM, Dick AJ, Raman VK, et al. Serial cardiac magnetic resonance imaging of injected mesenchymal stem cells. Circulation 2003;108:1009–14.
16. Gibson CM, Ryan K, Sparano A, et al. Angiographic methods to assess human coronary angiogenesis. Am Heart J 1999;137:169–79.
17. Kamihata H, Matsubara H, Nishiue T, et al. Improvement of collateral perfusion and regional function by implantation of peripheral blood mononuclear cells into ischemic hibernating myocardium. Arterioscler Thromb Vasc Biol 2002;22:1804–10.
18. Gorge G, Schmidt T, Ito BR, Pantely GA, Schaper W. Microvascular and collateral adaptation in swine hearts following progressive coronary artery stenosis. Basic Res Cardiol 1989;84:524–35.
19. van't Hof AW, Liem A, Suryapranata H, Hoorntje JC, de Boer MJ, Zijlstra F. Angiographic assessment of myocardial reperfusion in patients treated with primary angioplasty for acute myocardial infarction: myocardial blush grade. Zwolle Myocardial Infarction Study Group. Circulation 1998;97:2302–6.
20. Gibson CM, Cannon CP, Murphy SA, et al. Relationship of TIMI myocardial perfusion grade to mortality after administration of thrombolytic drugs. Circulation 2000;101:125–30.

21. Gibson CM, de Lemos JA, Murphy SA, et al. Methodologic and clinical validation of the TIMI myocardial perfusion grade in acute myocardial infarction. J Thromb Thrombolysis 2002;14:233–7.
22. Kang HJ, Kim HS, Zhang SY, et al. Effects of intracoronary infusion of peripheral blood stem-cells mobilised with granulocyte-colony stimulating factor on left ventricular systolic function and restenosis after coronary stenting in myocardial infarction: the MAGIC cell randomised clinical trial. Lancet 2004;363:751–6.
23. Khurana R, Zhuang Z, Bhardwaj S, et al. Angiogenesis-dependent and independent phases of intimal hyperplasia. Circulation 2004;110: 2436–43.
24. Edelman ER, Nugent MA, Smith LT, Karnovsky MJ. Basic fibroblast growth factor enhances the coupling of intimal hyperplasia and proliferation of vasa vasorum in injured rat arteries. J Clin Invest 1992;89:465–73.
25. Inoue M, Itoh H, Ueda M, et al. Vascular endothelial growth factor (VEGF) expression in human coronary atherosclerotic lesions: possible pathophysiological significance of VEGF in progression of atherosclerosis. Circulation 1998;98:2108–16.
26. Celletti FL, Waugh JM, Amabile PG, Brendolan A, Hilfiker PR, Dake MD. Vascular endothelial growth factor enhances atherosclerotic plaque progression. Nat Med 2001;7:425–9.
27. Kornowski R, Hong MK, Leon MB. Comparison between left ventricular electromechanical mapping and radionuclide perfusion imaging for detection of myocardial viability. Circulation 1998;98:1837–41.
28. Perin EC, Silva GV, Sarmento-Leite R, et al. Assessing myocardial viability and infarct transmurality with left ventricular electromechanical mapping in patients with stable coronary artery disease: validation by delayed-enhancement magnetic resonance imaging. Circulation 2002;106: 957–61.
29. Botker HE, Lassen JF, Hermansen F, et al. Electromechanical mapping for detection of myocardial viability in patients with ischemic cardiomyopathy. Circulation 2001;103:1631–7.
30. Keck A, Hertting K, Schwartz Y, et al. Electromechanical mapping for determination of myocardial contractility and viability. A comparison with echocardiography, myocardial single-photon emission computed tomography, and positron emission tomography. J Am Coll Cardiol 2002;40: 1067–74; discussion 1075–8.
31. Vale PR, Losordo DW, Milliken CE, et al. Left ventricular electromechanical mapping to assess efficacy of phVEGF(165) gene transfer for therapeutic angiogenesis in chronic myocardial ischemia. Circulation 2000;102:965–74.
32. Tse HF, Kwong YL, Chan JK, Lo G, Ho CL, Lau CP. Angiogenesis in ischaemic myocardium by intramyocardial autologous bone marrow mononuclear cell implantation. Lancet 2003;361:47–9.
33. Losordo DW, Vale PR, Hendel RC, et al. Phase 1/2 placebo-controlled, double-blind, dose-escalating trial of myocardial vascular endothelial growth factor 2 gene transfer by catheter delivery in patients with chronic myocardial ischemia. Circulation 2002;105:2012–18.
34. Ten Cate FJ, Drury JK, Meerbaum S, et al. Myocardial contrast two-dimensional echocardiography: experimental examination at different coronary flow levels. J Am Coll Cardiol 1984;3: 1219–26.
35. Feinstein SB, Shah PM, Bing RJ, et al. Microbubble dynamics visualized in the intact capillary circulation. J Am Coll Cardiol 1984;4:595–600.
36. Wei K, Jayaweera AR, Firoozan S, Linka A, Skyba DM, Kaul S. Quantification of myocardial blood flow with ultrasound-induced destruction of microbubbles administered as a constant venous infusion. Circulation 1998;97:473–83.
37. Ito H, Tomooka T, Sakai N, et al. Lack of myocardial perfusion immediately after successful thrombolysis. A predictor of poor recovery of left ventricular function in anterior myocardial infarction. Circulation 1992;85:1699–705.
38. Villanueva FS, Abraham JA, Schreiner GF, et al. Myocardial contrast echocardiography can be used to assess the microvascular response to vascular endothelial growth factor-121. Circulation 2002; 105:759–65.
39. Fujii H, Tomita S, Nakatani T, et al. A novel application of myocardial contrast echocardiography to evaluate angiogenesis by autologous bone marrow cell transplantation in chronic ischemic pig model. J Am Coll Cardiol 2004;43: 1299–305.
40. Bodi V, Sanchis J, Lopez-Lereu MP, et al. [Myocardial echocardiography with intracoronary injection of contrast in post-infarction patients. Implications and comparison with angiography and magnetic resonance imaging]. Rev Esp Cardiol 2004;57:20–8.
41. Giordano FJ. Angiogenesis: mechanisms, modulation, and targeted imaging. J Nucl Cardiol 1999; 6:664–71.
42. Marzullo P. Nuclear imaging after cell implantation. Int J Cardiol 2004;95(Suppl 1):S53–4.
43. Shaw LJ, Hachamovitch R, Berman DS, et al. The economic consequences of available diagnostic and prognostic strategies for the evaluation of stable angina patients: an observational assessment of the value of precatheterization ischemia. Economics of Noninvasive Diagnosis (END) Multicenter Study Group. J Am Coll Cardiol 1999;33:661–9.

44. Losordo DW, Vale PR, Symes JF, et al. Gene therapy for myocardial angiogenesis: initial clinical results with direct myocardial injection of phVEGF165 as sole therapy for myocardial ischemia. Circulation 1998;98:2800–4.
45. Rosengart TK, Lee LY, Patel SR, et al. Angiogenesis gene therapy: phase I assessment of direct intramyocardial administration of an adenovirus vector expressing VEGF121 cDNA to individuals with clinically significant severe coronary artery disease. Circulation 1999;100:468–74.
46. Bax JJ, Wijns W, Cornel JH, Visser FC, Boersma E, Fioretti PM. Accuracy of currently available techniques for prediction of functional recovery after revascularization in patients with left ventricular dysfunction due to chronic coronary artery disease: comparison of pooled data. J Am Coll Cardiol 1997;30:1451–60.
47. Underwood SR, Bax JJ, vom Dahl J, et al. Imaging techniques for the assessment of myocardial hibernation. Report of a Study Group of the European Society of Cardiology. Eur Heart J 2004; 25:815–36.
48. Duff SE, Li C, Garland JM, Kumar S. CD105 is important for angiogenesis: evidence and potential applications. FASEB J 2003;17:984–92.
49. Sipkins DA, Cheresh DA, Kazemi MR, Nevin LM, Bednarski MD, Li KC. Detection of tumor angiogenesis in vivo by $\alpha_V\beta_3$-targeted magnetic resonance imaging. Nat Med 1998;4:623–6.
50. Aicher A, Brenner W, Zuhayra M, et al. Assessment of the tissue distribution of transplanted human endothelial progenitor cells by radioactive labeling. Circulation 2003;107:2134–9.
51. Brenner W, Aicher A, Eckey T, et al. ^{111}In-labeled $CD34^+$ hematopoietic progenitor cells in a rat myocardial infarction model. J Nucl Med 2004; 45:512–18.
52. Rickers C, Gallegos R, Seethamraju RT, et al. Applications of magnetic resonance imaging for cardiac stem cell therapy. J Interv Cardiol 2004; 17:37–46.
53. Wu KC, Lima JA. Noninvasive imaging of myocardial viability: current techniques and future developments. Circ Res 2003;93:1146–58.
54. Stuber M, Botnar RM, Fischer SE, et al. Preliminary report on in vivo coronary MRA at 3 tesla in humans. Magn Reson Med 2002;48:425–9.
55. Semelka RC, Tomei E, Wagner S, et al. Interstudy reproducibility of dimensional and functional measurements between cine magnetic resonance studies in the morphologically abnormal left ventricle. Am Heart J 1990;119:1367–73.
56. Baer FM, Voth E, Schneider CA, Theissen P, Schicha H, Sechtem U. Comparison of low-dose dobutamine-gradient-echo magnetic resonance imaging and positron emission tomography with [^{18}F]fluorodeoxyglucose in patients with chronic coronary artery disease. A functional and morphological approach to the detection of residual myocardial viability. Circulation 1995;91: 1006–15.
57. Muhling OM, Wang Y, Jerosch-Herold M, et al. Improved myocardial function after transmyocardial laser revascularization according to cine magnetic resonance in a porcine model. J Thorac Cardiovasc Surg 2004;128:391–5.
58. Wesbey GE, Higgins CB, McNamara MT, et al. Effect of gadolinium-DTPA on the magnetic relaxation times of normal and infarcted myocardium. Radiology 1984;153:165–9.
59. Lima JA. Myocardial viability assessment by contrast-enhanced magnetic resonance imaging. J Am Coll Cardiol 2003;42:902–4.
60. Wilke NM, Jerosch-Herold M, Zenovich A, Stillman AE. Magnetic resonance first-pass myocardial perfusion imaging: clinical validation and future applications. J Magn Reson Imaging 1999; 10:676–85.
61. Kim RJ, Fieno DS, Parrish TB, et al. Relationship of MRI delayed contrast enhancement to irreversible injury, infarct age, and contractile function. Circulation 1999;100:1992–2002.
62. Kim RJ, Chen EL, Lima JA, Judd RM. Myocardial Gd-DTPA kinetics determine MRI contrast enhancement and reflect the extent and severity of myocardial injury after acute reperfused infarction. Circulation 1996;94:3318–26.
63. Wu E, Judd RM, Vargas JD, Klocke FJ, Bonow RO, Kim RJ. Visualisation of presence, location, and transmural extent of healed Q-wave and non-Q-wave myocardial infarction. Lancet 2001; 357:21–8.
64. Britten MB, Abolmaali ND, Assmus B, et al. Infarct remodeling after intracoronary progenitor cell treatment in patients with acute myocardial infarction (TOPCARE-AMI): mechanistic insights from serial contrast-enhanced magnetic resonance imaging. Circulation 2003;108:2212–18.
65. Pearlman JD, Hibberd MG, Chuang ML, et al. Magnetic resonance mapping demonstrates benefits of VEGF-induced myocardial angiogenesis. Nat Med 1995;1:1085–9.
66. Wilke N, Kroll K, Merkle H, et al. Regional myocardial blood volume and flow: first-pass MR imaging with polylysine-Gd-DTPA. J Magn Reson Imaging 1995;5:227–37.
67. Wilke N, Simm C, Zhang J, et al. Contrast-enhanced first pass myocardial perfusion imaging: correlation between myocardial blood flow in dogs at rest and during hyperemia. Magn Reson Med 1993;29:485–97.
68. Muhling OM, Wang Y, Panse P, et al. Transmyocardial laser revascularization preserves regional

myocardial perfusion: an MRI first pass perfusion study. Cardiovasc Res 2003;57:63–70.
69. Jerosch-Herold M, Wilke N, Stillman AE. Magnetic resonance quantification of the myocardial perfusion reserve with a Fermi function model for constrained deconvolution. Med Phys 1998;25:73–84.
70. Wilke N, Jerosch-Herold M, Wang Y, et al. Myocardial perfusion reserve: assessment with multisection, quantitative, first-pass MR imaging. Radiology 1997;204:373–84.
71. Zhang Z, van den Bos EJ, Wielopolski PA, de Jong-Popijus M, Duncker DJ, Krestin GP. High-resolution magnetic resonance imaging of iron-labeled myoblasts using a standard 1.5-T clinical scanner. Magma 2004;17:201–9.
72. Weber A, Pedrosa I, Kawamoto A, et al. Magnetic resonance mapping of transplanted endothelial progenitor cells for therapeutic neovascularization in ischemic heart disease. Eur J Cardiothorac Surg 2004;26:137–43.

chapter 13

Clinical Utilization of Stem Cell Therapy in Acute Myocardial Infarction

Francisco Fernández-Avilés, Pedro L Sánchez, José Alberto San Román, Luis de la Fuente, Ana Sánchez, Manuel Gómez-Bueno, Javier García-Sancho, María Jesús Peñarrubia, and Javier García-Frade

Introduction

Many of the therapies available today, including thrombolysis and urgent revascularization, have significantly improved the prognosis of patients with acute myocardial infarction (AMI).[1–3] However, currently fewer than 50% of patients with ST-segment elevation acute coronary syndrome, which involves ongoing myocardial necrosis, achieve adequate epicardial and microvascular reperfusion before irreversible damage to the supplied myocardial tissue occurs.[4] Moreover, neither medications nor procedures have so far shown any efficacy in increasing the resistance of the jeopardized myocardium to severe ischemia or in replacing necrosed myocardium with functional contractile tissue.[5] As a result, a high proportion of survivors of myocardial infarction are still at risk of developing heart failure due to left ventricular (LV) remodeling, a process characterized by mechanical expansion of the scarred, infarcted wall followed by progressive LV dilatation and dysfunction.[6]

Since the main underlying cause of postinfarction LV remodeling and dysfunction is irreversible damage to the infarcted wall,[7] the development of treatments aimed at regenerating its muscular and vascular components is now considered a major therapeutic challenge. The rationale for such an approach includes recent evidence demonstrating the remarkable ability of adult stem cells to produce differentiated cells from embryologically unrelated tissues,[8] as well as convincing data supporting the fact that the heart has a potent intrinsic regenerative capacity.[9] In fact, contrary to traditional thought, evidence has recently demonstrated the existence of cardiac stem cells able to regenerate myocytes and vasculature after aging or damage.[10–12] In addition, recent data from investigations carried out in sex-mismatched heart transplant patients strongly suggest that dividing cardiac stem cells are myocytes derived from an extracardiac origin,[13,14] such as bone marrow.[15]

On this basis, the hypothesis that the natural capability of the mammalian heart to regenerate infarcted myocardium can be reinforced has led to several investigations suggesting that adult stem cell-based therapies could prevent postinfarction LV remodeling.[11] In particular, bone marrow-derived stem cells delivered locally, or mobilized by means of systemic administration of stimulating factors (e.g., cytokines), have been shown to home to the necrotic tissue, engraft in the border zone of the infarct, replicate, induce both myogenesis and angiogenesis, reduce the infarct size, and ameliorate cardiac function and survival after an acute myocardial infarction

(AMI) in mice and pigs.[16–19] In general, these observations have been interpreted as being due to metaplastic transformation of bone marrow-derived stem cells into myocytes and vascular cells (transdifferentiation). However, the mechanism through which bone marrow-derived stem cells benefit postinfarction LV remodeling is controversial, and other views include the proposal of cell fusion or a paracrine effect as the actual mechanism of tissue repair.[20,21] In addition, concerns regarding the risk of myocardial damage and progression of restenotic and "de novo" coronary lesions after postinfarction stem cell therapy have recently arisen.[22–26]

In spite of these doubts and concerns, the capability of adult stem cells to prevent postinfarction LV remodeling has been investigated in humans. In this chapter, we summarize the available evidence regarding the application of this therapy in patients with an ST-segment elevation AMI (STEMI), describe the type of cells and delivery methods already used, and discuss the safety and the efficacy of such an approach. In addition, we also speculate on the value of current clinical data for gaining an insight into the mechanism of stem cell-based cardiac repair and designing future clinical trials.

Stem Cell Delivery in Patients with STEMI: Timing and Method for Transplantation and Follow-Up

Before describing how to transplant stem cells in patients with STEMI, it must be pointed out that the procedure of choice in this setting is far from being settled. Theoretically, there are several potential routes of stem cell delivery for this purpose (Figure 13.1): direct intramyocardial injection through the epicardium during open-chest cardiac surgery,[27–30] catheter-based direct intramyocardial injection of the cells through the endocardium guided by fluoroscopy and/or electromechanical mapping,[31–34] intracoronary administration of the cells,[24,35–38] and "mobilization" of the bone marrow using pharmacologic agents able to stimulate the proliferation of stem cells inside the bone marrow and their liberation into the peripheral circulation.[24,39] Other routes under investigation are peripheral intravenous infusion of the cells and the transvenous approach through the coronary venous system. However, in spite of these theoretical possibilities, pharmacologic bone marrow mobilization and percutaneous catheter-based intracoronary infusion have so far been the only routes used for stem cell administration in patients with a recent myocardial infarction.

Hematopoietic cellular growth factors are glycoprotein hormones that regulate hematopoietic stem cell proliferation and differentiation. Recruitment of hematopoietic stem and progenitor cells from the bone marrow to the peripheral blood following the administration of growth factors is a process termed *mobilization*, which mimics the enhancement of the physiologic release of stem cells from the bone marrow in response to stress signals during tissue injury. Granulocyte colony-stimulating factor (G-CSF) belongs to this group of agents and has been shown to ameliorate the postinfarction LV outcome in animals.[17] Although the administration of G-CSF before bare stent-based repair of the infarct-related artery could induce more in-stent restenosis than expected,[24] preliminary clinical data show that the early subcutaneous administration of this agent (5–10 μg/kg/day during 4 days) in patients with a recent myocardial infarction is well tolerated and seems to prevent LV remodeling.[24]

Currently, intracoronary administration of hematopoietic progenitors represents the best tried method for stem cell therapy in patients with STEMI. The procedure described in this chapter has been empirically designed and is based upon our experience and that of others.[35–38] It is clear that the procedure described here will change in the future as new experimental and clinical evidence emerges. Basically, the procedure can be divided into three stages: (1) the standard care of a patient with an AMI; (2) the extraction and management of stem cells; and (3) the infusion of stem cells. Although the standard optimal management of a patient with STEMI is beyond the scope of this chapter, it should be stressed that a percutaneous coronary

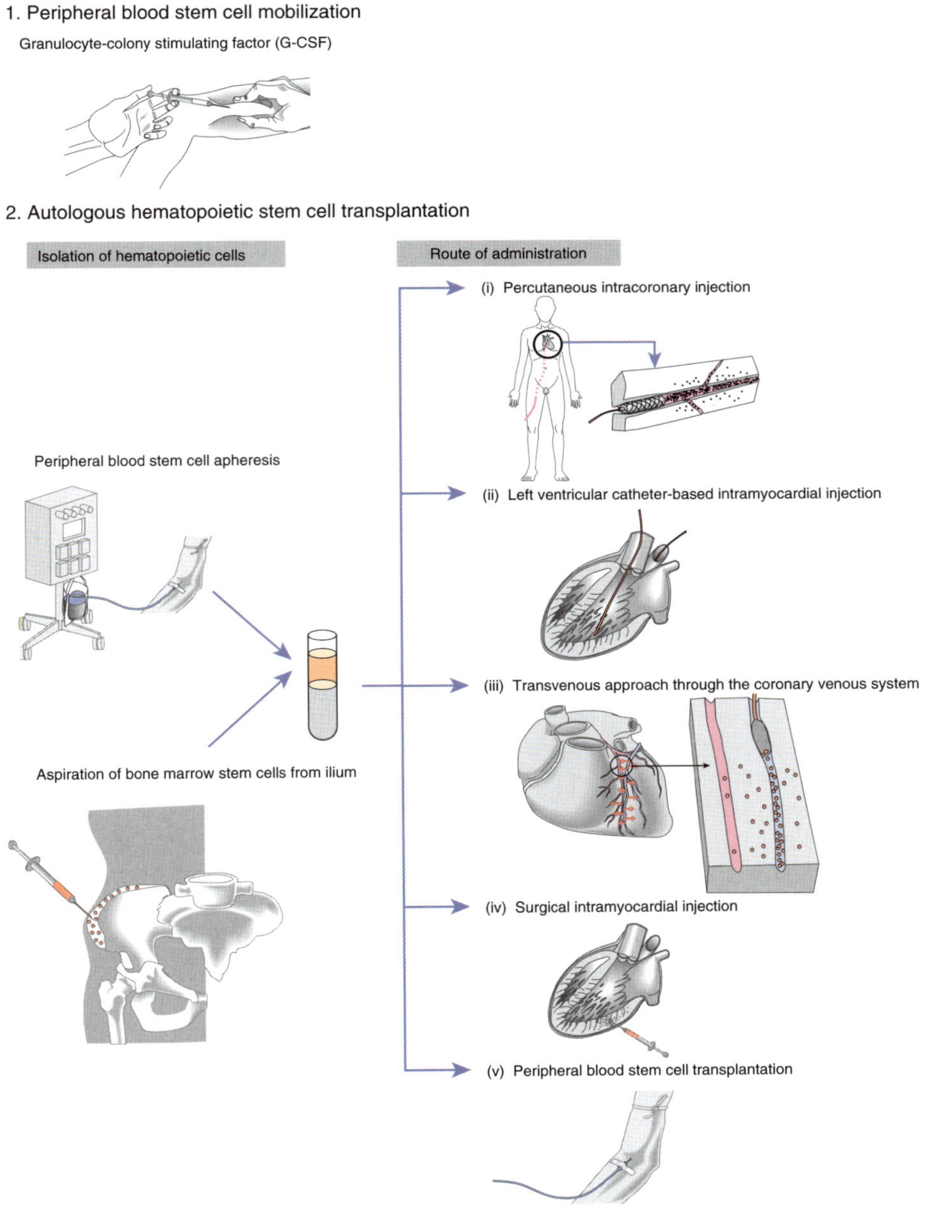

Figure 13.1 *Stem cell delivery in patients with an ST-segment elevation acute myocardial infarction (STEMI). Three types of stem cells have been used in cell regeneration studies: bone marrow-derived progenitor cells (harvested directly from the marrow), peripheral blood-derived progenitor cells (mobilized from the bone marrow using granulocyte colony-stimulating factor, (G-CSF), and skeletal myoblasts. In patients with STEMI, only the bone marrow- or peripheral blood-derived progenitor cells have been used. To date, only the percutaneous catheter-based intracoronary route of administration (i) has been employed in these patients. However, other means of administration are possible (including routes that have already been used in patients with ischemic cardiomyopathy, as well as approaches that are still under preclinical investigation): catheter-based direct intramyocardial injection through the endocardium under fluoroscopic and/or electromechanical mapping guidance (ii); a transvenous approach through the coronary venous system (iii); direct intramyocardial injection through the endocardium during coronary bypass surgery (iv); and infusion intravenously into the peripheral circulation (v).*

intervention in the culprit artery must be undertaken to ensure vascular access for the stem cells to be infused. Regarding the stem cell transplant procedure itself, the timing of percutaneous revascularization therapy (primary, facilitated, or delayed) makes no difference, provided that the culprit artery is opened wide.

Stem cells can be obtained from bone marrow. In this case, bone marrow is aspirated from the iliac crest under local anesthesia with an aspiration needle: 5 ml are obtained in every puncture, and the procedure is repeated until 50 ml of bone marrow has been obtained. The bone marrow is then filtered, and mononuclear cells are isolated by means of Ficoll density ultrafiltration. Then the erythrocytes are lysed with water. A small sample should be collected for typing. At this time, the cells can be injected[35,38] or can be cultivated overnight before being infused into the coronary artery.[36,37] It is not yet known whether all mononuclear cells or a specific subpopulation of previously selected cells should be given. The four clinical studies available utilized an unselected approach because several different fractions of mononuclear bone marrow cells may differentiate into myocytes and vessels. Therefore, not only hematopoietic and mesenchymal stem cells but also other mononuclear cells are infused into the necrotic area.[36–38]

Circulating progenitor cells can also serve as a source of stem cells.[35] In this case, peripheral venous blood (250 ml) is collected, mononuclear cells are purified and cultured ex vivo for 3 days, and these cells are then reinfused into the target artery. For intracoronary delivery of the cells, an over-the-wire angioplasty balloon is used. After being positioned in the previously stented infarct-related coronary segment, the balloon is inflated at 2–4 atm of pressure until a complete block of blood flow is achieved, to allow prolonged contact between the stem cells and the microcirculation and to avoid retrograde flow of the cells. Then the guidewire is withdrawn, and the central lumen of the balloon is used to infuse the cells. Intracoronary infusion of the cell suspension is carried out, manually or with a pump, periods of occlusion–infusion (2–3 minutes) and reperfusion (1–3 minutes) being alternated until the total dose has been given (Figure 13.2).

The timing of infusion of the stem cells is an unresolved issue. Theoretically, infusion could be performed as early as immediately after percutaneous coronary intervention, with a short delay to allow for bone marrow extraction and manipulation, or as late as 15–30 days after the acute phase. Although little evidence is available in this regard, there are some experimental data worth taking into account. An injection of fetal cardiomyocytes after 4 weeks of permanent coronary artery ligation in rats failed to reverse LV dilatation, suggesting that infusion at that time could have been too late to have any impact on cardiac remodeling.[40] One animal study was aimed at determining the optimum time for cardiomyocyte transplantation to enhance myocardial function after LV injury.[41] Rat hearts were cryoinjured, and fetal cardiomyocytes were transplanted immediately, at 2 weeks, and at 4 weeks. Histologic studies performed in the sacrificed animals showed that the inflammatory reaction was greatest during the first week and that scar size expanded at 4–8 weeks. Cardiomyocytes transplanted immediately after cryoinjury were not found at 8 weeks, and scar size and ventricular function were similar in control hearts. In contrast, cardiomyocytes transplanted at 2 and 4 weeks formed cardiac tissue within the scar, limited scar expansion, and led to better ventricular function than in control patients. The investigators concluded that cardiomyocyte transplantation was most successful after the inflammatory reaction had resolved but before scar expansion. In the clinical setting, it could be assumed that transplantation of stem cells too early or too late might result in their taking part in the inflammatory reaction or in the scar formation process, respectively, instead of forming functional myocytes or vessels. Clinical studies have infused stem cells 4–7 days after onset of pain.[35–38]

Follow-up of patients undergoing this treatment is of great importance. Two aspects have to be considered: safety and assessment of efficacy. Regarding safety, myocardial injury secondary to the procedure must be ruled out. Therefore,

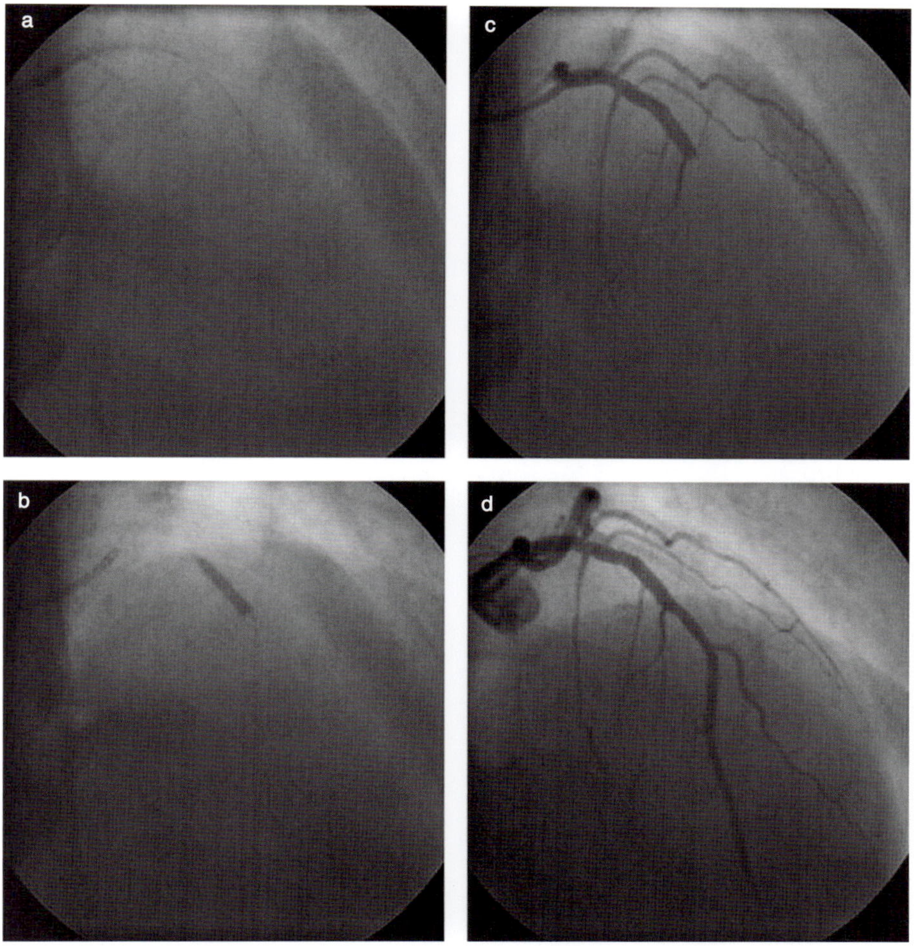

Figure 13.2 *Percutaneous intracoronary transplantation of bone marrow-derived stem cells. For intracoronary delivery of the cells, an over-the-wire angioplasty balloon catheter oversized by 0.5 mm is used (a, b). After positioning at the site of the former infarct-related coronary occlusion where the stent has been implanted, the balloon is inflated at low pressure (2–4 atm) to block blood flow (b). Then the guidewire is removed, and the bone marrow-derived stem cell suspension is infused through the internal lumen of the balloon under stop-flow conditions (c). The stem cells are infused with a pump at 1–2 ml/min, periods of 3 minutes of inflation and cell infusion alternating with 1 minute of de-inflation and reperfusion until the total dose of cells has been given to the patient. The integrity of the coronary artery used for transplantation and blood flow perfusion in the supplied myocardial area are checked after the procedure (d).*

electrocardiographic (ECG) and myocardial injury markers have to be periodically obtained within 24 hours after stem cell transplantation. Moreover, although arrhythmias have not been reported with bone marrow- or peripheral blood-derived stem cells, ECG monitoring for 24–48 hours is mandatory, as is ECG Holter monitoring at least 1 and 6 months after discharge.

The following parameters can be used to assess efficacy: global and regional function, viability, infarct size, thickness and thickening of the infarcted wall, contractile reserve, perfusion, and coronary reserve. Global and regional function can be calculated with angiography, echocardiography, and magnetic resonance imaging (MRI). In our opinion, MRI is the technique of choice for these patients. It is noninvasive has high temporal and spatial resolution, thus high reproducibility. Furthermore, exposure to ionizing radiation is avoided. Finally, given its tomographic nature, MRI is more accurate than echocardiography or cine angiography in assessing remodeling, because it does not make assumptions regarding ventricular geometry. This is crucial in distorted postinfarction ventricles. When assessing regional function, the wall motion score index must be calculated.[42] Viability is another parameter to be measured: this can be done with low-dose dobutamine echocardiography, scintigraphic techniques, or MRI using late hyperenhancement sequences following gadolinium administration. MRI also allows an accurate measurement of infarct size. Several investigations have demonstrated that thickness and thickening of the infarcted wall calculated by MRI or echocardiography correlate well with viability.[43,44] Contractile reserve, defined as the potential of the myocardium to increase its contractility after inotropic stimulation, can be assessed by echocardiographic or MRI monitoring of the response of the ventricle to dobutamine administration at low doses (from 5 to 10 or 20 μg/kg/min). Positron emission tomography (PET) and scintigraphic techniques permit an accurate estimate of myocardial perfusion. Lastly, coronary flow reserve and fractional flow reserve are measured in the infarct and in a noninfarct reference vessel by using an intracoronary Doppler or thermodilution wire and infusion of adenosine through the guiding catheter.[45]

To demonstrate any benefit of stem cell transplantation, a basal and a follow-up study must be compared. To rule out myocardial stunning, which could lead to confusing results, this follow-up examination should not be performed until at least 3 months after the acute event.

A proposed algorithm for intracoronary stem cell transplantation and follow-up in patients with STEMI is shown in Figure 13.3.

Results of Clinical Studies

The evidence that stem cells can reconstitute necrotic myocardium and improve cardiac function in animals has led to the initiation of clinical studies, which have been focused mainly on addressing the feasibility and the safety of this therapy. The main differences between these studies lie in the type of cell employed and the type of patient. Most patients suffered from ischemic heart disease at different stages. The methods of measurement differed, as it is not yet certain what is the best system in these settings. The principal endpoint was to assess whether stem cell transplantation improved LV function. In cell regeneration studies, three types of stem cells have been used: bone marrow-derived progenitor cells (harvested directly from the marrow), peripheral blood-derived progenitor cells (mobilized with G-CSF) and skeletal myoblasts. However, in patients with STEMI, only bone marrow- and peripheral blood-derived progenitor cells have been used (Table 13.1).

Assmus et al[35] randomly allocated 20 patients with reperfused STEMI to receive intracoronary infusion of either bone marrow-derived (9 patients) or peripheral blood-derived (11 patients) progenitor cells into the infarct-related artery 4.3 ± 1.5 days after STEMI. There were no differences in any measured parameter between the two groups of progenitor cells. Transplantation of progenitor cells was associated with a significant increase in the global LV ejection fraction (LVEF), improved regional wall motion in the infarct zone, and a profoundly reduced LV end-systolic volume (LVESV) at 4 months of follow-up. Coronary blood flow reserve was increased in the infarct-related artery. Quantitative [^{18}F]fluorodeoxyglucose (FDG)-PET revealed an increase in myocardial viability in the infarct zone.

Strauer et al[36] transplanted 10 patients with autologous bone marrow-derived mononuclear stem cells into 10 patient via a balloon catheter placed into the infarct-related artery during balloon dilatation 5–9 days after an AMI. After 3 months of follow-up, the infarct region had decreased significantly and showed significant improvement in the stroke volume index, LVESV, and contractility and myocardial perfusion.

Kang et al[24] studied the evolution of 11 patients with reperfused STEMI who were randomly allocated to conventional therapy (1 patient), intracoronary transplantation of peripheral blood-derived progenitor cells after bone marrow

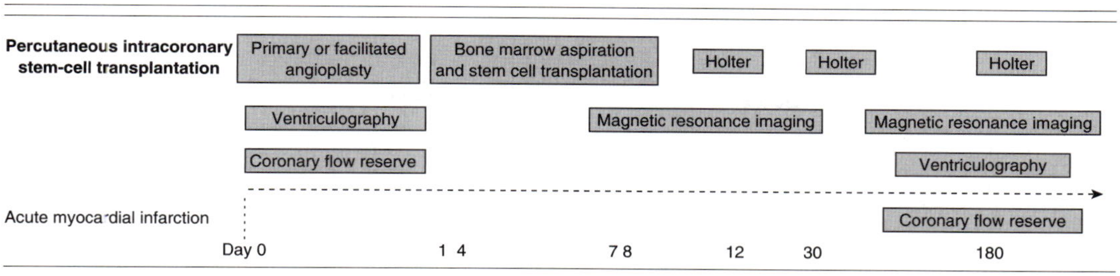

Figure 15.3 *Algorithm for intracoronary stem cell transplantation and follow-up in acute myocardial infarction.*

Table 13.1 Summary of studies in stem cell therapy in acute myocardial infarction

Authors	*Patients*	*Method of transplantation*	*Follow-up (months)*	*Endpoint*	*Results*	*Complications*
Strauer et al[36]	10 BMMNC	Intracoronary	3	ΔLVEF LVESV Improved myocardial perfusion	NS −15 ml Yes	No
Assmuss et al[35]	9 BMPC 11 PBPC	Intracoronary	4	ΔLVEF LVESV Improved myocardial viability	8.5% −13.9 ml Yes	No
Kang et al[24]	7 PBPC/G-CSF 3 G-CSF alone 1 conventional therapy	Intracoronary	6	ΔLVEF Improved myocardial perfusion	6.4% Yes	70% intrastent restenosis
Fernández-Avilés et al[37]	20 BMMNC	Intracoronary	6	ΔLVEF LVESV Δ(infarct wall thickness)	5.8% −9.6 ml 0.9 mm	No
Wollert et al[38]	30 BMPC 30 conventional therapy	Intracoronary	6	ΔLVEF LVESV	6.7% NS	No
Kuethe et al[39]	5 G-CSF	Subcutaneous	3	ΔLVEF Improved myocardial perfusion	9.4% Yes	No

BMMNC, bone marrow-derived mononuclear cells; BMPC, bone marrow-derived progenitor cells; G-CSF, granulocyte colony-stimulating factor; LVEF, left ventricular ejection fraction; LVESV, left ventricular end-systolic volume; NS, not significant; Δ, increment; PBPC, peripheral blood-derived progenitor cells.

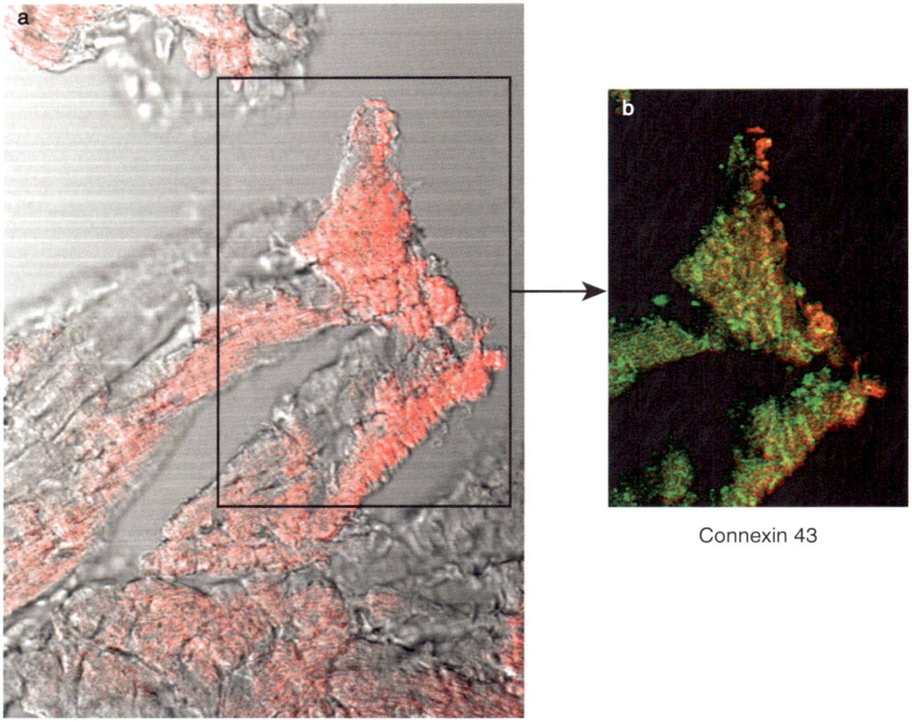

Figure 13.4 Culture of human mononuclear bone marrow-derived cells on cryoinjured mouse heart slices. Bone marrow-derived cells (stained in red with DiI) integrate into cardiac tissue (a) and express connexin 43 (green, b).

mobilization with G-CSF (7 patients), or mobilization alone (3 patients). Importantly, in this study the patient allocated to conventional therapy underwent bare stent-based repair of the infarct-related artery 4 days after randomization. Similarly, the patients treated with G-CSF alone or in combination with intracoronary infusion of peripheral blood-derived progenitor cells underwent stenting after being treated with G-CSF during 4 days. At 6 months of follow-up, myocardial perfusion and LVEF improved significantly in the patients who received cell infusion. However, enrollment was stopped because those patients randomized to G-CSF alone or in combination with progenitor cell transplantation before stenting had an unexpectedly high rate of in-stent restenosis.

Fernández-Avilés et al[37] used bone marrow mononuclear cells from 20 patients with STEMI to assess both the cells' myocardial regenerative capability in vitro and their effect on postinfarction LV remodeling. Human bone marrow-derived stem cells grafted into cryoinjured mice heart slices acquired a cardiomyocyte phenotype and expressed cardiac proteins after 1 week (Figure 13.4). In the clinical trial, an average of $78 \pm 41 \times 10^6$ bone marrow mononuclear cells per patient were transplanted via the intracoronary route 13.5 ± 5.5 days after infarction, with no adverse effects on microvascular function or myocardial injury. No major cardiac events occurred at up to 11 ± 5 months. At 6 months, MRI showed a decrease in the LVESV, an improvement in regional and global LV function,

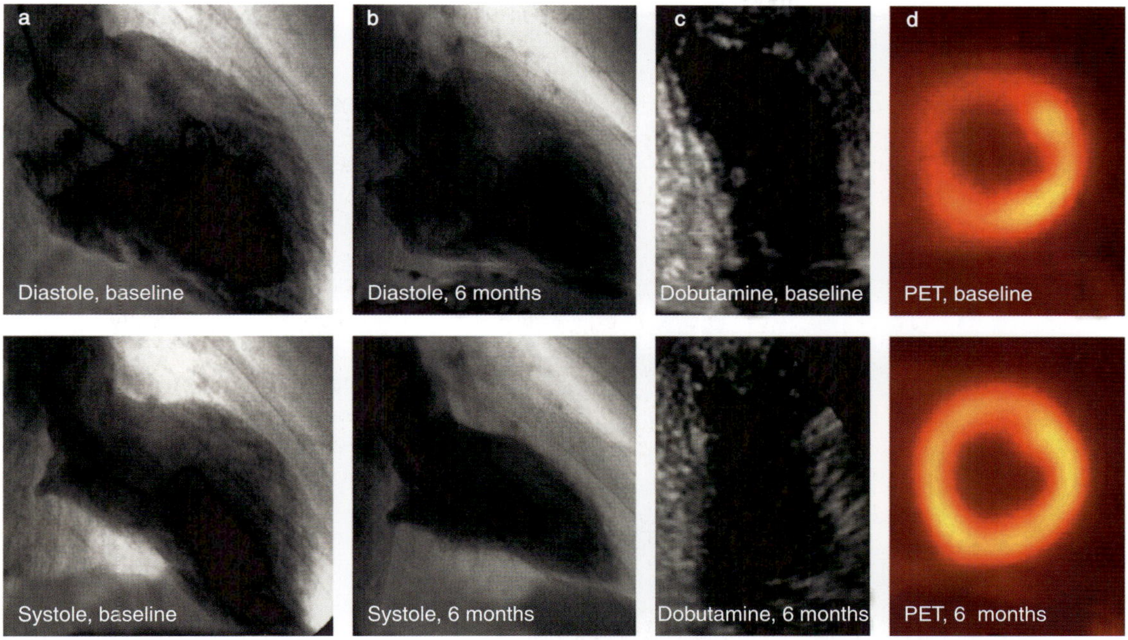

Figure 13.5 *(a, b) Improvement in angiographic left ventricular outcome in a patient undergoing cell therapy, with clear reductions in end-diastolic and end-systolic volumes, as well as complete normalization of anterior left ventricular systolic wall motion at 6 months. (c, d) In the same patient, the low-dose dobutamine echocardiogram and positron-emission tomogram (PET) 6 months after cell transplantation show marked improvements in anterior and apical contractility and in metabolism, respectively, suggesting recovery of viability not seen in the baseline studies.*

and increased thickness of the infarcted wall, while the coronary restenosis rate was only 15%. Angiographic follow-up confirmed the benefit on the LV outcome (Figure 13.5). Concordantly, PET and low-dose dobutamine stress echocardiography showed recovery of viability in the infarcted wall (Figure 13.5). No changes were found in a nonrandomized contemporary control group. Thus, according to these findings, intracoronary transplantation of autologous bone marrow-derived stem cells after an AMI is feasible and safe in the short and mid term, prevents LV remodeling, leads to significant recovery of cardiac function, and seems to regenerate myocardial tissue.

Wollert et al[38] included 60 patients who had had a myocardial infarction and had undergone primary angioplasty. They allocated patients randomly to receive standard therapy (30 patients) versus intracoronary infusion of unselected bone marrow progenitor cells (30 patients). Bone marrow cell transplantation was performed under a protocol similar to that used by Strauer et al,[28] and all patients were evaluated by MRI, with a basal study 3.5 days after primary angioplasty and another at 6 months. There was a significant improvement in LVEF within the cell therapy group. It is important to point out that this improvement concerned all groups of patients, especially those reperfused late. An electrophysiological study was carried out for exhaustive arrhythmia analysis at 6 months: no malignant arrhythmias were induced.

Kuethe et al[39] analyzed cardiac function and perfusion in 5 patients with AMIs, who were treated only with G-CSF in addition to a standard therapeutic regimen. After 3 months of follow-up, the global LVEF (determined by radionuclide ventriculography) increased significantly; the wall motion score and the wall perfusion score (determined by electrocardiographically gated single photon emission computed tomography, SPECT) decreased, indicating a significant improvement in myocardial function and perfusion. No severe side effects of G-CSF treatment or malignant arrhythmias were observed.

Stem Cell Therapy for AMI in Perspective

Much excitement has surrounded recent breakthroughs in the field of adult stem cell research and their implications for cell therapy in patients with acute ischemic heart disease. However, further proofs of the efficacy and safety of this therapy for AMI are necessary.

Available clinical data show that in patients with recent STEMI, intracoronary transplantation of autologous bone marrow-derived stem cells is a feasible and safe procedure that seems to diminish significantly the extent of LV remodeling and to promote a significant recovery of both global and segmental cardiac function. Moreover, although the mechanism of this putative beneficial effect remains to be elucidated, data from animal studies and from our parallel clinical and in vitro experiments strongly suggest that bone marrow cell therapy for STEMI might regenerate contractile myocardial tissue. Therefore, altogether, these results demonstrate a favorable risk–benefit ratio for early intracoronary administration of hematopoietic progenitors in patients with AMIs, which opens the way to the development of randomized large-scale clinical trials in this area. These trials should be compatible with simultaneous mechanistic clinical and basic research aimed at addressing some crucial questions that are still unsettled.

- How do adult stem cells contribute to repair in the setting of an AMI? At least six different mechanisms might be proposed: transdifferentiation, dedifferentiation, transdetermination, cell fusion, true pluripotent stem cell behavior, and the production of trophic factors. It is likely that our current knowledge of cell markers is inadequate to define cell populations accurately, so it is possible that cells with true multipotency may have contaminated experiments previously reported as examples of transdifferentiation.
- What is the ideal source of adult stem cells in patients with an AMI? Bone marrow stem cells seem to be simple to use, cheap, and apparently widely applicable.
- What is the best route of administration? So far, only percutaneous intracoronary delivery and mobilization of stem cells with G-CSF have been tested.
- When should cell transplantation be performed? Experimental studies suggest that stem cell transplantation is most successful after the inflammatory reaction has resolved but before scar expansion.
- How many times should cell transplantation be performed? Several clinical studies have demonstrated that stem cells can improve cardiac function in patients with an old myocardial infarction: therefore, compared with single autologous stem cell transplantation in the acute phase, successive transplantations may improve the benefit of this therapy.

We are optimistic that stem cell transplantation is likely to be of future benefit to all patients with AMIs and that new tools (e.g., MRI) will help to refine patient selection and lead to a better assessment of results. Finally, lessons from the past suggest that in this field, close collaboration between clinical and nonclinical scientists is of the utmost importance.

References

1. British Heart Foundation. Coronary Heart Disease Statistics. BHF Statistics Database, 2002: www.bhf.org.uk.
2. Reddy KS. Global perspective on cardiovascular disease. In: Yusuf S, Cairns JA, Camm AJ, Fallen EL, Gersh BJ (eds). Evidence-based Cardiology, 2nd, edn. BMJ Books, London, 2003:91–102.
3. Antman EM, Van de Werf F. Pharmacoinvasive therapy. The future of treatment for ST-elevation myocardial infarction. Circulation 2004;109: 2480–6.

4. Eagle KA, Goodman SG, Avezum A, Budaj A, Sullivan CM, Lopez-Sendon J. GRACE Investigators. Practice variation and missed opportunities for reperfusion in ST-segment-elevation myocardial infarction: findings from the Global Registry of Acute Coronary Events (GRACE). Lancet 2002; 359:373–7.
5. Ryan TJ, Antman EM, Brooks NH, et al. 1999 update: ACC/AHA guidelines for the management of patients with acute myocardial infarction: Executive summary and recommendations: a report of the American College of Cardiology/American Heart Association Task Force on Practice Guidelines (Committee on Management of Acute Myocardial Infarction). Circulation 1999;100:1016–30.
6. Pfeffer MA, Braunwald E. Ventricular remodeling after myocardial infarction: experimental observations and clinical implications. Circulation 1990;81:1161–72.
7. Bolognese L, Carrabba N, Parodi G, et al. Impact of microvascular dysfunction on left ventricular remodeling and long-term clinical outcome after primary coronary angioplasty for acute myocardial infarction. Circulation 2004;109:1121–6.
8. Tosh D, Slack JMW. How cells change their phenotype. Nat Rev Mol Cell Biol 2002;3:187–94.
9. Beltrami AP, Barlucchi L, Torella D, et al. Adult cardiac stem cells are multipotent and support myocardial regeneration. Cell 2003;114:763–76.
10. Beltrami AP, Urbanek K, Kajstura J, et al. Evidence that human cardiac myocytes divide after myocardial infarction. N Engl J Med 2001;344:1750–7.
11. Anversa P, Nadal-Ginard B. Myocyte renewal and ventricular remodeling. Nature 2002;415:240–3.
12. Nadal-Ginard B, Kajstura J, Leri A, Anversa P. Myocyte death, growth, and regeneration in cardiac hypertrophy and failure. Circ Res 2003;92: 139–50.
13. Quaini F, Urbanek K, Beltrami AP, et al. Chimerism of the transplanted heart. N Engl J Med 2002; 346:5–15.
14. Thiele J, Varus E, Wickenhauser C, Kvasnicka HM, Metz KA, Beelen DW. Regeneration of heart muscle tissue: quantification of chimeric cardiomyocytes and endothelial cells following transplantation. Histol Histopathol 2004;19:201–9.
15. Deb A, Wang S, Skelding KA, Miller D, Simper D, Caplice NM. Bone marrow-derived cardiomyocytes are present in adult human heart: a study of gender-mismatched bone marrow transplantation patients. Circulation 2003;107:1247–9.
16. Orlic D, Kajstura J, Chimenti S, et al. Bone marrow cells regenerate infarcted myocardium. Nature 2001;410:701–5.
17. Orlic D, Kajstura J, Chimenti S, et al. Mobilized bone marrow cells repair the infarcted heart, improving function and survival. Proc Natl Acad Sci USA 2001;98:10344–9.
18. Mangi AA, Noiseux N, Kong K, et al. Mesenchymal stem cells modified with Akt prevent remodeling and restore performance of infarcted hearts. Nat Med 2003;9:1195–201.
19. Tomita S, Mickle DA, Weisel RD, et al. Improved heart function with myogenesis and angiogenesis after autologous porcine bone marrow stromal cell transplantation. J Thorac Cardiovasc Surg 2002; 123:1132–40.
20. Balsam LB, Wagers AJ, Christensen JL, Kofidis T, Weissman IL, Robbins RC. Haematopoietic stem cells adopt mature haematopoietic fates in ischaemic myocardium. Nature 2004;428:668–73.
21. Murry CE, Soonpaa MH, Reinecke H, et al. Haematopoietic stem cells do not transdifferentiate into cardiac myocytes in myocardial infarcts. Nature 2004;428:664–8.
22. Vulliet PR, Greeley M, Halloran M, MacDonald A, Kittelson MD. Intra-coronary arterial injection of mesenchymal stromal cells and microinfarction in dogs. Lancet 2004;363:783–4.
23. Silvestre JS, Gojova A, Brun V, et al. Transplantation of bone marrow-derived mononuclear cells in ischemic apolipoprotein E-knockout mice accelerates atherosclerosis without altering plaque composition. Circulation 2003;108:2839–42.
24. Kang HJ, Kim HS, Zhang SY, et al. Effects of intracoronary infusion of peripheral blood stem-cells mobilized with granulocyte-colony stimulating factor on left ventricular systolic function and restenosis after coronary stenting in myocardial infarction: the MAGIC cell randomized clinical trial. Lancet 2004;363:751–6.
25. Chien KR. Lost in translation. Nature 2004;428: 607–8.
26. Matsubara H. Risk to the coronary arteries of intracoronary stem cell infusion and G-CSF cytokine therapy. Lancet 2004;363:746–7.
27. Hamano K, Nishida M, Hirata K, et al. Local implantation of autologous bone marrow for therapeutic angiogenesis in patients with ischemic heart disease: clinical trial and preliminary results. Jpn Circ J 2001;65:845–7.
28. Herreros J, Prosper F, Perez A, et al. Autologous intramyocardial injection of cultured skeletal muscle-derived stem cells in patients with nonacute myocardial infarction. Eur Heart J 2003;24: 2012–20.
29. Pagani FD, DerSimonian H, Zawadzka A, et al. Autologous skeletal myoblasts transplanted to ischemia-damaged myocardium in humans. Histological analysis of cell survival and differentiation. J Am Coll Cardiol 2003;41:879–88.
30. Galinanes M, Loubani M, Davies J, Chin D, Pasi J, Bell PR. Autotransplantation of unmanipulated bone marrow into scarred myocardium is safe and enhances cardiac function in humans. Cell Transplant 2004;13:7–13.

31. Smits PC, van Geuns RJ, Poldermans D, et al. Catheter-based intramyocardial injection of autologous skeletal myoblasts as a primary treatment of ischemic heart failure: clinical experience with six-month follow-up. J Am Coll Cardiol 2003;42: 2063–9.
32. Tse HF, Kwong YL, Chan JK, Lo G, Ho CL, Lau CP. Angiogenesis in ischaemic myocardium by intramyocardial autologous bone marrow mononuclear cell implantation. Lancet 2003;361:47–9.
33. Perin EC, Dohmann HF, Borojevic R, et al. Transendocardial, autologous bone marrow cell transplantation for severe, chronic ischemic heart failure. Circulation 2003;107:2294–302.
34. Fuchs S, Satler LF, Kornowski R, et al. Catheter-based autologous bone marrow myocardial injection in no-option patients with advanced coronary artery disease. A feasibility study. J Am Coll Cardiol 2003;41:1721–4.
35. Assmus B, Schächinger V, Teupe C, et al. Transplantation of Progenitor Cells and Regeneration Enhancement in Acute Myocardial Infarction (TOPCARE-AMI). Circulation 2002;106:3009–17.
36. Strauer BE, Brehm M, Zeus T, et al. Repair of infarcted myocardium by autologous intracoronary mononuclear bone marrow cell transplantation in humans. Circulation 2002;106:1913–18.
37. Fernández-Avilés F, San Román JA, García-Frade J, et al. Experimental and clinical regenerative capability of human bone marrow cells after myocardial infarction. Circ Res 2004;95:742–8.
38. Wollert KC, Meyer GP, Lotz J, et al. Intracoronary autologous bone-marrow cell transfer after myocardial infarction: the BOOST randomised controlled clinical trial. Lancet 2004;364:141–8.
39. Kuethe F, Figulla HR, Voth M, et al. Mobilization of stem cells by granulocyte colony-stimulating factor for the regeneration of myocardial tissue after myocardial infarction. Dtsch Med Wochenschr 2004;129:424–8.
40. Sakakibara Y, Tambara K, Lu F, et al. Cardiomyocyte transplantation does not reverse cardiac remodelling in rats with chronic myocardial infarction. Ann Thorac Surg 2002;74:25–30.
41. Li RK, Mickle DA, Weisel RD, Rao V, Jia ZQ. Optimal time for cardiomyocyte transplantation to maximize myocardial function after left ventricular injury. Ann Thorac Surg 2001;72: 1957–63.
42. Cerqueira MD, Weissman NJ, Dilsizian V, et al. Standardized myocardial segmentation and nomenclature for tomographic imaging of the heart. Circulation 2002;105:539–42.
43. Baer FM, Voth E, Scheneider CA, Theissen P, Schicha H, Sechtem U. Comparison of low-dose dobutamine-gradiente-echo magnetic resonance imaging and positron emission tomography with [^{18}F]fluorodeoxyglucose in patients with chronic coronary artery disease. Circulation 1995;91: 1006–15.
44. Cwajg JM, Cwajg E, Nagueh SF, et al. End-diastolic wall thickness as a predictor of recovery of function in myocardial hibernation: relation to rest-redistribution Tl-201 tomography and dobutamine stress echocardiography. J Am Coll Cardiol 2000;35:1152–61.
45. Barbato E, Aarnoudse W, Aengevaeren WR, et al. Week 25 study group. Validation of coronary flow reserve measurements by thermodilution in clinical practice. Eur Heart J 2004;25:219–23.

chapter 14

Clinical Utilization of Skeletal Myoblasts

Marco Valgimigli, Tomasz Siminiak, Maciej Kurpisz, Willem J van der Giessen, and Patrick W Serruys

Clinical and Scientific Background

The current pharmacotherapy for congestive heart failure,[1] including neurohormonal inhibition, with angiotensin-converting enzyme (ACE) inhibitors and β-blockers, improves the clinical outcome, but fails to stop the progression of the disease. Similarly, despite the best available treatment, the cumulative incidence of mortality and heart failure increases time-dependently in patients with a previous myocardial infarction.[2] Therefore, novel treatment methods that improve cardiac function and prevent heart failure are in demand. The mechanisms leading to congestive heart failure after an acute myocardial infarction are only partially understood,[3] and, according to current belief, a progressive decrease in the number of viable myocytes after an acute myocardial infarction could at least partially explain this transition. Therefore, myocardial infarction and subsequent heart failure can be viewed as a disease of cellular deficiency.[4]

Until recently, it was thought that adult mammalian cardiomyocytes were terminally differentiated and therefore could not divide. This dogma has been recently revisited in light of pathologic studies performed in patients with ischemic and dilated cardiomyopathies, which showed that some cells can actually reenter a mitotic cycle.[5,6] However, the magnitude of this self-repair mechanism is far too limited to compensate for the massive loss of cardiomyocytes resulting from a large infarct. Although it is intellectually provocative, genetically induced conversion of in-scar fibroblasts into myogenic cells has little clinical applicability, the only practical perspective being an exogenous supply of cells for effectively repopulating injured areas.

Historically, the proof of the principle was established by experiments using fetal (and neonatal) cardiomyocytes. Experiments with these cells have consistently shown that they are able to successfully engraft into infarcted myocardium, express gap junction proteins (thus allowing them to couple with host cardiomyocytes), survive for long periods of time, and improve left ventricular function.[7–9] From a clinical perspective, however, the use of fetal tissue is fraught with major challenges, including availability, immunogenicity, and ethical issues, and researchers have turned to autologous skeletal muscle and bone marrow stem cells as more realistic sources of cells for myocardial grafting. The goal of this chapter is to provide an updated overview on the use of skeletal myoblasts to treat overt or impeding heart failure from a clinical perspective.

Rationale for Myoblast Transplantation

Mature skeletal muscle originates from undifferentiated, mononucleated progenitor cells, which are termed myoblasts. Myoblasts proliferate in response to local mitogens, such as fibroblast growth factor (FGF) family members. When local growth factors are depleted, myoblasts withdraw irreversibly from the cell cycle, activate expression of muscle-specific genes (e.g., actins, myosins, and creatine kinase), and fuse to form multinucleated cells called myotubes. Myotubes undergo progressive maturation and hypertrophy to form differentiated myofibers characteristic of adult skeletal muscle. Not all myoblasts fuse into myotubes, however. Rather, some become quiescent stem cells, or satellite cells, residing in close apposition to the muscle fiber. Satellite cells can reenter the cell cycle in response to muscle injury and are responsible for the ability of skeletal muscle to regenerate. Therefore, skeletal myoblasts (i.e., satellite cells) are mononucleated, unipotent progenitor cells, located at the basal lamina of the adult skeletal muscle, which can be expanded in vitro (Figure 14.1). They are highly resistant to ischemia, and they multiply after injury. However, due to the fact that their proliferative capacity is not unlimited,[10] their stem cell nature has frequently been questioned. However, a considerable advantage of skeletal myoblasts is their wide availability: they can be easily and minimally invasively retrieved from a muscular biopsy (generally from the femoral quadriceps under local anesthesia) and, after 10–21 days of cultural expansion, injected into myocardium.

Moreover, despite concerns raised regarding the real number of injected myoblasts that will finally survive the transplantation procedure, engraftment of skeletal cells with subsequent myotube formation in the human myocardium has recently been demonstrated by two different groups.[11,12] These grafted cells acquire a fatigue-resistant slow-twitch muscle phenotype that is better suited to perform a cardiac-type workload. These findings have greatly supported the notion that the injected cells can actually contribute to cellular replenishment in the failing human heart.

Both surgical and percutaneous myoblast transplants have been undertaken, and several single or multicenter evaluations are ongoing in this new and promising field.

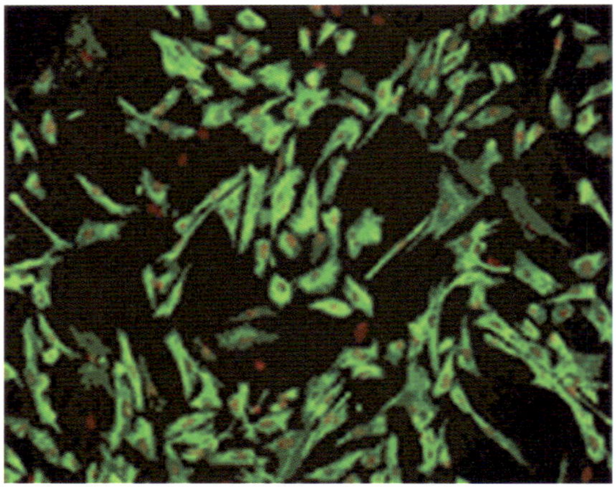

Figure 14.1 *Human skeletal myoblasts in in vitro culture. Courtesy of Bioheart, Inc.*

Myoblast Transplantation During Open-Chest Cardiac Surgery

The first human autologous skeletal myoblast transplantation during open-chest cardiac surgery was performed by Menasché, followed by phase I clinical trials performed both in Paris and in Poznań.[13–15] The trials were carried out in patients in whom direct intramyocardial injections could be performed during coronary artery bypass grafting (CABG).

In the first case to be described,[13] several injections of the cell suspensions into areas of postinfarction injury within the inferior wall of the left ventricle (LV) were performed. Five months later, significant improvement in clinical status was observed, including decrease of symptoms of heart failure by one New York Heart Association (NYHA) class, increase in segmental contractility and ejection fraction on echocardiography, and increase in tracer activity on positron emission tomography (PET), suggesting a new onset of metabolic activity in the previously nonviable scar area.[13,14] An independent phase I clinical trial of autologous skeletal myoblast transplantation in patients undergoing CABG[15–17] was performed in Poznań. Myocardial infarction survivors, with an akinetic area of the LV and scheduled for CABG, were screened by means of dobutamine stress echocardiography (DSE) and were included in the study when no viable myocardium was detected. A skeletal myocardial biopsy was obtained in all patients from the vastus lateralis. The biopsy sample was digested, and myoblasts (satellite cells) were isolated. The cells were cultured for 3 weeks to increase the number of cells to be implanted. Myoblast injections into the akinetic area were performed after constriction of the anastomoses during the CABG procedure. An increase in segmental contractility was seen in all patients 2–3 months after the procedure, and this effect was maintained throughout a 36-month follow-up period.

However, 3 years after combined myoblast transplantation and CABG, in almost every third case in the Poznań series, end-diastolic LV diameter increased, suggesting that cell transplantation did not prevent LV remodeling or that the number of cells transplanted was not sufficient to prevent LV dilatation.

A US multicenter phase I clinical trial aimed at evaluation of myoblast transplantation during CABG has also been reported.[18] Eleven patients underwent myoblast transplantation combined with CABG. Echocardiography, PET, and magnetic resonance imaging (MRI) scans showed evidence of increased viability in the area of grafted scar. The mean left ventricular ejection fraction (LVEF) improved from 22.7% to 35.9%. Another phase I study evaluating myoblast injections during CABG has been reported by Herreros et al,[19] suggesting safety and feasibility of the method as well as indicating its possible efficacy in increasing contractile LV performance. Recently, the same group published results regarding CABG in 20 patients for whom the mean follow-up time was 14 ± 5 months with no mortalities, no malignant cardiac arrythmias, and LVEF improvement from $28 \pm 3\%$ to $52 \pm 4.7\%$ ($p = 0.03$). Further, the wall motion score index (WMSI) improved from 3.1 to 1.4 ($p = 0.04$) in cell-treated segments.[20]

Also, Menasché and colleagues have reported preliminary safety information regarding their experience in the phase II MAGIC trial, in which 42 patients received myoblast transplantation in conjunction with CABG under MADIT II-type inclusion criteria (Menasché P, oral communication at the 2004 American Heart Association meeting, available at www.sessionsscienceon-demand.org). To date, there have been four reports of ventricular tachycardia (all late – as amiodarone use is prescribed shortly before and after myoblast transplantation), with a mean follow-up period of 8 months.

Despite all of its advantages, including good visualization of the target site and possible delivery of large amounts of cells per unit area, the direct transepicardial approach may incur an additional risk related to surgery. It should be noted that possible candidates for cell transplantation usually have a history of multiple infarctions, with significant LV dysfunction and clinical symptoms of severe heart failure, and are high-risk candidates for open-chest surgery. Furthermore, the open-chest approach does not provide ready access to the septal wall, which frequently is affected by postinfarction injury.

However, it should be recognized that the effect of revascularization (CABG) and cellular transplantation performed at the same time cannot easily be distinguished. Despite the use of careful inclusion criteria aimed at selection of patients with no viable myocardium within the target postinfarction area, the possible effect of skeletal myoblast transplantation may be enhanced by myocardial revascularization. Large ongoing clinical trials evaluating the efficacy of myoblast injections during CABG may allow evaluation of the cell effect independently of blood flow restoration.

Clinical Experience with Percutaneous Myoblast Transplantation

In order to avoid the trauma of open-chest surgery, several attempts have been made to effectively deliver progenitor cells via different percutaneous techniques. Although the intracoronary route has been tested successfully in animals, the transendocardial and transvenous approaches have been primarily employed in humans.

Intraventricular approach

A pilot safety and feasibility study of the percutaneous transplantation of autologous skeletal myoblasts via transendocardial injection (as a stand-alone procedure) in five patients with ischemic heart failure has been reported by our group.[21]

Only symptomatic patients in NYHA functional class ≥II under optimal medical therapy were selected. All patients were known to have experienced prior anterior wall myocardial infarction and depressed LV function (LVEF between 20% and 45% by radionuclide radiography). The myocardial infarction had to be >4 weeks old at the time of cell implantation. The presence and location of a myocardial scar were defined by akinesia or dyskinesia at rest during echocardiography, LV angiography, and MRI; no contractile reserve during DSE; and hyperenhancement by gadolinium on MRI.

Patients with a target wall region thickness <5 mm by echocardiography or MRI or with a history of syncope or sustained ventricular tachycardia or fibrillation were excluded.

Biopsy of the quadriceps muscle was performed under local anesthesia. On average, 8.4 g (range 5–13 g) of muscle was excised through a 10 cm long surgical incision. All biopsy procedures were uneventful and done on an outpatient basis. The culture period was an average of 17 days (range 14–19 days).

After a coronary and biplane LV angiogram was obtained, an outline of the LV chamber was drawn on transparent tabloids that were taped to the fluoroscopy monitors. Then an electromechanical NOGA map (Figure 9.2) of the LV was obtained using a 7F NOGASTAR catheter (F-curve) connected to the NOGA console (Biosense-Webster, Waterloo, Belgium). Areas exhibiting low voltages and linear local shortening (unipolar voltage <4 mV and linear local shortening <4%) on the NOGA map were considered the target areas of treatment if these areas were geographically concordant with the scar areas assessed by the preprocedural DSE, MRI, and LV angiogram. The investigators refrained from transendocardial injections into areas with a known wall thickness <5 mm by MRI. With an 8F Myostar (Biosense-Webster) injection catheter, 16±4 (mean±SD; range 9–19) transendocardial injections were made.

Injections of 0.3 ml (16.6×10^6 cells) were accomplished under NOGA and transparent tabloid guidance so that the spacing between injection sites was approximately 1 cm (Figure 14.2).

No procedural complications occurred. Only one patient experienced minor elevation of the creatine kinase MB fraction (<2 times upper level), and troponin T (0.16 µg/l) was noted after the procedure. During follow-up, one patient required hospitalization 6 weeks after the procedure due to progressive heart failure and long asymptomatic runs of nonsustained ventricular tachycardia (NSVT) on Holter monitoring. After recompensation, telemetry still showed NSVT, and an implantable cardioverter–defibrillator (ICD) was implanted prophylactically. In the other four patients, no adverse events or ventricular arrhythmias were observed.

Compared with baseline, the angiographic LVEF at 3 months increased from 36±11% to 41±9% ($p=0.009$). This increase in LVEF, however, was not observed by nuclear or MRI assessment at 3-month follow-up. At 6-month follow-up, both angiographic and nuclear assessments showed a trend toward an increased LVEF [36±11% to 45±8% ($p=0.23$) and 38±8% to 45±11% ($p=0.07$), respectively]. MRI analysis of regional wall thickening showed a clear shift toward more regional wall thickening in the target segments and less regional wall thickening in the remote hyperkinetic segments. By comparing the marked injection sites on the NOGA map and the fluoroscopy sheets with the MRI segments, 87 of the 304 MRI segments (all five patients) were identified as injected segments. Paired analysis of these injected segments showed significantly increased wall thickening at follow-up (0.9±2.3 mm at baseline vs. 1.8±2.4 mm at 3-month follow-up, $p=0.008$).

In the light of these preliminary favorable results, a multicenter European uncontrolled investigation was started and has recently been completed. Overall, 15 patients were been enrolled and treated with transendocardial skeletal myoblast injections using both the Myostar and MyoCath (Bioheart, Inc.) needle-injection

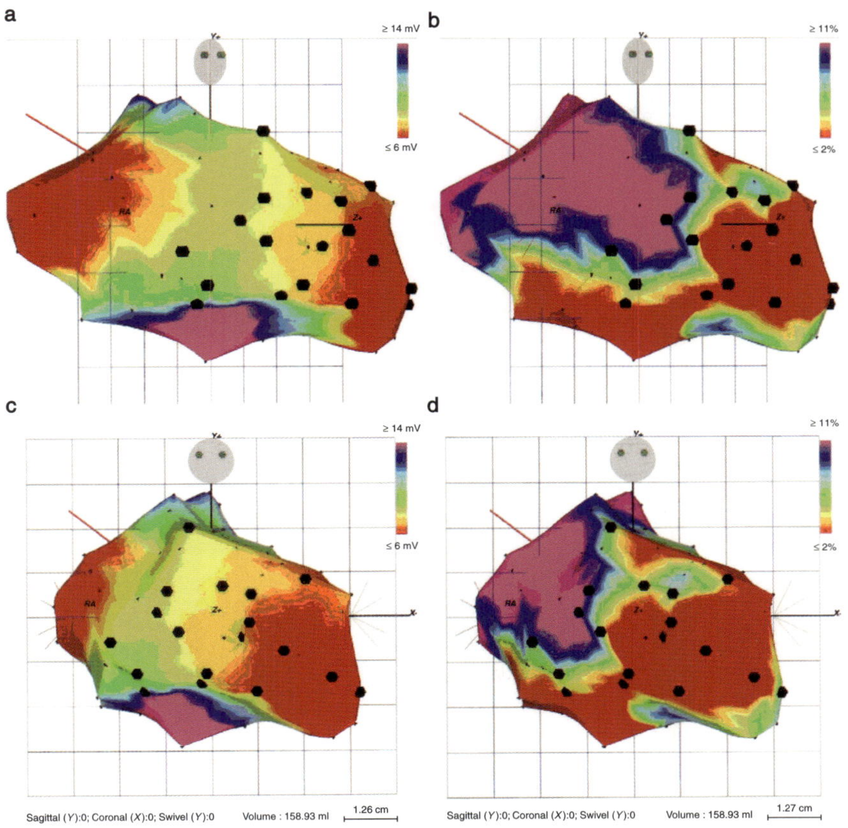

Figure 14.2 *NOGA maps in the right anterior oblique (a, b) and anteroposterior (c, d) views of a patient after 19 injections with autologous skeletal myoblasts in the anteroseptal and anterior myocardial scar and border zone: (a, c) unipolar voltage maps; (b, d) linear local shortening maps. The myocardial scar is indicated in red on the unipolar voltage maps (<6 mV) and the local linear shortening maps (<2%). The black dots indicate the transendocardial injection sites. Reproduced from Smits P, J Am Coll Cardiol 2003;42:2363–9*[21] *with permission from The American College of Cardiology Foundation.*

catheters. The results of this study will be published soon, and they have contributed tremendously to the understanding of the safety and potentiality of the skeletal myoblast-based cell therapy in these high-risk heart failure patients. Based on these phase I investigations, a phase II open-label randomized controlled multicenter trial, the SEISMIC [Safety and Effects of Implanted (Autologous) Skeletal Myoblasts (MyoCell) using an Injection Catheter] trial, recently began enrolling patients. Total study enrollment is anticipated within the next 6 months, with 6 months' follow-up for both the treatment and control arms. The study will recruit patients previously fitted with an ICD. Forty six patients will be recruited for the study, with patients randomly assigned to a treatment group ($n=30$) or a control group ($n=16$) after meeting the baseline enrollment criteria. For patients assigned to the treatment group, a skeletal muscle biopsy will be obtained for myoblast isolation, expansion, and culture.

At screening, all randomized patients will be prescribed amiodarone, which will be taken until 1 month post procedure. The flowchart of the protocol is shown in Figure 14.3.

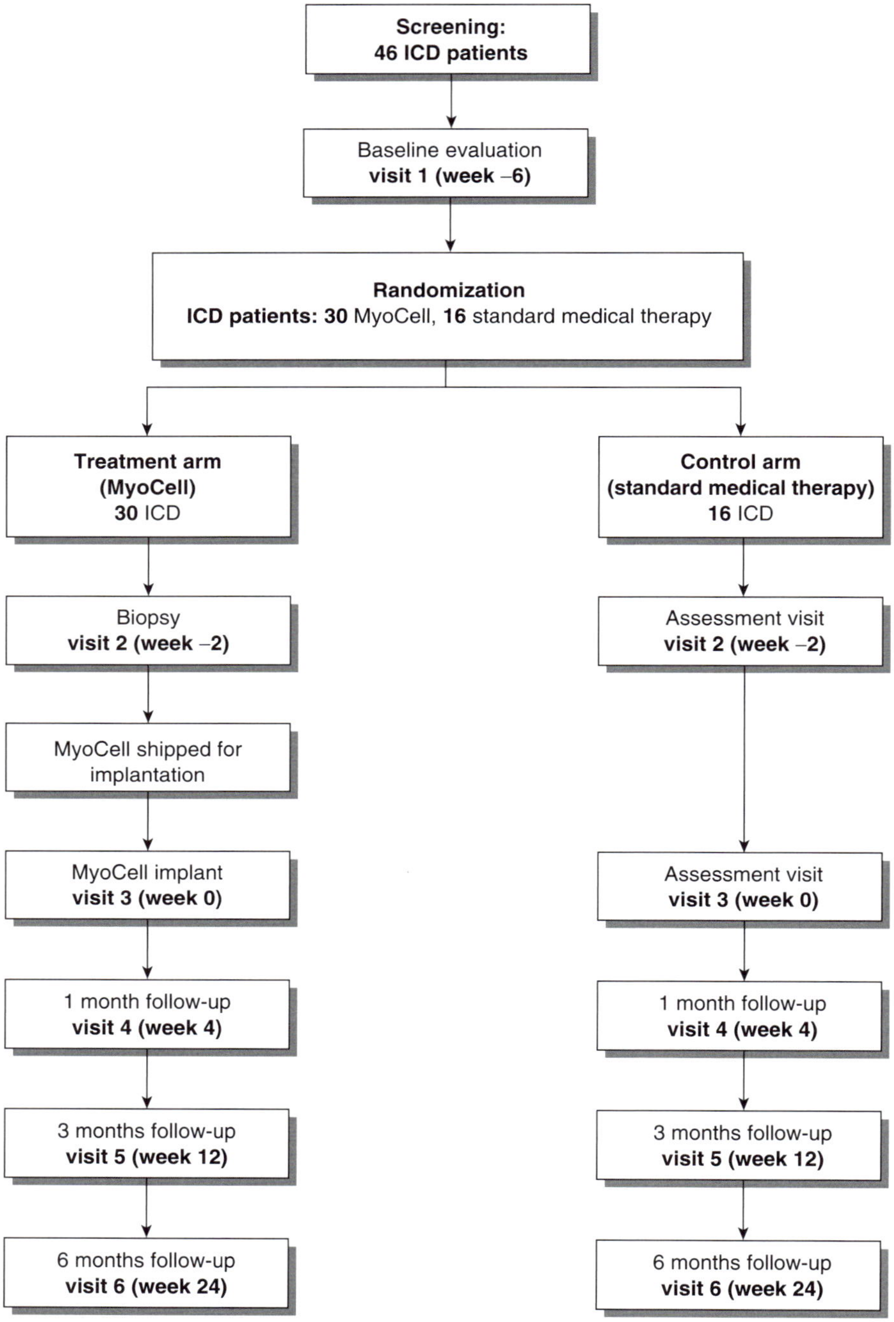

Figure 14.3 SEISMIC study flowchart. ICD, implantable cardioverter-defibrillator.

Transvenous approach

Endoventricular catheter systems, currently utilized for intramyocardial injections of therapeutic agents, have limited stability, since the catheter does not follow heart movements. Furthermore, the injection pressure with endoventricular systems can be destabilizing and can cause expulsion of the needle tip from the injection site. The puncture site after needle withdrawal from a short injection channel may cause therapeutic agent leakage back into the ventricle. Such a backflush of cells to be transplanted may lead to the presence of graft cells in the systemic circulation and/or a diminished number of cells delivered to the target area. Moreover, for endoventricular systems in which the needle is directed perpendicular to the inner surface of the cardiac muscle wall, a relatively thin postinfarction scar is currently a contraindication (see above).

A novel catheter-based endovascular system for direct myocardial injection using intravascular ultrasound (IVUS)-guided needle punctures via the coronary venous system (TransAccess; TransVascular Inc.) has been developed.[22,23] Briefly, the TransAccess catheter (Figure 14.4) is a monorail composite catheter system combining a phased-array IVUS and a preshaped nitinol needle. After the TransAccess system is placed in the target coronary vein, through the coronary sinus, intravascular orientation is performed using the corresponding artery, pericardium, and ventricular myocardium as landmarks with IVUS imaging. After confirmation of the appropriate TransAccess catheter position, the nitinol needle is extended into the myocardium and a microinfusion catheter (IntraLume; TransVascular Inc.) is then advanced through the needle deep into the myocardium with simultaneous cell injection.

The potential advantages of the TransAccess system are that it moves with the heart wall (residing deep within the coronary vein) and allows for advancement of the micro lumen injection catheter in a tangential direction with the myocardial tissue. In such a way, cells may be injected in long tracks in the target area, and less cell loss is anticipated with injections that are of a length measured in centimeters rather than

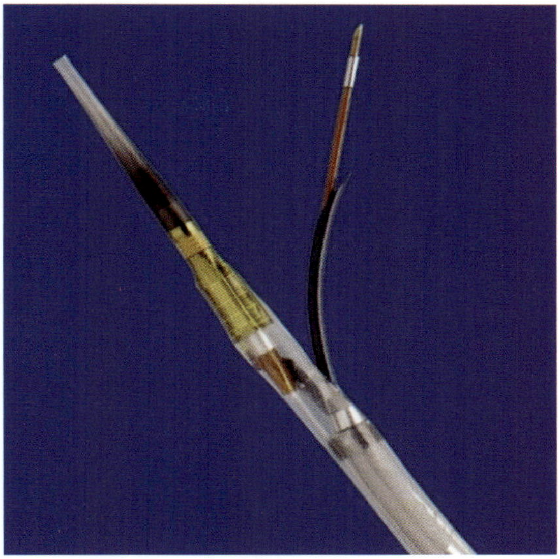

Figure 14.4 *TransAccess (TransVascular Inc.) catheter tip. Note the intravascular ultrasound transducer at the end of the catheter and the preshaped needle with an IntraLume microcatheter tip advanced through the needle.*

millimeters. Clinical experience with the device indicates that deep (up to 4 cm) channels are created during injections to deliver the cells to the target area (Figures 14.5 and 14.6). This was easily performed with minimal myocardial trauma, reflected by an absence of significant troponin elevation.[24,25] It is believed that injections during the advancement of the micro-lumen catheter form a channel produced by liquid pressure, which limits myocardial trauma. Furthermore, a thin postinfarction scar is not a contraindication for the TransAccess system, as the injections are parallel to the ventricular wall.

Although coronary sinus catheterization requires additional training even for an experienced interventionalist, it seems that IVUS-guided needle injection (Figure 14.7) provides appropriate accuracy for intramyocardial advancement of the micro-lumen injection catheter.

Initial clinical experience, including that obtained from the POZNAN trial,[24] shows that in the majority of cases, it is possible to perform intramyocardial injections using the TransAccess

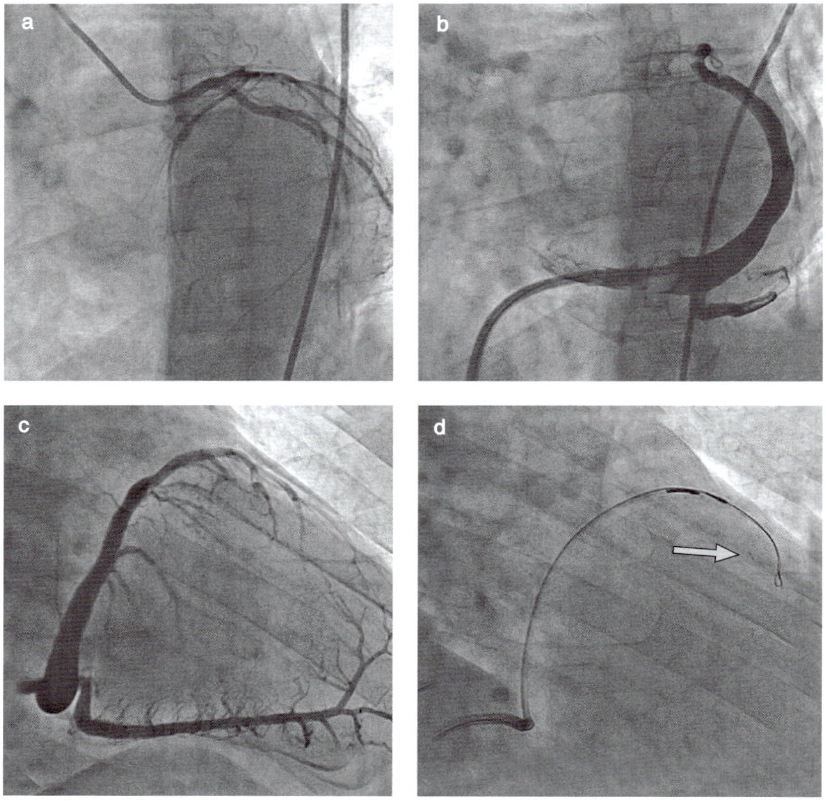

Figure 14.5 Procedural steps. (a) Coronary artery visualization in the left anterior oblique (LAO) 30° view. (b) Administration of contrast medium via a guiding catheter placed in the coronary sinus in the LAO 30° view. Note the balloon inflated at the tip of the guiding catheter to slow the outflow of the contrast medium. (c) Coronary venogram in the right anterior oblique (RAO) 40° view. (d) Placement of the TransAccess catheter system in the anterior interventricular vein and injection of the cell suspension via the IntraLume microcatheter into the anterior wall myocardium (the arrow indicates the microcatheter tip).

system. The visibility of the coronary artery parallel to the target coronary vein is good and allows safe intramyocardial needle injections with limited risk of artery puncture. Simultaneously recorded coronary angiograms, serving as landmarks, allow precise advancement of the micro-lumen catheter in the remote target area up to 4 cm deep within the injured myocardium. It should be noted that use of the middle cardiac vein, parallel to the posterior descending coronary artery, is also possible (Figure 14.6). In the POZNAN trial, in four cases, the TransAccess system was advanced closer to the apical segments of the LV with the middle vein rather than the anterior interventricular vein.[24] Lack of procedural success in one patient, related to an inability to position the guiding catheter appropriately across the venous valve present at the bifurcation of the great cardiac vein, suggests a need for better coronary sinus guiding catheter design (10 Fr guiding catheters were used). It may be speculated that newer and probably smaller guiding catheters will allow smooth crossing of the coronary venous valves.

In the POZNAN trial, two to four intramyocardial injections 1.5–4.5 cm deep were performed in each patient, delivering up to 10^8 cells in 0.6–2.5 ml of saline. During 6 months' follow-up,

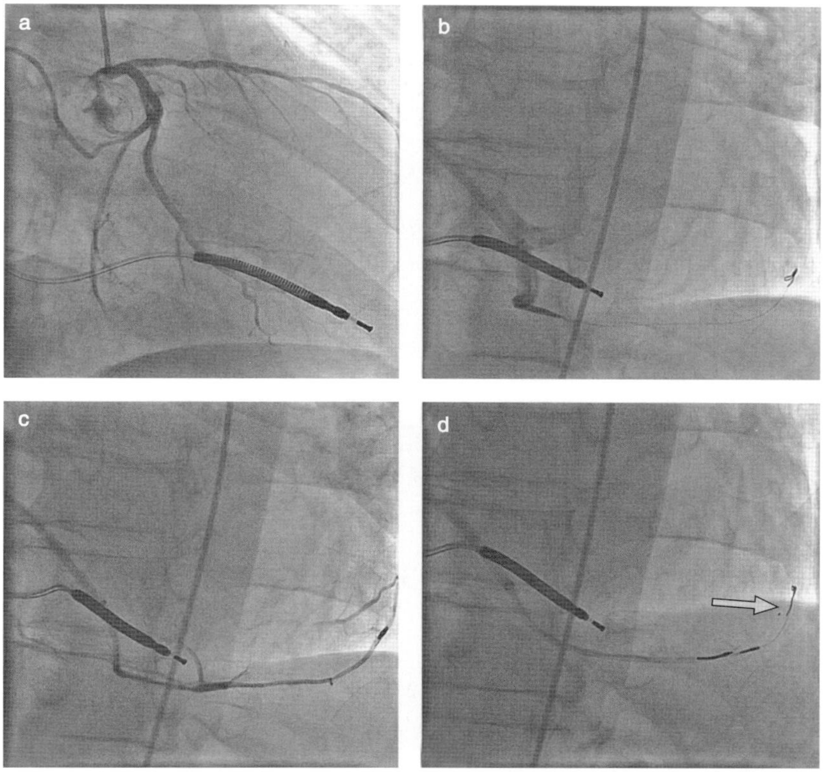

Figure 14.6 Procedural steps. (a) Coronary artery visualization in the right anterior oblique (RAO) 30° view. (b) The guiding catheter is placed in the coronary sinus and oriented to the middle cardiac vein with the guidewire advanced along the vein. (c) Administration of contrast medium to evaluate the anatomy of the proximal part of the middle cardiac vein. (d) Advancement of the needle from the TransAccess catheter placed in the middle cardiac vein and further advancement of the IntraLume microcatheter via the needle into the myocardium, with its tip (arrow) being placed in the apex.

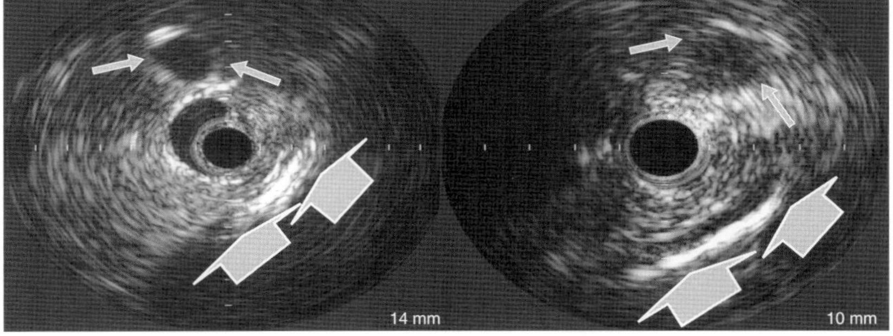

Figure 14.7 Intravascular ultrasound images obtained from the cardiac venous site. Note the visibility of the pericardium (large arrows) and the coronary artery parallel to the vein (small arrows), enabling orientation of the TransAccess catheter system.

the NYHA class improved in all patients and the LVEF increased 3–8% in six out of nine cases.[24,25]

At the Thoraxcenter, Rotterdam, three patients have been successfully treated with intramyocardial skeletal myoblast injections using the transvenous approach, and it is planned that other patients will soon follow. This technique of delivery appears to be safe and feasible. However, many more studies are needed to clarify the clinical advantages of the transvenous versus the endocardial route.

Myoblast Safety Issues: Focus on Arrhythmia

It is well known that the composition and electromechanical properties of myocardial and skeletal muscle tissues differ significantly. Cardiac cells, having specialized cell–cell junctions, even though separated from one another, act together in synchronization. Junctions, represented morphologically by intercalated disks, contain adherens and gap junctions for mechanical and electrical coupling. Cardiac tissue gap junctions contain the connexin 43 transmembrane protein by which an electrical current can be rapidly and freely conducted.[26] Although certain data suggest that skeletal myoblasts may acquire a few characteristics of cardiomyocytes,[12,27] it can generally be assumed that the grafted cells do not transdifferentiate and that they retain morphologic and electrophysiologic properties of skeletal muscle. It is speculated that satellite cells are not able to form intercellular junctions characteristic of cardiomyocytes.

On the other hand, it has been shown that the lack of junctions between grafted cells and host tissue does not preclude improvement in LV contractile function.[27] This positive effect on contractility seems to last over time and is correlated with the number of implanted cells.[28] Results of experimental studies performed on myocardial wound strips have shown that skeletal myoblast grafts do contract when exogenously stimulated.[29] Reinecke et al[30] showed that cardiomyocytes and skeletal myoblasts, when placed in coculture, form a synchronous beating network. On microscopy, these researchers even revealed the presence of N-cadherin- and connexin 43-mediated junctions between skeletal myoblasts and cardiomyocytes, allowing them to induce synchronous beating. Although encouraging, it must be emphasized that these results were obtained in cultured myoblasts, which are less differentiated than in vivo graft cells. Cultured myoblasts still express a low level of connexin 43, which is undetectable in more mature in vivo cells.[31] It has been suggested that transplanted cells can contract synchronously even in the absence of connections between cells, because a simple stretch may initiate contraction.[32]

In discussing the issue of connections between host and transplanted cells, it should be observed that scar tissue has the potential to isolate any kind of injected cells. The scar in itself forms a physical barrier, which impedes electromechanical coupling. Therefore, for any kind of cell therapy based on excitation of graft by host tissue, regardless of any special cell–cell junction, this issue needs to be addressed.

The inability of skeletal myoblasts to transdifferentiate into cardiomyocytes and to form junctions with neighboring cells may create a substrate for ventricular reentry arrhythmia. Indeed, current experimental and clinical data suggest a possibility of increased risk of arrhythmogenicity.

Menasché et al[14] implanted automatic ICDs (AICDs) in 4 out of 10 patients undergoing autologous skeletal myoblast transplantation due to sustained episodes of ventricular tachycardia. In the first European multicenter trial, one death occurred due to arrhythmia soon after the procedure. As a consequence, enrollment was stopped and the protocol amended so that all patients scheduled, before treatment, would have undergone AICD implantation. In a patient treated in Rotterdam a second death occurred 2 weeks after the procedure due to an electrical storm. The patient was resistant to multiple AICD shocks. The fact that, for this trial, end-stage cardyomyopathy was carefully selected for treatment makes it very difficult to draw clear conclusions from any these arrhythmic events: were these events related to the natural history of the disease or were they related to the procedure in itself? Further, it appears that the prophylactic use of amiodarone significantly helps reduce arrhythmic events in all patients, and, for those without an ICD, external defibrillators are also available as a precautionary measure.

In the POZNAN CABG phase I experience,[15,16] episodes of sustained ventricular tachycardia were observed in two patients during the early postoperative period, but prophylactic amiodarone administration in other patients prevented episodes of ventricular tachycardia, and no amiodarone treatment was continued later than 6 weeks during follow-up. This corresponds to the experience of Menasché et al. Later, during the follow-up period, only one of the four AICD patients experienced asymptomatic episodes of ventricular tachycardia. On the other hand, observations from the percutaneous series in the POZNAN trial, indicate successful prevention of cell transplantation-related ventricular arrhythmia by prophylactic amiodarone administration, perhaps suggesting that AICD implantations are not necessary in all patients undergoing myoblast transplantations.[24,25]

On the basis of published data from clinical studies, including our own experience, we believe that the possible arrhythmogenic effect of myoblast transplantation is present only in the initial weeks after the procedure. It may be speculated that this arrhythmogenic effect is more probably related to the mechanics of transplantation, including myocardial puncture and the inflammatory response to transplanted cells, some of which die after injection, than to possible problems with electromechanical coupling between newly developed myocytes and cardiomyocytes. Possible electromechanical coupling problems would result in late arrhythmia as cells differentiate (downregulation of connexin 43 and N-cadherin) – a situation that has not been observed in clinical trials thus.

However, it should be noted that no arrhythmic events have been reported so far in patients receiving bone marrow or circulating progenitor cells, possibly suggesting that the type of cells, rather than the methods employed to deliver them into the myocardium, could play a role in the genesis of arrhythmias.

At present, considering the small numbers of patients who have undergone autologous skeletal myoblast transplantations, it is difficult to predict whether these cells are really arrhythmogenic; this is especially so considering that patients with ischemic LV dysfunction frequently develop ventricular arrhythmia as part of their natural history. Nevertheless, future studies of cell transplantation in patients with postinfarction heart failure will have to focus on the potential arrhythmogenic effect of these cells. A clear overview of the safety profile of this new therapy is necessary in order to plan randomized investigations powered to assess efficacy.

References

1. Black HR. The burden of cardiovascular disease: following the link from hypertension to myocardial infarction and heart failure. Am J Hypertens 2003;16:4S–6S.
2. Lewis EF, Moye LA, Rouleau JL. Predictors of late development of heart failure in stable survivors of myocardial infarction: the CARE study. J Am Coll Cardiol 2003;42:1446–53.
3. Valgimigli M, Merli E, Malagutti P, et al. Hydroxyl radical generation, levels of tumor necrosis factor-alpha, and progression to heart failure after acute myocardial infarction. J Am Coll Cardiol 2004;43: 2000–8.
4. Kostin S, Pool L, Elsasser A, et al. Myocytes die by multiple mechanisms in failing human hearts. Circ Res 2003;92:715–24.
5. Beltrami AP, Urbanek K, Kajstura J, et al. Evidence that human cardiac myocytes divide after myocardial infarction. N Engl J Med 2001;344:1750–7.
6. Beltrami AP, Barlucchi L, Torella D, et al. Adult cardiac stem cells are multipotent and support myocardial regeneration. Cell 2003;114:763–76.
7. Leor J, Patterson M, Quinones MJ, Kedes LH, Kloner RA. Transplantation of fetal myocardial tissue into the infarcted myocardium of rat. Circulation 1996;94(Suppl II):II332–6.
8. Scorsin M, Hagège AA, Marotte F, et al. Does transplantation of cardiomyocyte improve function of infarcted myocardium? Circulation 1997;96(Suppl II):II188–93.
9. Müller-Ehmsen J, Peterson KL, Kedes L, et al. Long term survival of transplanted neonatal rat cardiomyocytes after myocardial infarction and effect on cardiac function. Circulation 2002;105:1720–6.
10. Chiu RCJ, Zibaitis A, Kao RL. Cellular cardiomyoplasty: myocardial regeneration with satellite cell implantation. Ann Thorac Surg 1995;60:12–18.

11. Hagege AA, Carrion C, Menasché P. Viability and differentiation of autologous skeletal myoblast grafts in ischaemic cardiomyopathy. Lancet 2003; 361:491–2.
12. Pagani FD, DerSimonian H, Zawadzka A, et al. Autologous skeletal myoblast transplantation to ischemia-damaged myocardium in humans. Histological analysis of cell survival and differentiation. J Am Coll Cardiol 2003;41:879–88.
13. Menasché P, Hagege AA, Scorsin M, et al. Myoblast transplantation for heart failure. Lancet 2001;357: 279–80.
14. Menasché P, Hagege AA, Vilquin JT, et al. Autologous skeletal myoblast transplantation for severe postinfarction left ventricular dysfunction. J Am Coll Cardiol 2003;41:1078–83.
15. Siminiak T, Kalawski R, Kurpisz M. Myoblast transplantation in the treatment of postinfarction myocardial contractility impairment. Kardiol Pol 2002;56:131–7.
16. Siminiak T, Kalawski R, Fiszer D, et al. Transplantation of autologous skeletal myoblasts in the treatment of patients with postinfarction heart failure. Circulation 2002;106(Suppl II):II-636 (abst).
17. Siminiak T, Kurpisz M. Myocardial replacement therapy. Circulation 2003;108:1167–71.
18. Dib N, McCarthy P, Campbell A, et al. Safety and feasibility of autologous myoblast transplantation in patients undergoing coronary artery bypass grafting: results from the United States experience. J Am Coll Cardiol 2003;41(Suppl):380A (abst).
19. Herreros J, Prósper F, Perez A, et al. Autologous intramyocardial injection of cultured skeletal muscle-derived stem cells in patients with non-acute myocardial infarction. Eur Heart J 2003;24: 2012–20.
20. Chachques JC, Herreros J, Trainini J, et al. Autologous human serum for cell culture avoids the implantation of cardioverter-defibrillators in cellular cardiomyoplasty. Int J Cardiol 2004; 95(Suppl 1):S29–33.
21. Smits P, van Geuns RJM, Poldermans D et al. Catheter-based intramyocardial injection of autologous skeletal myoblasts as a primary treatment of ischemic heart failure. Clinical experience with six-month follow-up. J Am Coll Cardiol 2003; 42:2363–9.
22. Thompson C, Oesterle S. Biointerventional cardiology: the future interface of interventional cardiovascular medicine and bioengineering. Vasc Med 2002;7:135–40.
23. Thompson CA, Nasser BA, Makower J, et al. Percutaneous transvenous cellular cardiomyoplasty. A novel nonsurgical approach for myocardial cell transplantation. J Am Coll Cardiol 2003;41:1964–71.
24. Siminiak T, Fiszer D, Jerzykowska O, Kurpisz M. Percutaneous transvenous transplantation of autologous myoblasts in the treatment of postinfarction heart failure. The POZNAN trial. Late Breaking Clinical Trial, Annual Scientific Session, American College of Cardiology, March 2004, New Orleans.
25. Siminiak T, Fiszer D, Jerzykowska O, et al. Percutaneous transvenous transplantation of autologous myoblasts in the treatment of postinfarction heart failure – the POZNAN trial. Eur Heart J 2004; 25(Suppl):264 (abst).
26. Beyer EC, Paul DL, Goodenough DA. Connexin43: a protein from rat heart homologous to a gap junction protein from liver. J Cell Biol 1987;105: 2621–9.
27. Taylor DA, Atkins BZ, Hungspreugs P, et al. Regenerating functional myocardium: improved performance after skeletal myoblast transplantation. Nat Med 1998;4:929–33.
28. Scorsin M, Hagege A, Vilquin J, et al. Comparison of the effects of fetal cardiomyocytes and skeletal myoblasts transplantation on post-infarct left ventricular function. J Thorac Cardiovasc Surg 2000;119:1169–75.
29. Murry CE, Wiseman RW, Schwartz SM, Hauschka SD. Skeletal myoblast transplantation for repair of myocardial necrosis. J Clin Invest 1996;98(11): 2512–23.
30. Reinecke H, Zhang M, Bartosek T, Murry CE. Electromechanical coupling between skeletal and cardiac muscle. Implications for infarct repair. J Cell Biol 2000;149:731–40.
31. Serruys PW, Smits P, van der Giessen W, Haimes HB, Harvey JM, Green JL. Challenges of myogenesis and repair of the heart. In: Kipshidze NN, Serruys PW (eds). Handbook of Cardiovascular Cell Transplantation, pp 225–40. 2004, London: Martin Dunitz.
32. Hagege AA, Vilquin JT, Bruneval P, Menasché P. Regeneration of the myocardium. A new role in the treatment of ischemic heart disease? Hypertension 2001;38:1413–15.

chapter 15

Angiogenesis and Cell Therapy for Peripheral Arterial Disease

Veerappan Subramaniyam, Andrew Zurick, and Arshed A Quyyumi

Introduction

Peripheral arterial disease (PAD) affects approximately 8–10 million people in the USA. Intermittent claudication, the most common symptom of PAD, affects approximately one-third to one-half of those with the disease. Critical limb ischemia is a severe manifestation of PAD in which the viability of the limb is threatened because the resting metabolic needs of the tissue are not met by the available blood supply. Patients develop pain, ulcers, or necrosis of the most distal parts of the limb. Approximately 10% of people with claudication progress to critical limb ischemia within 5 years, and roughly 25% of patients with critical limb ischemia require a major amputation.[1]

Current Therapy

Therapy directed specifically at PAD will not improve the patient's life expectancy, which is shortened by coronary and cerebral arterial disease. However, improving functional independence, not just the length of life, is an important element in promoting the health of this group. Currently available therapeutic options for the management of intermittent claudication include exercise, pharmacologic therapy, and mechanical revascularization.

Multiple controlled trials have demonstrated that both the initial walking distance until onset of claudication and the absolute claudication distance improve in patients who receive supervised exercise rehabilitation.[2,3] Pentoxifylline and cilostazol are the only Food and Drug Administration (FDA)-approved drugs for the treatment of intermittent claudication in the USA. Pentoxifylline, a methylxanthine with favorable rheologic effects, may benefit some patients with claudication, although results are conflicting.[4] Cilostazol, a specific inhibitor of cyclic adenosine monophosphate (cAMP) phosphodiesterase in platelets and vascular smooth muscle cells, has vasodilator and antiplatelet properties. Several controlled trials have found that compared with a placebo, cilostazol produces a modest increase (about 40 meters) in walking distances.[4]

Indications for mechanical revascularization include limb-threatening ischemia and disabling claudication refractory to medical therapy. Endovascular repair is the treatment of choice in unifocal stenoses without total occlusion. Stenting is especially effective in the iliac artery, success rates exceeding 90% in all series. Major complications occur in less than 6% of all endovascular procedures: 0.2% mortality, 2.5% need for surgery, and 0.2% limb loss. For more complex, multifocal and totally occluded lesions, surgical intervention is needed. The combined mortality and amputation rate is approximately 2.2% for aortofemoral, 1.4% for femoropopliteal, and 2.0% for distal reconstructions.[5] A substantial number of patients are not candidates for revascularization procedures because of unsuitable anatomy or medical comorbidities. Still others would prefer not to subject themselves to the risks of revascularization procedures if relief of symptoms could be obtained through other means.

Therapeutic Angiogenesis

Angiogenic growth factors

In the last several years, there has been significant interest in developing angiogenic therapies to provide novel approaches for the treatment of limb ischemia. A variety of different growth factors have been identified to promote angiogenesis by stimulating endothelial and smooth muscle cell proliferation and migration, as well as tissue degradation. Two of these growth factors, acidic/basic fibroblast growth factor (FGF) and vascular endothelial growth factor (VEGF), have been well studied clinically. Despite promising results from the initial animal and phase I clinical studies of FGF and VEGF,[6,7] phase II trials have failed to extrapolate those results into the therapeutic realm.[8] The TRAFFIC study was a randomized, double-blind, placebo-controlled study of intra-arterial recombinant basic FGF (bFGF, also known as FGF-2) in patients with intermittent claudication. Subjects received a placebo on days 1 and 30, or bFGF on day 1 and a placebo on day 30, or bFGF on days 1 and 30. The primary finding was that compared with a placebo, a single dose of bFGF increased the peak walking time by 1.17 minute at 90 days. There was no difference, however, between the placebo and a double dose of bFGF at 90 days and no difference between any of the groups in peak walking time at 180 days. Additionally, there was no intergroup difference in the pain-free walking time at any time point, and only a marginal increase in the ankle–brachial index was documented at 90 days in the bFGF-treated group. This an effect did not persist at 180 days.[9]

The RAVE trial was a phase II, randomized, double-blind, placebo-controlled study of adenoviral VEGF gene transfer in patients with intermittent claudication. Patients were randomized to low-dose VEGF, high-dose VEGF, or a placebo, administered as an intramuscular injection into the more ischemic leg. The primary efficacy endpoint, a change in peak walking time at 12 weeks, did not differ between the placebo, low-dose, and high-dose groups. Secondary measures of the ankle–brachial index and claudication onset time were also similar among the groups at 12 and 26 weeks.[10] The disappointing results of these and other large trials of growth factor-induced angiogenesis dampened the enthusiasm for its potential therapeutic application. However, newer therapeutic approaches that enhance the formation of collaterals have since been recognized.[8]

Bone marrow cell therapy

Embryonic blood vessel development is believed to originate as a "blood island" comprising angioblasts at the periphery and hematopoietic stem cells (HSCs) at the center. In addition to this spatial association, angioblasts and HSCs share certain antigenic determinants, including CD34 and VEGF receptor 2 (VEGFR-2, also known as FLK-1/KDR), and HSCs from peripheral blood can provide sustained hematopoietic recovery. Unifying these concepts, Asahara et al[11] hypothesized that peripheral blood contains cells that can differentiate into endothelial cells (ECs). These reseachers exploited two antigens that are shared by angioblasts and HSCs to isolate putative angioblasts from the leukocyte fraction of peripheral blood. CD34 is expressed by all HSCs but is lost by hematopoietic cells as they differentiate. Many cells, including most activated ECs in the adult, also express CD34. VEGFR-2 is also expressed by both early HSCs and ECs but ceases to be expressed during hematopoietic differentiation.

$CD34^+$ mononuclear blood cells isolated from human peripheral blood and plated on fibronectin became attached and spindle-shaped and proliferated for 4 weeks. Attached cells were generally not observed among $CD34^-$ mononuclear blood cells. However, co-incubation of $CD34^+$ and $CD34^-$ populations increased the proliferation rate to more than 10 times that of $CD34^+$ cells plated alone. These clusters comprised round cells centrally and sprouts of spindle-shaped cells at the periphery, resembling blood island-like cell clusters. $CD34^+$ cells progressed to an endothelial phenotype, expressing CD34, CD31, VEGFR-2, Tie-2, and E-selectin, and possessed endothelial constitutive nitric oxide synthase (eNOS).[11]

To determine if $CD34^+$ cells contribute to angiogenesis in vivo, Asahara et al[11] used animal models of hind-limb ischemia. Two days after unilateral hind-limb ischemia was surgically induced, 5×10^5 labeled human $CD34^+$ or $CD34^-$ cells were injected into the tail vein of immunodeficient mice. Histologic examination 1–6 weeks later revealed numerous labeled cells in the neovascularized ischemic hind limb. Nearly all labeled cells appeared integrated into capillary vessel walls. In $CD34^+$-injected mice, 13.4% of all $CD31^+$ capillaries contained labeled cells, compared with 1.6% in $CD34^-$- injected mice. By 6 weeks, labeled cells were clearly arranged into capillaries among preserved muscle structures. Similar findings were observed with VEGFR-2^+ cells. Taken together, these experiments suggest the presence of a circulating endothelial progenitor cell (EPC) within the $CD34^+$ or VEGFR-2^+ fraction of peripheral blood mononuclear cells (PBMNCs).

Subsequently, Asahara et al[12] employed bone marrow transplantation models to demonstrate that these $CD34^+$VEGFR-2^+ EPCs originated from the bone marrow. Immunodeficient mice underwent bone marrow transplantation from transgenic mice constitutively expressing β-galactosidase (*lacZ*) transcriptionally regulated by an EC-specific promoter, VEGFR-2, or Tie-2. Reconstitution of the transplanted bone marrow yielded mice in which expression of *lacZ* was restricted to bone marrow cells expressing endothelial cell markers. *lacZ* expression was used to assess the contribution of bone marrow-derived EPCs in various physiologic and pathologic neovascularization models. In a murine model of hind-limb and myocardial ischemia, *lacZ*$^+$ EPC colonies were observed in tissue stroma at sites of ischemia and were incorporated into capillaries among myocytes.

Ischemia mobilizes EPCs from the bone marrow into the peripheral circulation. Takahashi et al[13] assayed EPC kinetics for frequency and differentiation during severe tissue ischemia using mouse and rabbit models. The EPC-enriched population in circulating blood and EPC colony formation increased after the onset of ischemia, peaking at day 7. The effect on neovascularization of ischemia-induced EPC mobilization was assessed by the mouse cornea micropocket assay. Fluorescent photomicrographs 7 days after ischemia showed that neovascularization of avascular mouse corneas was greater in mice with hind-limb ischemia than in nonischemic sham-operated control mice ($p<0.05$).

The mechanism by which circulating EPCs "home" to the ischemic bed is complex and not yet completely understood. Among the many substances proclaimed to play a role in this process, VEGF is believed to be vital, because it is released by ischemic tissues, increases EPC activity and differentiation, and chemoattracts EPCs through VEGFR-2. The CXCR4 receptor found on EPCs also appears to have an important function in guiding these cells to the ischemic area via its interaction with stromal cell-derived factor 1α (SDF-1α), a chemokine upregulated in ischemic tissues.[14,15] Recent reports also suggest roles for β_2 integrins and the protease cathepsin L in the homing process.[16,17]

Finally, some recent studies suggest that bone marrow-derived cells do not directly incorporate into growing vasculature, but rather may mediate their effects by creating a favorable milieu for angiogenesis. They have been hypothesized to be the source of growth factors, cytokines, and various proteinases. Ziegelhoeffer et al[18] used high-resolution laser scanning confocal microscopy in a bone marrow transplantation/hind-limb ischemia mouse model and failed to colocalize labeled bone marrow cells with endothelial or smooth muscle cells in neovasculature. These researchers did, however, observe a threefold increase in the accumulation of labeled bone marrow cells adjacent to growing collateral arteries versus in the nonoccluded limb. Other researchers have corroborated this view. Kinnaird et al[19] further examined the role of paracrine mechanisms in bone marrow cell therapy. Normal human bone marrow stromal cells (BMSCs) were cultured under normoxic or hypoxic conditions, and their gene expression profile was determined. A wide array of arteriogenic cytokine genes were expressed at baseline, and several were induced >1.5-fold by hypoxic stress. After removal of the cells, the culture media from these experiments promoted in vitro proliferation and migration of endothelial and smooth muscle cells in a dose-dependent manner; anti-VEGF and anti-FGF antibodies only partially attenuated these effects. In a murine hind-limb ischemia model, murine BMSC culture media enhanced collateral flow recovery and remodeling, improved limb function, reduced the incidence of auto-amputation, and attenuated muscle atrophy compared with control media. These data imply that paracrine signaling may be an important mediator of bone marrow cell therapy in tissue ischemia and that cell incorporation into vessels is not a prerequisite for their effects.

EPCs may play a role in vascular homeostasis by contributing to ongoing endothelial repair, as well. The relationship between cardiovascular risk profile, endothelial dysfunction, and circulating EPC activity was examined in a study of 45 healthy male subjects. Endothelial function was measured using flow-mediated vasodilatation of the brachial artery, and EPC activity was assessed according to the number of colonies formed by PBMNCs plated on fibronectin. The magnitude of endothelial dysfunction correlated with reduced EPC activity ($r=0.6$, $p<0.001$). In fact, EPC activity was a stronger predictor of endothelial function than was the Framingham cardiovascular risk score. Analysis of the subgroup with a high risk score revealed that endothelial function was depressed only in those with low EPC counts and that the group with a high risk score and high EPC activity had preserved endothelial function.[20]

Despite the controversy regarding how bone marrow cells mediate neovascularization and endothelial repair, there is strong evidence for the therapeutic potential of these cells. Indeed, many groups have investigated the potential of bone marrow cell therapy in various ischemic vascular diseases. Two main approaches have been employed: transplantation of bone marrow (-derived) cells and mobilization of bone marrow cells. Here, we will explore these two approaches as applied to the treatment of limb ischemia.

Cell transplantation

Preclinical studies

There is considerable evidence to support cell transplantation for induction of therapeutic angiogenesis in animal models of hind-limb ischemia. Various types of cells and routes of administration have been utilized. The types of cells studied can be divided into two broad categories: ex vivo-expanded EPCs and freshly isolated EPC-enriched populations. The ex vivo-expanded EPCs are typically isolated by culture of mononuclear cells from peripheral blood, cord blood, or bone marrow. The EPC-enriched populations are obtained by various cell separation techniques, including flow cytometry and density gradient centrifugation of peripheral blood or bone marrow. Cell populations believed to be rich in EPCs include peripheral blood $CD34^+$ or $VEGFR\text{-}2^+$ cells, bone marrow mononuclear cells (BMMNCs), and BMSCs. Some of these subsets also contain other cells that may play supporting roles in the process of neovascularization. Intravenous, intraarterial, intracardiac, and intramuscular routes of administration have been used.

Based on the findings reported by Asahara et al,[11,12] Schatteman et al[21] showed that human $CD34^+$ cells could accelerate the rate of blood flow restoration in diabetic mice undergoing neovascularization due to hind-limb ischemia. Murohara et al[22] showed that transplantation of EPCs isolated by culture of $CD34^+$ mononuclear cells from human umbilical cord blood and adult peripheral blood augmented neovascularization and blood flow in the ischemic hind limb. Kalka et al[23] confirmed that transplantation of ex vivo-expanded human EPCs resulted in blood flow recovery and reduced the rate of limb loss in mouse models. One day after operative excision of one femoral artery, athymic nude mice received an intracardiac injection of 5×10^5 culture-expanded EPCs. By day 28, the ratio of ischemic/normal blood flow had improved by approximately twofold in EPC-transplanted mice compared with control mice, and the rate of limb salvage was six- to sevenfold higher.

These experiments demonstrated that EPCs isolated by culture of mononuclear cells are effective in enhancing blood flow. Shintani et al[24] took the next logical step and performed direct local transplantation of autologous BMMNCs instead of culture-isolated EPCs. Unilateral hind-limb ischemia was surgically induced in 27 rabbits, and autologous BMMNCs (6.9×10^6 cells/animal) or bone marrow fibroblasts (6.5×10^6 cells/animal) or saline were injected at six different points in the ischemic thigh muscles on postoperative day 7. Four weeks after transplantation, the BMMNC-transplanted group had more angiographically detectable collateral vessels, a higher capillary density, and a greater laser Doppler Sperfusion index than the controls. Subsequently, numerous studies have supported the concept of BMMNC transplantation in ameliorating blood flow in ischemic hind-limb models.[25,26]

BMSCs, which include EPCs and are considered to be present in the monocytoid and/or lymphocytoid fractions of BMMNCs, have also been evaluated for their angiogenic potential. Three weeks after ligation of the common iliac artery, 5×10^6 autologous BMSCs were injected into the ischemic thighs of male rats. BMSCs were found to differentiate into endothelium, vascular smooth muscle, skeletal muscle, and adipocytes. Four to six weeks after cell transplantation, the BMSC-treated limbs had greater vascular and arteriolar density, a greater ischemic/normal femoral artery flow index, and higher angiographic collateral reconstitution of the femoral artery.[27]

As discussed previously, the mechanism by which bone marrow cells enhance blood flow restoration is not clearly defined, and some investigators have suggested that paracrine effects may be important. PBMNCs, platelets, and polymorphonuclear leukocytes are known to synthesize and release high levels of various angiogenic substances but contain a low frequency of $CD34^+$ cells. Iba et al[28] have demonstrated that implantation of PBMNCs and platelets into ischemic limbs can also effectively induce collateral vessel formation, but these findings were not confirmed by earlier studies that used these cells as controls. Implantation of 10^6 or 10^5 human marrow $CD34^+$ cells (an EPC-enriched population) led to incorporation into some capillaries, whereas implantation of 10^4 $CD34^+$ cells did not cause any detectable incorporation. Iba et al[28] compared the angiogenic potential of BMMNCs and PBMNCs isolated from patients with peripheral arterial disease. BMMNCs contained approximately 100-fold greater numbers of $CD34^+$ cells (2.4%) than did PBMNCs (0.02%), and when implanted in equal numbers (10^7 cells) into ischemic rat limbs, the angiogenic effect of BMMNCs was about 50% higher. Taken together, these observations suggest that the paracrine signaling mechanisms of transplanted cells may play a greater role in mediating their angiogenic effect than their ability to incorporate into growing vessels.

EPC transplantation using gene-modified EPCs has been attempted to enhance the angiogenic effect. Iwaguro et al[29] investigated the impact of human VEGF-transduced EPC administration on neovascularization in a murine model of hind-limb ischemia. One day after excision of one femoral artery, athymic nude mice received an intravenous injection of 1.5×10^4 VEGF-EPCs or nontransduced EPCs. The ratio of ischemic/normal hind-limb blood flow and the rate of limb salvage were significantly higher in mice transplanted with VEGF-transduced EPCs.

Clinical studies

Based on these preclinical observations, preliminary clinical studies have been performed. Tateishi-Yuyama et al[30] administered autologous BMMNCs into ischemic muscles of patients with critical limb ischemia, including those with non-healing ulcers (22%) and gangrene (40%). In their initial unmasked pilot study, these researchers injected 25 patients who had unilateral limb ischemia with BMMNCs in the more ischemic leg and saline in the less ischemic leg. The cells were administered into 40 sites over a 3×3 cm area in the gastrocnemius muscle. The limbs injected with BMMNCs showed improvements in the ankle–brachial index, transcutaneous oxygen pressure, and rest pain score at 4 and 24 weeks of follow-up, while the saline-injected limbs showed no changes (Table 15.1). The pain-free walking time increased by 3.5 minutes at 24 weeks. The second part of this study had a randomized, controlled, double-blinded design. Twenty-two patients with bilateral leg ischemia were injected with BMMNCs in one leg and PBMNCs in the other leg as a control. The authors considered PBMNCs to be a more appropriate cell control than saline, since BMMNCs are contaminated by peripheral blood (about 10% of marrow cells) during the marrow aspiration procedure, and the number of $CD34^+$ cells, including EPCs, is at least

Table 15.1 Clinical studies of cell transplantation in limb ischemia

Study	*n*	*Study design*	*Cell type*	*No. of cells*	*Follow-up (weeks)*	*ABI*	*TcO$_2$ (mmHg)*	*PFWT (min)*
Tateishi-Yuyama et al[30] (group A)	25	Controlled, unblinded	BMMNC vs saline	1.6×10^9	24	↑0.11 ($p<0.001$)	↑16 ($p<0.001$)	↑3.5 ($p<0.001$)
Tateishi-Yuyama et al[30] (group B)	20	Controlled, blinded	BMMNC vs PBMNC	1.5×10^9	24	↑0.09 ($p<0.001$)	↑12 ($p<0.001$)	↑1.4 ($p<0.001$)
Esato et al[33]	8	Uncontrolled	BMMNC	4×10^8 – 1.5×10^{10}	4	No change	NA	NA
Higashi et al[31]	7	Uncontrolled	BMMNC	1.6×10^9	24	↑0.06 ($p=0.06$)	↑8 ($p=0.03$)	↑2.1 ($p=0.02$)
Miyamoto et al[32]	12	Uncontrolled	BMMNC +platelets	4.0×10^9	4	↑0.08 ($p=0.055$)	NA	↑5.2 ($p=0.034$)

↑, increased; All studies used autologous cells and an intramuscular route of administration. ABI, ankle-brachial index; BMMNC, bone marrow mononuclear cells; NA, not available; PBMNC, peripheral blood mononuclear cells, used as a control; PFWT, pain-free walking time; TcO$_2$, transcutaneous oxygen pressure.

100-fold lower in PBMNCs than in BMMNCs. Two patients discontinued the study due to clinical worsening before the 4-week follow-up. In the BMMNC-treated legs, 4 weeks after transplantation, the ankle–brachial index, transcutaneous oxygen pressure, and angiographic scores for new collateral vessel formation increased significantly (Table 15.1). In the PBMNC group, there was no significant change in these measures. Subjectively, the rest pain score improved by 2.2 units on a 0–4 scale in the BMMNC limbs and by 1.4 units ($p<0.03$) in the PBMNC limbs; the pain-free walking time increased significantly (by 1.2 minutes), and the improvement persisted for 24 weeks post transplantation. Interestingly, ischemic ulceration or gangrene was improved in just under half of all limbs, allowing successful salvage of these legs. No adverse events were reported.

Higashi et al[31] examined the value of cell therapy for improving endothelial dysfunction in addition to the standard markers of PAD such as the ankle–brachial index, transcutaneous oxygen pressure, and pain-free walking time in seven patients with rest pain and/or nonhealing ulcers. Leg blood flow was measured by strain-gauge plethysmography, and endothelial function was measured by the leg blood flow response to intrafemoral acetylcholine. Intramuscular BMMNC transplantation ameliorated the group's average basal leg blood flow from 1.7 to 2.0 ml/min per 100 ml of tissue after 24 weeks and enhanced endothelial function in response to acetylcholine. The transcutaneous oxygen pressure and pain-free walking time also improved, but the ankle–brachial index did not change significantly (Table 15.1).

Miyamoto et al[32] investigated the safety and efficacy of autologous BMMNCs plus platelets in 12 patients with severe chronic PAD, including those with non-atherosclerotic vasculitic conditions. Nineteen limbs and hands with severe ischemia were injected with an average of 4.0×10^9 cells and followed for 4 weeks. Rest pain improved in 11 of the 12 patients. Technetium-99m (^{99m}Tc)-tetrofosmin perfusion scintigraphy demonstrated an improvement in proximal limb perfusion, and there was an improvement in the pain-free walking time and a trend toward improvement in the ankle–brachial index (Table 15.1). Esato et al[33] studied autologous BMMNC transplantation in eight patients with advanced PAD in whom traditional treatments had failed. Four of the patients had arteriosclerosis obliterans and the other four had thromboangiitis obliterans. All but one of them had rest pain or ischemic ulcers. Nine limbs received intramuscular administration of 4×10^8–1.5×10^{10} BMMNCs in multiple sites within the affected area. At 4 weeks, subjective symptoms were improved in 7 of the 8 patients, without an appreciable change in the ankle–brachial index. Although the small sample size precludes a definitive conclusion, the outcomes in this study seem to correlate with the number of cells implanted. No relative toxicity was observed in any of the patients.

All of these studies have employed small numbers of patients. Many of the studies have been uncontrolled and can only be considered preliminary in their conclusions. However, there are some promising trends in these early clinical investigations of bone marrow cell transplantation for limb ischemia. Large, randomized, placebo-controlled studies should be pursued to confirm these findings.

Cell mobilization

Mobilization of endogenous EPCs from the bone marrow may be an alternative strategy for induction of therapeutic angiogenesis. Cytokines such as granulocyte–macrophage colony-stimulating factor (GM-CSF), granulocyte colony-stimulating factor (G-CSF), and erythropoietin (Epo); growth factors such as VEGF, placental growth factor, and angiopoietin-1; chemokines such as SDF-1; hormones such as estrogens; statins, and exercise have all been shown to mobilize EPCs. G-CSF and GM-CSF are the most powerful, but also the most inflammatory, of these mobilizing agents.[34]

Preclinical studies

Takahashi et al[13] showed that in rabbits with surgically induced hind-limb ischemia, circulating bone marrow-derived EPCs were augmented after pretreatment with GM-CSF compared with saline, with a corresponding improvement in hind-limb neovascularization. Subcutaneous GM-CSF pre treatment at 50 μg/day for 7 days resulted in almost a twofold increase in the circulating EPC-enriched cell population (measured by lack of expression of mature lymphocyte and monocyte markers) and a fourfold increase in EPC colony-forming units on assay ($p < 0.01$ for both). Seven days after the induction of ischemia, capillary density analysis by histologic examination with alkaline phosphatase staining showed 70% greater neovascularization in the GM-CSF group compared with the control group ($p < 0.01$). There was also significant improvement in the ischemic/normal hind-limb blood pressure ratio (GM-CSF vs control, 0.71 vs 0.49; $p < 0.01$).

Clinical studies

In patients with coronary artery disease, subcutaneous G-CSF at 10 μg/kg/day for 5 days led to a >30-fold rise in the EPC-enriched population of $CD34^+$ $CD133^+$ cells, a response similar to that observed in healthy subjects. Indices of platelet and coagulation activation were not changed, but C-reactive protein (CRP) increased from 4.5 to 8.6 mg/l ($p = 0.017$). Two out of 16 patients experienced serious adverse events potentially related to G-CSF administration: one fatal and one nonfatal myocardial infarction. There was no objective evidence of improvement in myocardial ischemia at 3 months.[35] Interestingly, a placebo-controlled study of 42 patients receiving G-CSF after adjunctive chemotherapy for breast cancer showed improved endothelial function despite a concomitant rise in CRP levels.[36] G-CSF has also been associated with an increased rate of restenosis in some studies, although results are conflicting.[37,38] When compared with G-CSF,[39–41] GM-CSF appears to produce a less robust mobilization of $CD34^+$ cells but with a greater number of more primitive cells. A placebo-controlled study of GM-CSF in 10 patients with coronary artery disease demonstrated significantly improved collateral flow without any complications.[42] Epo mobilizes EPCs, increases capillary density, and improves cardiac function in rats with post-myocardial infarction heart failure.[43] Erythropoietin has also been shown to mobilize $CD34^+$ $CD45^+$ circulating EPCs in humans and may be preferable due to its lower pro-inflammatory profile.[34] Finally, well-accepted therapies such as statins and exercise have now been shown to mobilize EPCs, invoking a possible mechanism for their beneficial effects beyond that attributable to lipid lowering.[44–47]

Two recent studies have examined bone marrow cell mobilization for the treatment of chronic limb ischemia. Van Royen and colleagues[48] studied, in a placebo-controlled manner, the effects of subcutaneous GM-CSF (10 mcg/kg qod for 14 days) in 40 patients with moderate to severe intermittent claudication. Although GM-CSF resulted in mobilization of $CD34^+$ mononuclear cells, the change in walking time, which was the primary endpoint of the study, was not different between the placebo and treated groups. No change in ankle–brachial index was found with GM-CSF treatment at day 14 or at day 90. Interestingly, laser doppler flowmetry measurements showed a significant decrease in microcirculatory flow reserve in the control group but no change in the GM-CSF group. The authors concluded that this study did not support the use of GM-CSF for the treatment of intermittent claudication.

However, we demonstrated more promising results in our study of a similar population of patients.[49] Forty-five subjects with unrevascularizable PAD were randomized, in a double-blind fashion, to either placebo or subcutaneous GM-CSF thrice weekly for 2 weeks. GM-CSF increased circulating $CD34^+$ mononuclear cells by 46%, $CD34^+CD133^+$ cells by 77% and EPC colonies by 31% at 2 weeks. Endothelial function, measured as brachial artery flow-mediated dilation, improved by 59% at 12 weeks after GM-CSF therapy. Ankle–brachial index remained unchanged in both groups. Pain-free walking time improved by 38 seconds and total walking time increased by 55 seconds at 12 weeks in the GM-CSF group but did not change in the placebo group.

Cell mobilization can be followed by peripheral collection of progenitor cells and local implantation. This combined strategy would offer an advantage if the mobilized cells were to have reduced homing capacity. Although there have been no published investigations employing this approach in limb ischemia, studies utilizing this approach are currently underway.

Summary of Therapeutic Angiogenesis

Therapeutic angiogenesis for the treatment of chronic limb ischemia (and other ischemic conditions) has gained momentum with the introduction of bone marrow cell therapy. Of the two approaches discussed here, cell transplantation has received more attention and, hence, has accumulated greater evidence of therapeutic potential. Patients with unrevascularizable critical limb ischemia, who would otherwise require an amputation, have the greatest potential to benefit from a trial of autologous BMMNC transplantation. In general, however, direct cell transplantation is still in its infancy, and large well-controlled trials with extended follow-up are needed before this approach can enter clinical practice. Future studies should include a careful evaluation of safety endpoints, especially given the reports of atherosclerotic plaque progression following EPC transplantation in experimental models.[50] Also, patients with stable intermittent claudication need to be evaluated separately from those with critical limb ischemia. Preliminary investigations suggest that cytokine mobilization of bone marrow is safe and may be effective in the treatment of intermittent claudication. Head-to-head trials comparing cell transplantation with cell mobilization need to be performed in order to determine whether the systemic increase in circulating EPC levels is preferable to a local injection of progenitor cells. In light of the evidence suggesting a paracrine mechanism rather than direct incorporation for the observed effects of cell therapy, administration of a "cocktail" of cytokines and/or factors produced by bone marrow cells is another approach warranting further investigation. The possibility of identifying more potent, yet safe, mobilizing agents with targeted mobilization capability and the prospect of combining genetic engineering with bone marrow cell therapy keep the future bright for therapeutic angiogenesis.

References

1. Creager MA. Medical management of peripheral arterial disease. Cardiol Rev 2001;9:238–45.
2. Gardner AW, Poehlman ET. Exercise rehabilitation programs for the treatment of claudication pain. A meta-analysis. JAMA 1995;274:975–80.
3. Leng GC, Fowler B, Ernst E. Exercise for intermittent claudication. Cochrane Database Syst Rev 2000;(2):CD000990.
4. Jacoby D, Mohler ER 3rd. Drug treatment of intermittent claudication. Drugs 2004;64:1657–70.
5. Dormandy JA, Rutherford RB. Management of peripheral arterial disease (PAD). TASC Working Group. TransAtlantic Inter-Society Concensus (TASC). J Vasc Surg 2000;31:S1–296.
6. Comerota AJ, Throm RC, Miller KA, et al. Naked plasmid DNA encoding fibroblast growth factor type 1 for the treatment of end-stage unreconstructible lower extremity ischemia: preliminary results of a phase I trial. J Vasc Surg 2002;35:930–6.
7. Lazarous DF, Unger EF, Epstein SE, et al. Basic fibroblast growth factor in patients with intermittent claudication: results of a phase I trial. J Am Coll Cardiol 2000;36:1239–44.
8. Heil M, Ziegelhoeffer T, Mees B, Schaper W. A different outlook on the role of bone marrow stem cells in vascular growth: bone marrow delivers software not hardware. Circ Res 2004;94:573–4.
9. Lederman RJ, Mendelsohn FO, Anderson RD, et al. Therapeutic angiogenesis with recombinant fibroblast growth factor-2 for intermittent claudication (the TRAFFIC study): a randomised trial. Lancet 2002;359:2053–8.
10. Rajagopalan S, Mohler ER 3rd, Lederman RJ, et al. Regional angiogenesis with vascular endothelial growth factor in peripheral arterial disease: a phase II randomized, double-blind, controlled study of adenoviral delivery of vascular endothelial growth factor 121 in patients with disabling intermittent claudication. Circulation 2003;108:1933–8.
11. Asahara T, Murohara T, Sullivan A, et al. Isolation of putative progenitor endothelial cells for angiogenesis. Science 1997; 275:964–7.
12. Asahara T, Masuda H, Takahashi T, et al. Bone marrow origin of endothelial progenitor cells responsible for postnatal vasculogenesis in physiological and pathological neovascularization. Circ Res 1999;85:221–8.
13. Takahashi T, Kalka C, Masuda H, et al. Ischemia- and cytokine-induced mobilization of bone marrow-derived endothelial progenitor cells for neovascularization. Nat Med 1999;5:434–8.
14. Hristov M, Weber C. Endothelial progenitor cells: characterization, pathophysiology, and possible clinical relevance. J Cell Mol Med 2004;8: 498–508.
15. Yamaguchi J, Kusano KF, Masuo O, et al. Stromal cell-derived factor-1 effects on ex vivo expanded endothelial progenitor cell recruitment for ischemic neovascularization. Circulation 2003;107:1322–8.
16. Chavakis E, Aicher A, Heeschen C, et al. Role of β_2-integrins for homing and neovascularization capacity of endothelial progenitor cells. J Exp Med 2005;201:63–72.
17. Urbich C, Heeschen C, Aicher A, et al. Cathepsin L is required for endothelial progenitor cell-induced neovascularization. Nat Med 2005;11:206–13.
18. Ziegelhoeffer T, Fernandez B, Kostin S, et al. Bone marrow-derived cells do not incorporate into the adult growing vasculature. Circ Res 2004;94:230–8.
19. Kinnaird T, Stabile E, Burnett MS, et al. Marrow-derived stromal cells express genes encoding a broad spectrum of arteriogenic cytokines and promote in vitro and in vivo arteriogenesis through paracrine mechanisms. Circ Res 2004;94:678–85.
20. Hill JM, Zalos G, Halcox JP, et al. Circulating endothelial progenitor cells, vascular function, and cardiovascular risk. N Engl J Med 2003;348:593–600.
21. Schatteman GC, Hanlon HD, Jiao C, Dodds SG, Christy BA, et al. Blood-derived angioblasts accelerate blood-flow restoration in diabetic mice. J Clin Invest 2000;106:571–8.
22. Murohara T, Ikeda H, Duan J, et al. Transplanted cord blood-derived endothelial precursor cells augment postnatal neovascularization. J Clin Invest 2000;105: 1527–36.
23. Kalka C, Masuda H, Takahashi T, et al. Transplantation of ex vivo expanded endothelial progenitor cells for therapeutic neovascularization. Proc Natl Acad Sci USA 2000;97:3422–7.
24. Shintani S, Murohara T, Ikeda H, et al. Augmentation of postnatal neovascularization with autologous bone marrow transplantation. Circulation 2001;103:897–903.
25. Ikenaga S, Hamano K, Nishida M, et al. Autologous bone marrow implantation induced angiogenesis and improved deteriorated exercise capacity in a rat ischemic hindlimb model. J Surg Res 2001;96:277–83.
26. Yoshida M, Horimoto H, Mieno S, et al. Intra-arterial bone marrow cell transplantation induces angiogenesis in rat hindlimb ischemia. Eur Surg Res 2003;35:86–91.
27. Al-Khaldi A, Al-Sabti H, Galipeau J, Lachapelle K. Therapeutic angiogenesis using autologous bone marrow stromal cells: improved blood flow in a

chronic limb ischemia model. Ann Thorac Surg 2003;75:204–9.
28. Iba O, Matsubara H, Nozawa Y, et al. Angiogenesis by implantation of peripheral blood mononuclear cells and platelets into ischemic limbs. Circulation 2002;106:2019–25.
29. Iwaguro H, Yamaguchi J, Kalka C, et al. Endothelial progenitor cell vascular endothelial growth factor gene transfer for vascular regeneration. Circulation 2002;105:732–8.
30. Tateishi-Yuyama E, Matsubara H, Murohara T, et al. Therapeutic angiogenesis for patients with limb ischaemia by autologous transplantation of bone-marrow cells: a pilot study and a randomised controlled trial. Lancet 2002;360:427–35.
31. Higashi Y, Kimura M, Hara K, et al. Autologous bone-marrow mononuclear cell implantation improves endothelium-dependent vasodilation in patients with limb ischemia. Circulation 2004; 109:1215–18.
32. Miyamoto M, Yasutake M, Takano H, et al. Therapeutic angiogenesis by autologous bone marrow cell implantation for refractory chronic peripheral arterial disease using assessment of neovascularization by ^{99m}Tc-tetrofosmin (TF) perfusion scintigraphy. Cell Transplant 2004;13:429–37.
33. Esato K, Hamano K, Li TS, et al. Neovascularization induced by autologous bone marrow cell implantation in peripheral arterial disease. Cell Transplant 2002;11: 747–52.
34. Aicher A, Zeiher AM, Dimmeler S. Mobilizing endothelial progenitor cells. Hypertension 2005; 45:321–5.
35. Hill JM, Syed MA, Arai AE, et al. Outcomes and risks of granulocyte colony-stimulating factor in patients with coronary artery disease. J Am Coll Cardiol 2005;46:1643–8.
36. Ikonomidis I, Papadimitriou C, et al. Treatment with recombinant granulocyte colony stimulating factor improves endothelial function despite concomitant C-reactive protein elevation. In: Proceedings of ACC Annual Scientific Sessions, 2005.
37. Kang HJ, Kim HS, Zhang SY, et al. Effects of intracoronary infusion of peripheral blood stem-cells mobilised with granulocyte-colony stimulating factor on left ventricular systolic function and restenosis after coronary stenting in myocardial infarction: the MAGIC cell randomised clinical trial. Lancet 2004;363:751–6.
38. Engelmann MG, Hennig C, et al. Bone-marrow stem cell mobilization induced by granulocyte-colony stimulating factor in patients undergoing delayed revascularization for ST-segment elevation myocardial infarction: early results from the G-CSF in STEMI trial. In: Proceedings of ACC Annual Scientific Sessions, 2005.
39. Fischmeister G, Kurz M, Haas OA, et al. G-CSF versus GM-CSF for stimulation of peripheral blood progenitor cells (PBPC) and leukocytes in healthy volunteers: comparison of efficacy and tolerability. Ann Hematol 1999;78:117–23.
40. Ho AD, Young D, Maruyama M, et al. Pluripotent and lineage-committed $CD34^+$ subsets in leukapheresis products mobilized by G-CSF, GM-CSF vs. a combination of both. Exp Hematol 1996;24: 1460–8.
41. Lane TA, Ho AD, Bashey A, et al. Mobilization of blood-derived stem and progenitor cells in normal subjects by granulocyte–macrophage- and granulocyte-colony-stimulating factors. Transfusion 1999;39:39–47.
42. Seiler C, Pohl T, Wustmann K, et al. Promotion of collateral growth by granulocyte–macrophage colony-stimulating factor in patients with coronary artery disease: a randomized, double-blind, placebo-controlled study. Circulation 2001;104: 2012–17.
43. Van der Meer P, Henning RH, et al. Erythropoietin increases capillary density and improves cardiac function in rats with heart failure after myocardial infarction. In: Proceedings of ACC Annual Scientific Sessions, 2005.
44. Llevadot J, Murasawa S, Kureishi Y, et al. HMG-CoA reductase inhibitor mobilizes bone marrow-derived endothelial progenitor cells. J Clin Invest 2001;108:399–405.
45. Rehman J, Li J, Parvathaneni L, et al. Exercise acutely increases circulating endothelial progenitor cells and monocyte-/ macrophage-derived angiogenic cells. J Am Coll Cardiol 2004;43: 2314–18.
46. Vasa M, Fichtlscherer S, Adler K, et al. Increase in circulating endothelial progenitor cells by statin therapy in patients with stable coronary artery disease. Circulation 2001;103:2885–90.
47. Walter DH, Rittig K, Bahlmann FH, et al. Statin therapy accelerates reendothelialization: a novel effect involving mobilization and incorporation of bone marrow-derived endothelial progenitor cells. Circulation 2002;105:3017–24.
48 van Royen N, Schirmer SH, Atasever B, et al. A pilot study on stimulation of arteriogenesis using subcutaneous application of granuloctyte-macrophage colony-stimulating factor as a new treatment for peripheral vascular disease. Circulation 2005;112:1040–46.
49 Subramaniyam V, et al. Stimulation of endothelial progenitor cells with granulocyte-macrophage colony stimulating factor improves endothelial dysfunction in patients with peripheral arterial disease. Presented at ACC 2006.
50. Silvestre JS, Gojova A, Brun V, et al. Transplantation of bone marrow-derived mononuclear cells in ischemic apolipoprotein E-knockout mice accelerates atherosclerosis without altering plaque composition. Circulation 2003;108:2839–42.

chapter 16

Concerns Regarding Stem Cell Therapy from the Clinical Perspective

Arjun Deb and Noel Caplice

Introduction

The traditional view of the heart as a postmitotic organ incapable of regeneration has been challenged by animal and human data demonstrating the presence of extracardiac progenitors.[1–6] These progenitors offer great hope for augmenting cardiac repair post myocardial infarction. Promising preliminary experimental data have been greeted with enthusiasm by the clinical community and have led to clinical trials of cell-based cardiac therapy. Although one or more definitive and pre-eminent cardiac progenitor cells remain to be identified, putative sources of such cells include bone marrow-derived progenitor cells of hematopoietic, angioblastic, and mesenchymal lineages and, more recently, resident cardiac stem cells.[7–9] Clinical trials of cell therapy in the heart so far have used cells of varying lineages, with differing endpoints determining efficacy. Moreover, many studies have used heterogeneous mixtures of cells rather than a purified or clonal population of a particular cell type. Nothwitstanding differing cell types, differing endpoints, and the uncontrolled nature of such clinical trials, cell-based therapy has shown universal improvement in cardiac function.[10–15]

Early clinical success has also led to questions regarding the mechanisms of action and the short- and long-term safety of cardiac cell therapy. Although many beneficial mechanisms have been postulated,[4,16–18] animal and human studies to date have failed to point to a specific mechanism underlying the improvement in cardiac performance. Initial enthusiasm about stem cell plasticity has also been tempered by recent animal data demonstrating a lack of transdifferentiation of hematopoietic progenitors following injection into an injured heart.[19–21] The lack of understanding of a precise mechanism has led some basic science researchers to propose slowing the pace of all clinical trials until the true risks and benefits of such therapy can be fully evaluated in more extensive animal studies. Unfortunately, experimental models are an imprecise predictor of subsequent clinical events, and, more importantly, unanticipated clinical adverse events may not always be detected in preclinical models. A compromise approach to further clinical trials of cell therapy may therefore be to proceed cautiously with larger, double-blinded, randomized, controlled clinical trials while adhering to the most rigorous safety standards applicable to pharmacologic clinical trials.

As the clinical community embarks on more widespread application of cell therapy, one area of particular concern is the appearance of previously unanticipated adverse effects. For instance, cell-based de novo angiogenesis may improve the contractile function of ischemic myocardium and lead to symptomatic improvement in the short term, but aberrant angiogenesis also has the

Table 16.1 Potential adverse effects and safety monitoring required following administration of stem cells

Potential adverse effects	*Monitoring required*
■ Arrhythmias ■ Aberrant angiogenesis and plaque growth ■ Thrombosis ■ Restenosis ■ Malignant transformation ■ Distant organ-seeding events	■ Symptom-related follow-up, event monitor/Holter ■ IVUS/MRI/CT to monitor plaque burden; exercise caution in patients with diabetes or occult tumors ■ Strict event-related follow-up of patients to determine rates of thrombosis and restenosis following PCI

IVUS/MRI/CT, intravascular ultrasound/magnetic resonance imaging/computed tomography; PCI, percutaneous coronary intervention.

potential to do long-term harm both in diseased vasculature and in the myocardium. Moreover, optimization of cell therapy, including determination of the type of cell used, the timing and route of infusion, and the establishment of rigorous safety monitoring criteria, may be difficult if the beneficial mechanisms of cell-based therapy remain unknown. For example, systemic infusion of cells may lead to improvement in myocardial performance but could have deleterious effects on other organs (multiorgan seeding). The clinical profile of the patient may also be critically important in determining the safety and efficacy of these cells. The safety profile of these cells in patients with ischemic cardiomyopathy may be entirely different from the profile in those with nonischemic cardiomyopathy. The interplay of cellular, patient, and disease factors may therefore determine not only the efficacy of therapy but also potential short- and long-term adverse consequences of treatment.

Importantly, clinical studies of cardiac cell therapy to date have been safe and have not reported any untoward adverse effects. However, long-term data are still unavailable. Moreover, therapeutic parameters regarding cell type, route and timing of administration, and indications for therapy in various disease states remain to be defined. This chapter will review safety concerns regarding cardiac cell therapy from a clinical perspective and will discuss the broad interplay of cellular factors, the clinical patient profile, and the disease environment in determining the potential adverse outcomes of cell-based cardiac therapy (Table 16.1).

Safety Concerns Regarding Cardiac Stem Cell Therapy

Adverse effects related to cell type

As the number of clinical trials increases and the spectrum of cells and indications for cardiac stem cell therapy widens, safety should remain a primary concern. Safety issues may relate to the cells used, the disease environment in which the cells are delivered, and the underlying clinical condition of the patient being treated. Cardiac stem cell therapy trials have used numerous cell types, including bone marrow-derived mononuclear cells (BMMNCs), endothelial progenitor cells (EPCs), and cells bearing specific cell surface markers, such as CD133 (AC133) (Table 16.1).[11]

Increased susceptibility to, or induction of, new arrhythmias following infusion of stem cells remains a potential risk. Early animal studies of skeletal myoblast implantation in a canine model of ventricular cryoablation demonstrated

Table 16.2 Specific safety concerns related to the type of cell used for cell therapy

Cell type	*Safety concerns*
Embryonic	Teratoma, uncontrolled proliferation, abnormal differentiation, immunogenicity, arrhythmias, cell fusion, chromosomal instability
Mesenchymal	Arrhthymias, immunogenicity
Endothelial progenitor	Plaque angiogenesis, worsening atherosclerosis
Total bone marrow mononuclear	Heterogeneous population, with difficulty in ascribing culpability of potential adverse effects to one particular cell; in-stent thromobosis; restenosis
$CD133^+$	Potential for unregulated growth

new myofiber formation but failed to show electrical integration of engrafted myoblasts with native myocytes.[22,23] The potential risk of arrhythmogenesis has been sufficiently demonstrated in clinical applications of skeletal myoblast therapy[24] that current trials utilizing skeletal myoblasts require prophylactic implantable cardioverter–defibrillator (ICD) placement.

The use of poorly characterized, undifferentiated BMMNCs (as in many stem cell therapy trials to date) raises the possibility of unexpected outcomes. A study by Yoon et al[25] demonstrated intramyocardial calcification in 28% of animals following injection of unfractionated cells in a rat model of myocardial infarction. If these results were replicated in humans, it is not difficult to conceive a situation in which calcium deposition within the myocardium could lead to depression of ventricular performance and act as a nidus for future arrhythmia propagation. Furthermore, calcification within the conduction system could lead to additional conduction disturbances that might necessitate pacemaker implantation. Such arrhythmogenic events or conduction disturbances may conceivably manifest days to months later, underlining the importance of close yet long-term follow-up of patients enrolled in these trials.

Stem cells have the ability to differentiate along a particular tissue lineage as well as to produce progeny that maintain multipotentiality.[21] Unregulated differentiation of stem cells following infusion in human subjects could have potentially deleterious consequences. The use of embryonic stem cells (ESCs) may lead to teratoma formation,[26] and mesenchymal and bone marrow-derived multipotent adult progenitor cells (MAPCs) have been shown to differentiate into various tissues belonging to different germ layers.[7,27] Aberrant and uncontrolled differentiation following infusion of these cells could potentially lead to formation of noncardiac tissue within the heart. For instance, differentiation of a cardiac stem cell into a cell of fibroblast lineage rather than a cardiomyocyte could have adverse consequences on ventricular performance and potentiate rather than retard scar formation. Aberrant fibroblast differentiation could also retard conduction, potentiating heart block. Because the local and systemic factors determining differentiation pathways of infused stem cells are largely unknown, we should remain cautiously alert when infusing heterogeneous populations of cells (e.g., BMMNCs) into an area of active inflammation and healing.

Uncontrolled proliferation of clonal cell populations within the heart may pose a specific risk of developing malignant tumors. In one study, stem cell antigen 1-positive ($Sca\text{-}1^+$) cells were isolated from the heart and injected into mice following a myocardial infarction.[9] Differentiation and cell fusion accounted equally for new cardiomyocyte formation. Cell fusion does not occur naturally in the heart, and multiploid nuclei could potentially lead to chromosomal instability and oncogenic transformation. This theoretical risk in human subjects may warrant surveillance with sophisticated imaging modalities to detect the presence of tumors in subjects treated with clonally expanded cell populations. The discovery of a $CD133^+$ brain tumor stem cell in medulloblastomas suggests that additional caution should be applied in the systemic administration of these cell lines.[28]

Aberrant angiogenesis leading to worsening atherosclerosis is another potential concern when using vasculogenic precursor cells. Several animal studies have now demonstrated a link between mononuclear cell infiltration and angiogenesis-induced plaque growth in rodent models.[29] Moreover Moulton et al[29] have shown EPC infiltration in plaques in atherogenic mice following genetically tracked bone marrow transplantation. Thus, the current approach of infusing BMMNCs carries the theoretical risk of worsening atherosclerosis. Bone marrow-derived smooth muscle cells have also been detected in coronary artery plaques in both animals and humans.[30] These cells are enriched 100-fold in diseased versus undiseased segments of atherosclerotic vessels. Although the precise function of these cells is currently unknown, it is conceivable that infusion of bone marrow-derived precursors may lead to further smooth muscle infiltration and proliferation within the vessel wall, contributing to plaque growth. Monitoring plaque growth by intravascular ultrasound (IVUS), magnetic resonance imaging (MRI), or multislice computed tomography (CT) may be warranted in these patients. Indeed, it is important to consider the additional risk of promoting plaque instability by neovascularization of the adventitial and intimal layers of diseased vessels.[31–34] Some studies have used growth factors such as granulocyte colony-stimulating factor (G-CSF) for mobilization of cardiac progenitors from the bone marrow.[35] It is interesting to note here that gene therapy studies using growth factors such as vascular endothelial growth factor (VEGF) have shown worsening of atherosclerosis and angioma formation in some experimental settings.[36] The effects of mobilizing a heterogeneous population of cells by the use of growth factors or cytokines that are indiscriminate in activation and recruitment capacity may pose a similar risk. Recent data reported by Kang et al,[35] showing an increased incidence of restenosis in the setting of G-CSF and bone marrow cell administration in the setting of percutaneous coronary intervention (PCI) for acute myocardial infarction, underscore this concern regarding inappropriate endogenous cell recruitment and its potentially detrimental consequences.

Cardiac stem cell therapy has also been associated with an increased risk of thrombosis in at least one animal study. Following infusion of 5×10^5 mesenchymal stromal cells/kg in the circumflex artery of a dog, electrocardiographic (ECG) changes of acute myocardial injury were observed.[37] In this respect, it is interesting to bear in mind that cells of the monocytic lineage, as well as EPCs, express tissue factor and that systemic and local factors at the time of infusion and thereafter may lead to activation of tissue factor and the coagulation cascade. Moreover, the culture environment in which cells are grown prior to implantation may have a significant impact on the subsequent biology of these cells in vivo. For instance, it has recently been suggested that the use of fetal calf serum in myoblast culture media may in part explain the proarrhthymic effects of these cells when used in clinical trials.[38]

The effects of seeding of distant organs by exogenously administered stem cells are not known. In a study of sex-mismatched bone marrow transplant patients, bone marrow-derived tissue chimeric cells were found (albeit in very low levels) in the liver, kidney, and skeletal muscles.[5] Theoretically, injected cells may contribute to ectopic sites of vasculogenesis or differentiation. In particular, such effects on neovascularization could be of concern for patients with diabetes or occult cancer.

There are no long-term data regarding the survival of implanted progenitor cells following infusion, although preliminary data suggest that less than 10% of these cells survive more than 48 hours after implantation (N Caplice, unpublished data). It is conceivable that infusion of progenitor cells may initiate an immune response and lead to the early rejection and death of these cells. This is clearly the case for human ESCs and perhaps, to a lesser extent, for mesenchymal stem cells, both of which express major histocompatibility complex (MHC) class I molecules.[27,39] It has also been hypothesized that culture modification or differentiation of progenitor cells ex vivo may make them more immunogenic. Subsequent host-mediated attacks on newly engrafted cells may presage further inflammation and potentiation of injury to the recipient heart.

Adverse effects related to the patient and disease environment

The clinical status of the patient and the underlying disease substrate may also impact the short- and long-term safety profile of cell-based therapy. Patients with diabetes and risk factors for coronary disease are known to have decreased numbers of circulating EPCs.[31] It is not known whether this reduction is secondary to marrow exhaustion, the presence of circulating inhibitory cytokines, or growth signaling deficiencies in diabetic progenitor cells. The presence of circulating inhibitory factors would certainly limit the success of stem cell infusion, as the survival of these cells would potentially be severely compromised. Furthermore, lack of appropriate myocardial perfusion at sites of implantation in patients with acute and chronic myocardial ischemia may diminish the rates of survival of engrafted cells. Apoptosis or early necrosis of these cells within an already diseased and inflamed heart may augment inflammatory responses, further depressing myocardial performance.

The timing of cell delivery, especially in the setting of an acute myocardial injury, may be crucial. Early following an infarction, the myocardium is infiltrated with a number of inflammatory cells. Inflamed myocardium may not be the best substrate for stable engraftment of exogenously delivered cells. On the other hand, if the cells were infused weeks later, the presence of an evolving scar and thinning of the myocardium might negate the potential benefits of cell therapy. Therefore, a window of opportunity that is yet to be precisely defined may exist for maximizing myocardial performance. This may mirror the experience gained during more than a decade of research into thrombolytic therapy. Elucidation of this therapeutic window may be further enhanced by well-designed animal studies.

The optimal route of cell delivery requires further evaluation but may be an important determining factor for therapeutic success and safety. Direct myocardial injection of stem cells, particularly via a percutaneous approach, is technically challenging and requires specialist training, which may limit its use to tertiary care settings with electromechanical mapping capability. Intracoronary infusion of cells via an infarct-related artery after percutaneous revascularization has been adopted in several human studies and may be more widely applicable, but it has potential risks of in situ thrombosis and stent restenosis, depending on the cell type and adjunctive agents selected for therapy. Patients with a large burden of atherosclerosis or unstable lesions may also be at increased risk of disease potentiation.

No human data currently exist about the efficacy of cell therapy in the setting of nonischemic cardiomyopathy. Vastly differing outcomes and safety concerns may emerge from this patient cohort. Rigorous animal studies performed prior to implementing stem cell therapy in this group of patients may help to clarify these issues. Indeed, preliminary studies of skeletal myoblasts in experimental nonischemic cardiomyopathy suggest improvements in left ventricular function following cell therapy.[40]

In conclusion, precise definition of the mechanisms of cell therapy and determination of the optimal therapeutic parameters related to the cell, the recipient, and the underlying disease, along with appropriate assessment of outcomes in randomized, blinded, and controlled trials, have to be performed for successful, safe, and widespread translation of cell therapy from the bench to the bedside (Figure 16.1). Rigorous monitoring of short- and long-term safety has to be a priority in this worthy endeavor.

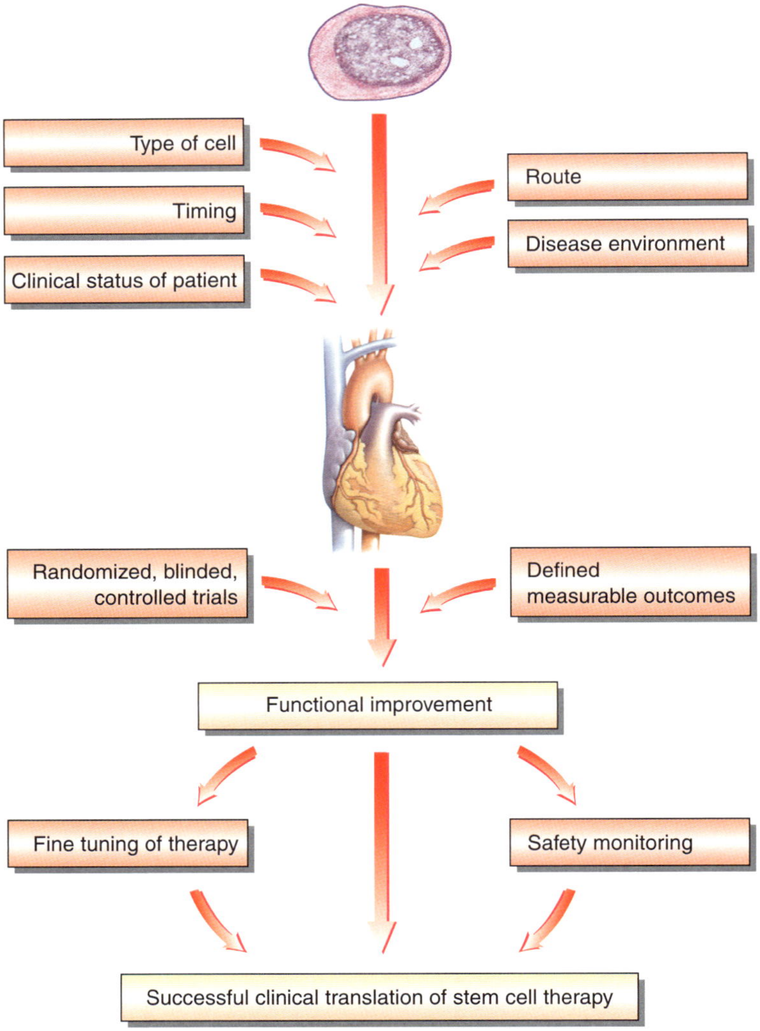

Figure 16.1 *Pathway to the successful translation of cardiac stem cell therapy from bench to bedside.*

References

1. Quaini F, Urbanek K, Beltrami AP, et al. Chimerism of the transplanted heart. N Engl J Med 2002;346:5–15.
2. Laflamme MA, Myerson D, Saffitz JE, Murry CE. Evidence for cardiomyocyte repopulation by extracardiac progenitors in transplanted human hearts. Circ Res 2002;90:634–40.
3. Muller P, Pfeiffer P, Koglin J, et al. Cardiomyocytes of noncardiac origin in myocardial biopsies of human transplanted hearts. Circulation 2002;106:31–5.
4. Jackson KA, Majka SM, Wang H, et al. Regeneration of ischemic cardiac muscle and vascular endothelium by adult stem cells. J Clin Invest 2001;107:1395–402.
5. Deb A, Wang S, Skelding KA, Miller D, Simper D, Caplice NM. Bone marrow-derived cardiomyocytes are present in adult human heart: a study of gender-mismatched bone marrow transplantation patients. Circulation 2003;107:1247–9.
6. Hruban RH, Long PP, Perlman EJ, et al. Fluorescence in situ hybridization for the Y-chromosome can be used to detect cells of recipient origin in

allografted hearts following cardiac transplantation. Am J Pathol 1993;142:975–80.
7. Jiang Y, Jahagirdar BN, Reinhardt RL, et al. Pluripotency of mesenchymal stem cells derived from adult marrow. Nature 2002;418:41–9.
8. Beltrami AP, Barlucchi L, Torella D, et al. Adult cardiac stem cells are multipotent and support myocardial regeneration. Cell 2003;114:763–76.
9. Oh H, Bradfute SB, Gallardo TD, et al. Cardiac progenitor cells from adult myocardium: homing, differentiation, and fusion after infarction. Proc Natl Acad Sci USA 2003;100:12313–18.
10. Saito T, Kuang JQ, Lin CC, Chiu RC. Transcoronary implantation of bone marrow stromal cells ameliorates cardiac function after myocardial infarction. J Thorac Cardiovasc Surg 2003;126: 114–23.
11. Melo LG, Pachori AS, Kong D, et al. Molecular and cell-based therapies for protection, rescue, and repair of ischemic myocardium: reasons for cautious optimism. Circulation 2004;109:2386–93.
12. Orlic D, Kajstura J, Chimenti S, Bodine DM, Leri A, Anversa P. Bone marrow stem cells regenerate infarcted myocardium. Pediatr Transplant 2003; 7(Suppl 3):86–8.
13. Strauer BE, Brehm M, Zeus T, et al. Repair of infarcted myocardium by autologous intracoronary mononuclear bone marrow cell transplantation in humans. Circulation 2002;106:1913–18.
14. Perin EC, Dohmann HF, Borojevic R, et al. Transendocardial, autologous bone marrow cell transplantation for severe, chronic ischemic heart failure. Circulation 2003;107:2294–302.
15. Assmus B, Schachinger V, Teupe C, et al. Transplantation of Progenitor Cells and Regeneration Enhancement in Acute Myocardial Infarction (TOPCARE-AMI). Circulation 2002;106:3009–17.
16. Condorelli G, Borello U, De Angelis L, et al. Cardiomyocytes induce endothelial cells to transdifferentiate into cardiac muscle: implications for myocardium regeneration. Proc Natl Acad Sci USA 2001;98:10733–8.
17. Orlic D, Kajstura J, Chimenti S, et al. Mobilized bone marrow cells repair the infarcted heart, improving function and survival. Proc Natl Acad Sci USA 2001;98:10344–9.
18. Orlic D, Kajstura J, Chimenti S, Bodine DM, Leri A, Anversa P. Transplanted adult bone marrow cells repair myocardial infarcts in mice. Ann NY Acad Sci 2001;938:221–9; discussion 229–30.
19. Murry CE, Soonpaa MH, Reinecke H, et al. Haematopoietic stem cells do not transdifferentiate into cardiac myocytes in myocardial infarcts. Nature 2004;428:664–8.
20. Balsam LB, Wagers AJ, Christensen JL, Kofidis T, Weissman IL, Robbins RC. Haematopoietic stem cells adopt mature haematopoietic fates in ischaemic myocardium. Nature 2004;428:668–73.
21. Wagers AJ, Weissman IL. Plasticity of adult stem cells. Cell 2004;116:639–48.
22. Chiu RC, Zibaitis A, Kao RL. Cellular cardiomyoplasty: myocardial regeneration with satellite cell implantation. Ann Thorac Surg 1995;60:12–18.
23. Reinecke H, MacDonald GH, Hauschka SD, Murry CE. Electromechanical coupling between skeletal and cardiac muscle. Implications for infarct repair. J Cell Biol 2000;149:731–40.
24. Menasche P, Hagege AA, Vilquin JT, et al. Autologous skeletal myoblast transplantation for severe postinfarction left ventricular dysfunction. J Am Coll Cardiol 2003;41:1078–83.
25. Yoon YS, Park JS, Tkebuchava T, Luedeman C, Losordo DW. Unexpected severe calcification after transplantation of bone marrow cells in acute myocardial infarction. Circulation 2004;109: 3154–7.
26. Heng BC, Haider H, Sim EK, Cao T, Ng SC. Strategies for directing the differentiation of stem cells into the cardiomyogenic lineage in vitro. Cardiovasc Res 2004;62:34–42.
27. Pittenger MF, Martin BJ. Mesenchymal stem cells and their potential as cardiac therapeutics. Circ Res 2004;95:9–20.
28. Singh SK, Clarke ID, Terasaki M, et al. Identification of a cancer stem cell in human brain tumors. Cancer Res 2003;63:5821–8.
29. Moulton KS, Vakili K, Zurakowski D, et al. Inhibition of plaque neovascularization reduces macrophage accumulation and progression of advanced atherosclerosis. Proc Natl Acad Sci USA 2003;100:4736–41.
30. Simper D, Wang S, Deb A, et al. Endothelial progenitor cells are decreased in blood of cardiac allograft patients with vasculopathy and endothelial cells of noncardiac origin are enriched in transplant atherosclerosis. Circulation 2003;108:143–9.
31. Hill JM, Zalos G, Halcox JP, et al. Circulating endothelial progenitor cells, vascular function, and cardiovascular risk. N Engl J Med 2003;348: 593–600.
32. Kawamoto A, Gwon HC, Iwaguro H, et al. Therapeutic potential of ex vivo expanded endothelial progenitor cells for myocardial ischemia. Circulation 2001;103:634–7.
33. Kawamoto A, Tkebuchava T, Yamaguchi J, et al. Intramyocardial transplantation of autologous endothelial progenitor cells for therapeutic neovascularization of myocardial ischemia. Circulation 2003;107:461–8.
34. Kocher AA, Schuster MD, Szabolcs MJ, et al. Neovascularization of ischemic myocardium by human bone-marrow-derived angioblasts prevents cardiomyocyte apoptosis, reduces remodeling and improves cardiac function. Nat Med 2001;7:430–6.
35. Kang HJ, Kim HS, Zhang SY, et al. Effects of intracoronary infusion of peripheral blood stem-cells

mobilised with granulocyte-colony stimulating factor on left ventricular systolic function and restenosis after coronary stenting in myocardial infarction: the MAGIC cell randomised clinical trial. Lancet 2004;363:751–6.

36. Carmeliet P. VEGF gene therapy: stimulating angiogenesis or angioma-genesis? Nat Med 2000; 6:1102–3.
37. Vulliet PR, Greeley M, Halloran SM, MacDonald KA, Kittleson MD. Intracoronary arterial injection of mesenchymal stromal cells and microinfarction in dogs. Lancet 2004;363:783–4.
38. Chachques JC, Herreros J, Trainini J, et al. Autologous human serum for cell culture avoids the implantation of cardioverter–defibrillators in cellular cardiomyoplasty. Int J Cardiol 2004; 95(Suppl 1):S29–33.
39. Caspi O, Gepstein L. Potential applications of human embryonic stem cell-derived cardiomyocytes. Ann NY Acad Sci 2004;1015:285–98.
40. Pouly J, Hagege AA, Vilquin JT, et al. Does the functional efficacy of skeletal myoblast transplantation extend to nonischemic cardiomyopathy? Circulation 2004;110:1626–31.

Index

N.B. Page numbers in *italic* denote material appearing in figures or tables but not in the main body of text.

B

C

D

E

F

G

H

I

K

L

M

T